OXFORD MONOGRAPHS ON MEDICAL GENETICS

General Editors
Arno G. Motulsky   Martin Bobrow   Peter S. Harper   Charles Scriver

Formal Editors
J. A. Fraser Roberts   C. O. Carter

16. C. R. Scriver and B. Childs: *Garrod's inborn factors in disease*
18. M. Baraitser: *The genetics of neurological disorders*
19. R. J. Gorlin, M. M. Cohen, Jr., and L. S. Levin: *Syndromes of the head and neck, third edition*
20. R. A. King, J. I. Rotter, and A. G. Motulsky: *The genetics basis of common diseases*
21. D. Warburton, J. Byrne, and N. Canki: *Chromosome anomalies and prenatal development: an atlas*
22. J. J. Nora, K. Berg, and A. H. Nora: *Cardiovascular diseases: genetics, epidemiology, and prevention*
24. A. E. H. Emery: *Duchenne muscular dystrophy, second edition*
25. E. G. D. Tuddenham and D. N. Cooper: *The molecular genetics of haemostasis and its inherited disorders*
26. A. Boué: *Fetal medicine*
27. R. E. Stevenson, J. G. Hall, and R. M. Goodman: *Human malformations*
28. R. J. Gorlin, H. V. Toriello, and M. M. Cohen, Jr.: *Hereditary hearing loss and its syndromes*
29. R. J. M. Gardner and G. R. Sutherland: *Chromosome abnormalities and genetic counseling, second edition*
30. A. S. Teebi and T. I. Farag: *Genetic disorders among Arab populations*
31. M. M. Cohen, Jr.: *The child with multiple birth defects*
32. W. W. Weber: *Pharmacogenetics*
33. V. P. Sybert: *Genetic skin disorders*
34. M. Baraitser: *Genetics of neurological disorders, third edition*
35. H. Ostrer: *Non-mendelian genetics in humans*
36. E. Traboulsi: *Genetic diseases of the eye*
37. G. L. Semenza: *Transcription factors and human disease*
38. L. Pinsky, R. P. Erickson, and R. N. Schimke: *Genetic disorders of human sexual development*
39. R. E. Stevenson, C. E. Schwartz, and R. J. Schroer: *X-linked mental retardation*
40. M. J. Khoury, W. Burke, and E. Thomson: *Genetics and public health in the 21st century*
41. J. Weil: *Psychosocial genetic counseling*
42. R. J. Gorlin, M. M. Cohen, Jr., and R. C. M. Hennekam: *Syndromes of the head and neck, fourth edition*
43. M. M. Cohen, Jr., G. Neri, and R. Weksberg: *Overgrowth syndromes*

OXFORD MONOGRAPHS ON MEDICAL GENETICS NO. 43

OVERGROWTH SYNDROMES

M. MICHAEL COHEN, JR., D.M.D., Ph.D.
*Departments of Oral and Maxillofacial Sciences,
Pediatrics, Community Health
and Epidemiology,
Health Services Administration,
Sociology and Social Anthropology
Dalhousie University
Halifax, Nova Scotia, Canada*

GIOVANNI NERI, M.D.
*Institute of Medical Genetics
Catholic University of the Sacred Heart
Rome, Italy*

ROSANNA WEKSBERG, M.D., Ph.D.
*Division of Clinical and Metabolic Genetics,
Department of Paediatrics and
Research Institute,
Hospital for Sick Children,
and Departments of Paediatrics and
Molecular and Medical Genetics
University of Toronto
Toronto, Ontario, Canada*

OXFORD
UNIVERSITY PRESS
2002

WS
104
C6780
2002

OXFORD
UNIVERSITY PRESS

Oxford   New York
Athens   Auckland   Bangkok   Bogotá   Buenos Aires   Calcutta
Cape Town   Chennai   Dar es Salaam   Delhi   Florence   Hong Kong   Istanbul
Karachi   Kuala Lumpur   Madrid   Melbourne   Mexico City   Mumbai
Nairobi   Paris   São Paulo   Shanghai   Singapore   Taipei   Tokyo   Toronto   Warsaw

and associated companies in
Berlin   Ibadan

Copyright © 2002 by Oxford University Press.

Published by Oxford University Press, Inc.,
198 Madison Avenue, New York, New York, 10016
http://www.oup-usa.org

Oxford is a registered trademark of Oxford University Press.

All rights reserved. No part of this publication may be reproduced,
stored in a retrieval system, or transmitted, in any form or by any means,
electronic, mechanical, photocopying, recording, or otherwise,
without the prior permission of Oxford University Press.

Library of Congress Cataloging-in-Publication Data
Cohen, M. Michael (Meyer Michael), 1937–
Overgrowth syndromes / M. Michael Cohen, Jr., Giovanni Neri, Rosanna Weksberg.
p. cm.— (Oxford monographs on medical genetics ; no. 41)
Includes bibliographical references and index.
ISBN 0-19-511746-8
1. Growth disorders. 2. Growth disorders—Genetic aspects.
3. Children—Growth. 4. Genetic disorders in children.
I. Neri, Giovanni. II. Weksberg, Rosanna. III.
Title. IV.
Series.
RJ482.G76 C64 2001   618.9290042—dc21   2001021060

1 2 3 4 5 6 7 8 9
Printed in the United States of America
on acid-free paper

Foreword

Overgrowth has excited human imagination and curiosity since antiquity. Giant humans are abundantly represented in mythology, fiction, circus sideshows and other public exhibitions, and their skeletal remains are found in museums worldwide. During the 7th century A.D., the first serious attempt at classification of monstrosities, by St. Isidore, Archbishop of Seville, included abnormally large size of all or part of the body among the fundamental categories of monstrosity. The concept of *monstra per excessum*, signifying either abnormally large size or duplication anomalies, has been included in virtually every classification of malformations since that time. However, significant progress toward understanding the causes and mechanisms of overgrowth was not made until late in the 19th century, when the recognition of pituitary tumors as a cause of certain cases of generalized somatic overgrowth led to the discovery and purification of human growth hormone.

Localized or *patterned* overgrowth, limited to specific organs, tissues, cell types, or body regions has proved far more elusive and complex than the generalized forms, but is now revealing important new insight into the biology of growth. *Patterns* of overgrowth have provided critical information concerning the existence and nature of targeted growth factors affecting specific organs, tissues, cell types, or developmental stages.

The recognition of the clinical and biological importance of "overgrowth syndromes," and the unifying concept under which they are collected together, is due largely to the efforts of Dr. Michael Cohen. His pioneering publications concerning specific overgrowth syndromes, and reviews of general aspects of the topic, have played a leading role in generating interest in this topic. It is no exaggeration to refer to Michael as the "guru of overgrowth syndromes." His ability to bridge the gap between clinic and basic science laboratory is abundantly demonstrated in the pages of the present volume.

Physicians and scientists in many disciplines will welcome this unique book. It represents the culmination of several years of close collaboration between Michael Cohen and two other leading students of overgrowth syndromes, Giovanni Neri and Rosanna Weksberg. The uncommon disorders it covers present remarkable clinical challenges by virtue of their complex and varied manifestations. Those who care for patients will appreciate the authoritative and detailed clinical information concerning these controversial and confusing entities. The association of many overgrowth disorders with susceptibility to specific neoplasms is among the most intriguing and provocative aspects of the topic, with the potential to provide significant clues to the pathogenesis of developmental neoplasms. Authoritative coverage of molecular and genetic aspects of many of these syndromes provides state-of-the-art reviews of a rapidly changing field.

I have long been a fascinated and frustrated observer of the complexities and conundrums encountered during genetic and molecular studies of the "Beckwith-Wiedemann Syndrome."

Dr. Weksberg, a leading investigator of this topic, provides in Chapter 2 the best review of this complex subject I have read to date We all assumed at the outset that there must be a "BWS gene," which would prove to be a growth-promoting factor active in the several organs and tissues that are usually hyperplastic in BWS patients. When early clues pointed to the p11.5 region as the locus for this gene, a lively international stampede to identify this gene ensued. Though the search has to date not revealed an acceptable candidate gene, a substantial body of new knowledge has resulted from the effort. *IGF2* or a closely related gene is clearly an important participant in the story. Since its function is modulated by an amazing array of other genes, many of them being expressed in a temporally and/or tissue-specific fashion, it is likely that several types of genetic or epigenetic abnormality that enhance the action of an IGF can lead to the clinical syndrome called BWS. Abnormalities of genomic imprinting have emerged as a significant factor in many, perhaps most, cases of BWS. This discovery has contributed significantly to increasing awareness of the role of loss of imprinting in many neoplastic diseases and other overgrowth disorders. As Dr. Weksberg's review indicates, a full understanding of the mechanisms involved in BWS remains for the future, but the search itself continues to yield valuable information.

This book contains gems in every chapter concerning a group of clinically challenging disorders that provide insight into fundamental problems of growth regulation in the developing organism. Drs. Cohen, Neri, and Weksberg have created a unique resource that will be appreciated by clinicians and investigators concerned with these confusing, fascinating, and biologically instructive abnormalities of growth control.

J. Bruce Beckwith, M.D., Hon. FRCPath(UK)
Emeritus Professor
Department of Pathology and Human Anatomy
Loma Linda University
Loma Linda, California

Preface

Overgrowth Syndromes presents a broad yet in-depth discussion of children who are large at birth or have excessive postnatal growth or some combination of increased weight, increased length, and/or increased head circumference. Many of these syndromes are associated with an increase in neoplasia.

Overgrowth syndromes have become more important in pediatrics and medical genetics. The subject has been highlighted at several recent medical genetics meetings. Papers on overgrowth were delivered at the plenary session of the Birth Defects Conference in San Antonio, Texas in 1996. The Manchester Birth Defects Conference held in Manchester, England in 1996 also had overgrowth syndromes as one major focus. The 1997 Robert J. Gorlin Conference on Dysmorphology was devoted entirely to overgrowth syndromes and the conference papers were published as an issue of the *American Journal of Medical Genetics* (1).

There were two reasons for writing this book: (a) the field is expanding, with an ever-increasing number of newly identified entities, and (b) molecular knowledge is progressing at a rapid pace, as, for example, with Beckwith-Wiedemann syndrome, Simpson-Golabi-Behmel syndrome, and Bannayan-Riley-Ruvalcaba syndrome. For each syndrome in this book, the clinical findings, natural history, genetics, molecular biology when relevant, associated neoplasms, and diagnosis are discussed. Each chapter is organized along its own lines according to the particular syndrome addressed.

We have been interested in overgrowth syndromes for many years and our own publications are cited in the reference sections of various chapters. In 1995, we began to collaborate on the study of overgrowth syndromes. Our purpose was threefold: (a) to discuss issues of overgrowth syndromes on an annual basis; (b) to start an International Registry for Overgrowth Syndromes (IROS); and (c) to write a book on overgrowth syndromes. Three IROS meetings have been held: Michael Cohen hosted the first one in Boston in 1995, Rosanna Weksberg hosted the second in Toronto in 1996, and Giovanni Neri, the third in Rome in 1997. We are always pleased to receive problem consultation cases. Pertinent clinical material and photographs can be sent to the Office of the International Registry for Overgrowth Syndromes (IROS), at the following address:

Giovanni Neri, MD
IROS Office
Institute of Medical Genetics
Catholic University of the Sacred Heart
Largo Francesco Vito, 1
00168 Rome, Italy

In this book Michael Cohen is responsible for 14 chapters: 1 (Perspectives on Overgrowth Syndromes), 3 (Hemihyperplasia), 6 (Sotos Syndrome), 7 (Weaver Syndrome), 8 (Bannayan-Riley-Ruvalcaba Syndrome), 9 (Proteus Syndrome), 10 (Klippel-Trenaunay Syndrome, Parkes Weber Syndrome, and Sturge-Weber

Syndrome), 11 (Maffucci Syndrome), 12 (Neurofibromatosis), 14 (Chromosomal Syndromes), 15 (Other Syndromes), 16 (Maternal and Endocrine Effects), 17 (Fetal Hydrops), and 19 (Miscellaneous Syndromes and Conditions with Overgrowth). Giovanni Neri is responsible for chapters 4 (Simpson-Golabi-Behmel Syndrome), 5 (Perlman Syndrome), 13 (Fragile X Syndrome), and 18 (Nonsyndromal Overgrowth). Rosanna Weksberg is responsible for chapter 2 (Beckwith-Wiedemann Syndrome).

The book fulfills the third mission of our collaborative endeavor on overgrowth syndromes. We hope it will be of interest to pediatricians, medical geneticists, oncologists, hematologists, pathologists, surgeons, dermatologists, nephrologists, and molecular biologists.

REFERENCE

1. Cohen MM Jr (ed.): The Gorlin Symposium on Overgrowth. Am J Med Genet 79:233–305, 1998.

Acknowledgments

M. MICHAEL COHEN, JR:

I would like to thank J. Bruce Beckwith for writing the foreword for this volume. I am also grateful to Jeffrey House, Vice President and Executive Editor of Oxford University Press, for helping to expedite the book. I have been collaborating with Leslie G. Biesecker (Genetics Disease Research Branch, National Human Genome Research Institute, National Institutes of Health, Bethesda, Maryland); we have been examining and studying a great many patients with Proteus syndrome, and, to date, this research has resulted in two publications (1,2). I am also grateful to Kathryn F. Peters (National Human Genome Research Institute, National Institutes of Health, Bethesda, Maryland) for her work with Proteus syndrome patients and her organizational skills. I admire Kimberly Hoag (Colorado Springs, Colorado) for her inspired founding and managing of the Proteus Syndrome Foundation. I would like to thank Paul Meltzer (Laboratory of Cancer Genetics, National Human Genome Research Institute, National Institutes of Health, Bethesda, Maryland) for his clinical and laboratory efforts on behalf of patients with Proteus syndrome. During my Seattle years, I was exposed to the brilliant thinking of J. Bruce Beckwith on a variety of topics including Wilms tumor, Beckwith-Wiedemann syndrome, human teratology, and pediatric pathology in general. I owe special thanks to Robert J. Gorlin (University of Minnesota, Minneapolis, Minnesota) for training me in pathology, which has allowed me to focus on neoplasms in overgrowth syndromes from both pathologic and genetic perspectives. I have learned a great deal about vascular anomalies from John B. Mulliken (Division of Plastic Surgery, Children's Hospital, Boston, Massachusetts) and about dermatologic disorders from Rudolf Happle (Department of Dermatology, University of Marburg, Marburg, Germany). I am particularly grateful to my able administrator Ruth E. MacLean (Dalhousie University, Halifax, Nova Scotia) for her organizational skills in arranging the material for this book. Finally, I would like to thank all the patients and their families for their participation in clinical research studies in Seattle and Halifax and at the National Institutes of Health.

GIOVANNI NERI:

I wish to express my deepest gratitude to all those who contributed their clinical and molecular expertise to my understanding of overgrowth syndromes: John Opitz, Angela Lin, and Giuseppe Pilia, for their knowledge of Simpson-Golabi-Behmel syndrome; John Opitz and my wife Maria Enrica Martini, for Perlman syndrome; Pietro Chiurazzi, for fragile X syndrome; and Marco Cappa and Katharina Steindl, for nonsyndromal overgrowth. I particularly appreciate the efforts and patience of my executive secretary, Luciana Amato. Finally, I would like to extend my thanks to all the patients and their families for participating in clinical and research studies.

ROSANNA WEKSBERG:

I would like to acknowledge the many colleagues who have been instrumental in elucidating the clinical and molecular underpinnings of the Beckwith-Wiedemann syndrome. I am particularly thankful to my collaborators, Jeremy Squire, Paul Sadowski, Madeline Li, and Cheryl Shuman, for their continued insights and critical appraisal of this very complex field of study. I wish to extend my appreciation to Yan-Ling Fei for her unusual technical expertise and patience and to Irfan Dhalla for his conscientious and masterful approach to data collection and synthesis. I thank Nancy Taylor for administrative assistance. Finally, I am indebted to all the families who participated in the clinical and research studies and to the National Cancer Institute of Canada for funding the studies that have led to our current understanding of overgrowth and tumor predisposition.

REFERENCES

1. Biesecker LG, Happle R, Mulliken JB, Weksberg R, Graham JM Jr, Viljoen DL, Cohen MM Jr: Proteus syndrome: Diagnostic criteria, differential diagnosis, and patient evaluation. Am J Med Genet 84:389–395, 1999.
2. Biesecker LG, Peters KF, Darling TN, Choyke P, Hill S, Schimke N, Cunningham M, Meltzer P, Cohen MM Jr: Clinical differentiation between Proteus syndrome and hemihyperplasia. Am J Med Genet 79:311–318, 1998.

Contents

1 **Perspectives on Overgrowth Syndromes, 1**
   Mythology of Overgrowth, 1
   Historical Perspective, 1
   Overgrowth, 2
   Overgrowth Syndromes, 2
   Infant Macrosomia, 2
   Mutations, 3
   Lumping and Splitting, 4
   Classification, 4
   Neoplasia, 4
   Vascular Involvement, 5
   Syndrome Designations, 7

2 **Beckwith-Wiedemann Syndrome, 11**
   Historical Perspective, 11
   Phenotype and Diagnostic Criteria, 11
   Molecular Genetics of Beckwith-Wiedemann Syndrome, 11
   Genomic Imprinting, 11
   Beckwith-Wiedemann Syndrome and Epigenetics, 12
   Beckwith-Wiedemann Syndrome Genetic and Epigenetic Subgroups, 14
   Imprinted Genes Implicated in Beckwith-Wiedemann Syndrome, 15
   Beckwith-Wiedemann Syndrome with Unknown Etiologies, 17
   A Model for Regulation of Imprinted Genes in the 11p15 Region, 17
   Beckwith-Wiedemann Syndrome, Imprinting, and Cancer, 17
   Diagnostic Testing and Recurrence Risk, 18
   Natural History, 18
   Prenatal Patient Evaluation, 24

Postnatal Patient Evaluation, 24
  Differential Diagnosis, 26

3 Hemihyperplasia (Hemihypertrophy), 32
  Nosology, 32
  Epidemiology, 32
  Etiologic Considerations, 32
  Tumors, 33

4 Simpson-Golabi-Behmel Syndrome, 38
  Historical Perspective, 38
  Etiology, 38
  Clinical Phenotype, 41
  Neoplasms, 43
  Diagnosis, 43
  Differential Diagnosis, 43

5 Perlman Syndrome, 47
  Historical Perspective, 47
  Etiology, 47
  Clinical Phenotype, 47
  Pathology, 48
  Differential Diagnosis, 49

6 Sotos Syndrome, 51
  Etiologic Considerations, 51
  Diagnostic Considerations, 52
  Growth and Skeletal Findings, 52
  Performance and Central Nervous System Abnormalities, 53
  Craniofacial Features, 54
  Other Findings, 54
  Neoplasms, 55
  Laboratory Findings, 56
  Differential Diagnosis, 56

7 Weaver Syndrome, 59
  Etiologic Considerations, 59
  Growth and Skeletal Findings, 59
  Performance and Central Nervous System, 60

Craniofacial Features, 60
Limbs, 61
Neoplasms, 61
Cardiovascular Anomalies, 62
Differential Diagnosis, 62

8   Bannayan-Riley-Ruvalcaba Syndrome, 66

Delineation and Nomenclature, 66
Molecular Biology of *PTEN*, 66
Mutations, 67
Phenotypic Features, 69
Differential Diagnosis, 71

9   Proteus Syndrome, 75

Phenotype, 75
Understanding Proteus Syndrome and Neurofibromatosis, Unmasking the Elephant Man, and Stemming Elephant Fever, 75
Etiologic Considerations, 81
Natural History, 84
Causes of Premature Death, 84
Clinical Features, 86
Clinical Aspects of Somatic Mosaicism, 100
Publications and the Diagnosis of Proteus Syndrome, 102
Diagnostic Criteria, Differential Diagnosis, and Patient Evaluation, 103

10 Klippel-Trenaunay Syndrome, Parkes Weber Syndrome, and Sturge-Weber Syndrome, 111

Klippel-Trenaunay Syndrome, 111
Parkes Weber Syndrome, 116
Sturge-Weber Syndrome, 116
Vascular Tumors and Vascular Malformations, 119
Kasabach-Merritt Phenomenon, 119
Diagnosis, 122
Differential Diagnosis, 122

11 Maffucci Syndrome, 125

Skeletal System, 125
Vascular Abnormalities, 125
Neoplasms, 125
Differential Diagnosis, 125

12 Neurofibromatosis, 130

Classification and Types of Neurofibromatosis, 130
Epidemiology of Neurofibromatosis, Type 1, 133
Molecular Biology of the *NF1* Gene 133
Mutations, 134
Pseudogenes, 135
Microdeletions, 135
Tumorigenesis, 135
Expressivity, 136
Neurofibromatosis, Type 1, 137
Neurofibromatosis, Type 2, 143
Diagnosis, 144
Differential Diagnosis, 145

13 Fragile X Syndrome, 152

Prevalence, 152
Genetics, 152
Clinical Phenotype, 154
Diagnosis, 156
Differential Diagnosis, 156
Guidelines for Health Supervision, 156

14 Chromosomal Disorders with Overgrowth, 161

dup(4)(p16.3), 161
dup(5p), 161
dup(12p), 161
Pallister Killian Syndrome [Mosaic i 12p), Mosaic Tetrasomy 12p], 162
dup(12)(q11 → q15), 162
dup(15)(q25–qter), 164
del(15)(q12), 164
del(22)(q13 → qter), 164

15 Other Syndromes, 166

Costello Syndrome, 166
Macrocephaly–Cutis Marmorata Syndrome, 169
Cantú Syndrome, 171
Nevo Syndrome, 173
Elejalde Syndrome, 175

16 Maternal and Endocrine Effects, 180

Infants of Diabetic Mothers, 180
Persistent Hyperinsulinemic Hypoglycemia of Infancy, 183
Infants of Psoriatic Mothers, 186

17 Fetal Hydrops, 189

18 Nonsyndromal Overgrowth, 191

Nosologic Considerations, 191
Phenotype, 191

19 Miscellaneous Syndromes and Conditions with Overgrowth, 193

Bakker-Hennekam Syndrome, 193
Bayoumi Syndrome, 193
Carpenter Syndrome, 193
Chorangioma, 193
Congenital Hypothyroid Gigantism, 194
Congenital Muscular Hypertrophy, Hypertonia, and Developmental Retardation, 194
Cranioectodermal Dysplasia, 194
Ectodermal Overgrowth Syndrome, 194
Homfray Syndrome, 194
Lipodystrophy, 194
Macrocephaly–Autism Syndrome, 195
Macrocephaly–Megalocornea Syndrome, 195
Marshall-Smith Syndrome, 195
MOMO Syndrome, 196
Ørstavik Macrocephaly Syndrome, 197
PEHO Syndrome, 197
Quattrin Syndrome, 197
Richieri-Costa Overgrowth Syndrome, 198
Siena Type Overgrowth, 198
Stevenson Syndrome, 198
Teebi Overgrowth–Microphthalmia Syndrome, 198
Transposition of the Great Vessels with Overgrowth, 198

Index, 201

Overgrowth Syndromes

Perspectives on Overgrowth Syndromes

MYTHOLOGY OF OVERGROWTH

Mythology about overgrowth is fascinating. The Cyclopes were a race of one-eyed giants who lived in Sicily. The occasional newborn of a diabetic mother can have both cyclopia and macrosomia and possibly may have served as an observation that became mythically transformed into cyclopian giants. A number of Greek myths deal with Athena, who sprang full-grown from Zeus's forehead, making her the most overgrown mythical newborn known. No information has been passed down to us, however, about Zeus's presumed brain contractions, throbbing headaches, or metopic suture as an alternative birth mode.

In his sixteenth-century French masterpiece, *Gargantua and Pantagruel*, Rabelais (66) relates how Gargantua, a gigantic infant, was born to his mother, Gargamelle, in a very strange fashion. After an "astringent" had been concocted for the mother-to-be, the nativity took place in the following manner (because of abruptio placentae, which precluded vaginal delivery):

> the infant, leaping up, entered the hollow vein and climbed over the diaphragm to her shoulder where the said vein divides into two parts and there he took the left hand path and came out by the left ear.

Almost 100 years later, Gargantua's own wife, Badebec, died in childbirth, the newborn Pantagruel being "so amazingly large and so heavy that he could not come into the world without suffocating his mother" (66).

These are tall tales, perhaps even overgrown. However, Beach (3) reported the birth of a gigantic male infant weighing 23 and 3/4 lb. The mother was a Nova Scotia giant, Anna Swan (2.29 meters tall), who was married to a Kentucky giant, Captain Martin Bates (2.3 meters tall). The infant was born at their home in Seville, Ohio, on January 18, 1879, and died 11 hours later. Other references to gigantic infants are found in Ballantyne (2) and in Gould and Pyle (38).

HISTORICAL PERSPECTIVE

Although problems of overgrowth were documented and appreciated in the nineteenth century and conditions such as the Beckwith-Wiedemann, Sotos, and other syndromes were delineated by the 1960s, the study of overgrowth syndromes as a clinical field of inquiry was set forth in the early 1980s (16). The subject has been reviewed extensively elsewhere (14,17,21) and, recently, an entire issue of the *American Journal of Medical Genetics* was devoted to overgrowth (13,18).

Historically, pediatricians and geneticists focused on intrauterine growth retardation (IUGR) and its many associated syndromes. In contrast, overgrowth syndromes are known to be far fewer in number, although a rapid increase in knowledge has occurred in the last two decades. With the recent molecular advances in research on several overgrowth syndromes, e.g., Beckwith-Wiedemann syndrome, Simpson-Golabi-Behmel syndrome, and Bannayan-Riley-Ruvalcaba syndrome, breakthroughs in other overgrowth syndromes can be anticipated in the near future (18).

OVERGROWTH

Most overgrowth results from (a) an increased number of cells, (b) hypertrophy, (c) an increase in the interstitium, most commonly excessive fluid as in fetal hydrops, or (d) some combination of these factors. In overgrowth syndromes such as Beckwith-Wiedemann syndrome or Weaver syndrome, excessive cellular proliferation predominates and can be demonstrated or inferred to have occurred (14,21). An expected consequence of cellular overgrowth is that cell cultures from affected persons manifest the growth excess. An example is Elejalde syndrome in which cultured fibroblasts complete the cell cycle in 63% of the normal time (28) (Fig. 1–1). However, in a preliminary study of the autosomal recessively inherited Perlman syndrome, cell growth rate was not increased in fibroblasts. Negative findings may be explained by (a) nonexpression in fibroblasts, (b) switching off of the mutant genes, or (c) possible expression of the mutant genes in some other way (62).

OVERGROWTH SYNDROMES

Infant macrosomia can be defined as a newborn birth weight exceeding 4000 g, which in some studies include approximately 5% of newborns. Certainly, the cutoff point for defining infant macrosomia is arbitrary (17). In pediatric assessment, birth length is usually considered before birth weight. With overgrowth syndromes, weight is as important as length. Other features of overgrowth syndromes may include malformations, mental deficiency, and neoplasia (14).

INFANT MACROSOMIA

In a large study of 104,000 deliveries (41), 5.3% of newborns exceeded 4000 g. The prevalence of birthweights over 4500 g varies from 0.4% to 0.9% in different reports (42). Many factors seem to be implicated in the etiology of large–birthweight infants. Large fetal weight reflects the genetic predisposition of the fetus and is also linked to excessive weight gain by the mother during pregnancy (57). Prepregnancy weight is also a factor. Overweight mothers are known to deliver macrosomic infants four times more often than underweight mothers (46,63). Large infants are born three times more frequently to multiparas than to primiparas, and male infants are usually heavier than female in-

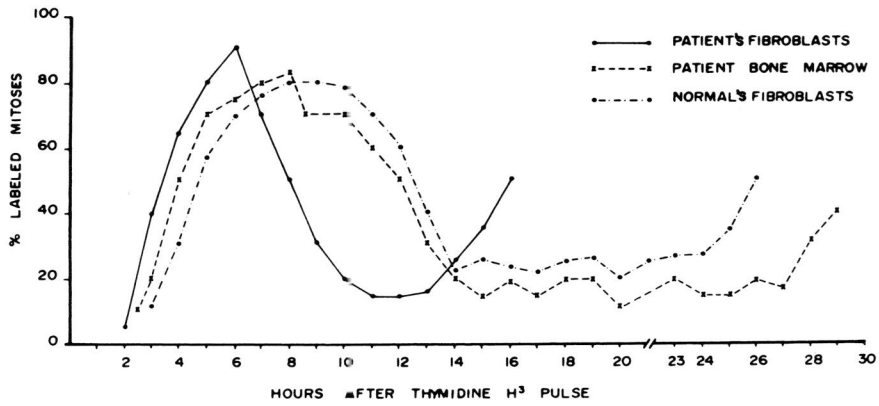

Figure 1–1 Elejalde syndrome. Results of cell kinetic studies. Bone marrow cells from Elejalde syndrome patient behave essentially like normal fibroblasts, taking approximately 37 hours to complete cell cycle. However, fibroblasts from Elejalde syndrome patient complete whole cycle in 16–18 hours (63% of normal time). From Elejalde et al. (28).

fants (39,54). Finally, birthweight is known to vary among different populations, but in most studies socioeconomic level is a confounding factor. In general, the highest mean birthweights are found in Swedish infants, and the lowest mean birthweights occur in indigent black populations (39).

Although many macrosomic infants are proportionately overgrown, infants of diabetic or gestational diabetic mothers may be disproportionately large with increased weight–length ratios (76). Other macrosomic infants may also have discrepancies between birthweight and body length. Some may have chorioangiomas of the placenta, heart failure in utero, or asphyxia; size is a reflection of increased extracellular fluid volume. By contrast, true somatic growth is always accompanied by placental growth, the total mass of the trophoblast limiting fetal size (74).

The optimum birthweight for the lowest perinatal mortality and morbidity is 3500–4000 g (47). As birthweight exceeds this level, the frequency of complications rises sharply. A predisposition to both asphyxia and trauma results from fetal macrosomia. Traumatic morbidity in newborns of diabetic mothers occurs in 3%–9% of vaginal deliveries (34,48,73). In a regional network databank study of 574 macrosomic infants weighing >4500 g and a control group of 18,739 infants weighing 2500–3499 g, Spellacy et al. (72) found that macrosomia had a higher frequency of birth trauma, especially of shoulder dystocia; higher death rates; a significantly greater number of males; and lower Apgar scores, especially in macrosomic infants weighing >5000 g. High-risk factors predisposing to macrosomia included obesity, diabetes, and postmaturity, which combined to give a macrosomic frequency of 5%–14%.

Elliott et al. (29) developed a macrosomia index by subtracting the biparietal diameter from the chest diameter. In their study of 23 macrosomic newborns, 87% had an index of ≥1.4 cm, and cesarean section of all fetuses with such an index would have reduced traumatic morbidity from 27% to 9%. Spellacy et al. (72) indicate that women at risk should be screened for macrosomic infants and, if found, should be delivered electively by cesarean section. Boyd et al. (9) noted that fetal macrosomia, regardless of cause, was rare at 37 weeks gestation and increasingly common thereafter. They suggested that fetal size assessment by ultrasound at 36–38 weeks gestation would permit induction of labor for the macrosomic infant before size became excessive or would make the obstetrician aware of the dangers that might arise during delivery.

Leonard (50), in evaluating abnormal pregnancies in a prenatal diagnosis program ($n = 413$), recognized 10 cases (2.4%) as large for gestation (Table 1–1). Further studies will not only identify other disorders that may be associated with fetal macrosomia but may also establish ultrasound patterns of growth in such fetuses (14).

Table 1–1 Prenatal Diagnosis of Large-for-Gestational Age Fetuses in a Series of 413 Abnormal Pregnancies

Disorder	No. of Cases
Infant of diabetic mother	2
Renal anomalies (nonlethal)	2
Congenital heart defect	1
Familial CNS disorder	1
Resolved choroid plexus cyst	1
Idiopathic nonimmune hydrops	1
Carpenter syndrome	1
Meckel syndrome	1
Total number (%)	10 (2.4)

Source: From Cohen (14). Adapted from data of Leonard (50).

MUTATIONS

Mutations in *GPC3*, a glypican gene, have been found for Simpson-Golabi-Behmel syndrome (65,80). *GPC3* maps to Xq26. However, another Simpson-Golabi-Behmel locus maps to Xp22 (11). Mutations in *PTEN* cause both Bannayan-Riley-Ruvalcaba and Cowden syndromes, which overlap phenotypically (55,56). The molecular basis of the Beckwith-Wiedemann syndrome, the classic overgrowth syndrome, is complex and not completely resolved at this time. Implicated are imprinted genes at the 11p15.5 domain, including *IGF2* and $p57^{KIP2}$ (40,51,52,79).

Molecular studies of fibroblast growth factor receptor 3 (*FGFR3*) provide an intriguing example of how a single gene can cause overgrowth or growth deficiency, depending on particular human mutations and on mouse model study. The function of *FGFR3* can be deduced from the $Fgfr3^{-/-}$ knockout mouse, which is overgrown with excessively long femora and elongated vertebrae, resulting in a long tail (18,25). Thus, the normal function of *FGFR3* is to regulate endochondral ossification by "putting the brakes" on growth. Mutations for short-limb skeletal dysplasias on *FGFR3* (hypochondroplasia, achondroplasia, and thanatophoric dysplasia) are gain-of-function mutations that "put the brakes" on growth even more to various degrees (61,78).

LUMPING AND SPLITTING

Until the anticipated molecular breakthrough occurs that may clarify many more overgrowth syndromes, clinical delineation remains essential. With dominantly inherited or chromosomally defined syndromes, clinical delineation is straightforward, but the problem of "lumping" and "splitting" will continue for sporadically defined overgrowth syndromes. Proteus syndrome is a case in point. Is the hemihyperplasia/multiple lipomatosis syndrome different from Proteus syndrome or is it a part of the same spectrum (7,8), as we assume to be the case for encephalocraniocutaneous lipomatosis (19)? Also, given that Proteus syndrome is thought to be caused by somatic mosaicism, lethal in the nonmosaic state, minimal mosaic involvement may result in truncated phenotypic expression that is nondiagnostic (19,71). Another example of partially sorted heterogeneity in sporadic cases is "hemihyperplasia" and its many subsets, both known and unknown (18) (Table 1–2).

CLASSIFICATION

There are a number of different ways to define and classify overgrowth syndromes. Classificatory systems have been proposed by Cohen (21), Beighton (6), and Weaver (77) (Table 1–3). Because of molecular advances, such classificatory

Table 1–2 Hemihyperplasia Subsets

Beckwith-Wiedemann syndrome
Trisomy 18 mosaicism
Diploid/triploid mosaicism
Translocation 7p;13q
Partial B and G monomy with B/G translocation
Hemihyperplasia/multiple lipomatosis syndrome
Many others

Source: From Cohen (18).

Table 1–3 Overgrowth Syndromes: Definition and Classification

Cohen (21)	Familial tall stature Prenatal onset overgrowth Postnatal onset overgrowth Intrinsic cellular hyperplasia vs. humorally mediated hyperplasia
Beighton (6)	Generalized overgrowth Obesity Localized overgrowth Digital overgrowth
Weaver (77)	Generalized overgrowth Regional overgrowth Parameter-specific overgrowth

Source: From Cohen (18).

schemes appear to be outmoded. At present, it is recommended that overgrowth definition and classification be loose, and simply serve as an organizing principle for review and discussion.

NEOPLASIA

The association of increased body size, particularly birthweight and neoplasia, has been documented by several authors (24,30,32,33,45,49, 53,64,67,75,81) (Table 1–4). The possibility that hepatoblastoma[a] and adult germ cell tumors, particularly testicular, may be associated with low birthweight has been explored by Ikeda et al. (44), Ross (68), and Brown et al. (10).

The relationship of neoplasia to overgrowth syndromes has been discussed by Cohen (14). Overgrowth syndromes not known to be associated with neoplasia may possibly be explained by (*a*) their rarity and/or too few case reports to establish a relationship or (*b*) a high infant mortality rate with insufficient time for tumor development.

In a study of precursors of Wilms tumor, Beckwith (4,5) distinguished two major nephrogenic rest patterns: perilobar and intralobar. In Wilms tumor, perilobar rests are more common in Beckwith-Wiedemann syndrome and hemihyperplasia (70%); intralobar rests are more common in WAGR[b] (84%) and Denys-Drash syndrome (91%).

[a]Except when associated with Beckwith-Wiedemann syndrome and/or hemihyperplasia.
[b]Wilms tumor, *a*niridia, *g*enitourinary abnormalities, and *r*etardation.

PERSPECTIVES ON OVERGROWTH SYNDROMES

Table 1–4 Increased Body Size and Neoplasia

Wilms tumor (increased birthweight)	Irving (45) Daling et al. (24) Lindblad et al. (53) Leisenring et al. (49) Olshan (64)
Leukemia (increased birthweight)	Fasal et al. (32) Wertelecki and Mantel (81) Daling et al. (24) Ross et al. (67)
Neuroblastoma (increased birthweight)	Daling et al. (24)
Astrocytoma (increased birthweight)	Emerson et al. (30)
Osteosarcoma (larger breeds of dogs) (taller, young humans)	Tjalma (75) Fraumeni (33)

Source: From Cohen (18).

In comparing Beckwith-Wiedemann syndrome, hemihyperplasia, and Sotos syndrome, Cohen (14) noted that tumors of the kidney and liver (Fig. 1–2) occurred in all three conditions and that adrenal neoplasms were found in two of the three. Both kidney and liver tumors occurred with low frequency in Sotos syndrome and with higher frequency in Beckwith-Wiedemann syndrome and hemihyperplasia. Tumors in these three disorders are listed in Table 1–5.

Cohen (14,19) further noted that some overgrowth syndromes had distinctive patterns of common and uncommon tumors. For example, in Proteus syndrome, lipomas and vascular malformations commonly occur, but tumors of the central nervous system, ovary, testis, and salivary gland are found with low frequency (19,35).

VASCULAR INVOLVEMENT

Many overgrowth syndromes have vascular lesions of various types. Mulliken and Glowacki (58) and Mulliken (59) made a distinction between hemangiomas and vascular malformations based on cellular kinetics and clinical behavior. Hemangiomas have endothelial hyperplasia with rapid postnatal growth followed by slow involution. In contrast, vascular malformations are characterized by flat endothelium, growth of the lesion being commensurate with growth of the child. The differences between hemangiomas and vascular malformations are contrasted in Table 1–6. In vascular malformations, a single type of channel anomaly may predominate or combined channel anomalies of various types may occur (Table 1–7).

Mulliken (59) noted that the "standard" terminology used for vascular lesions has led to confusion, improper diagnosis, illogical treatment, and misdirected research efforts (Fig. 1–3). The Mulliken classification, which is based on research and clinical behavior of vascular lesions, is now considered state of the art in plastic surgery. Significant inroads are also being made in dermatology and pathology. The distinction between hemangiomas and vascular malformations is particularly important in the phenotypic description and analysis of overgrowth syndromes.

Burns et al. (12) indicated that vascular components of various syndromes are commonly and incorrectly subsumed under the rubric of "hemangioma." The authors stated that on the basis of clinical and cellular criteria, vascular birthmarks can be properly classified as either a hemangioma, a malformation, or a macular stain.[c] Since hemangiomas occur in 10%–12% of

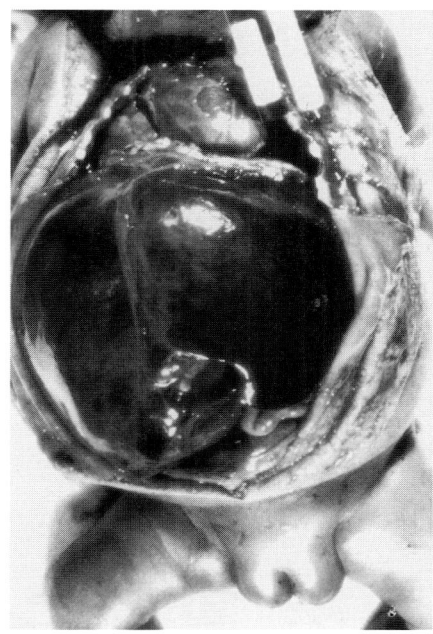

Figure 1–2 Beckwith-Wiedemann syndrome. Hepatoblastoma at autopsy.

[c]Macular stains are transient, flat, pink, and irregularly outlined. They are commonly known as nevus flammeus.

Table 1–5 Comparison of Reported Neoplasms Associated with Beckwith-Wiedemann Syndrome, Hemihyperplasia (Hemihypertrophy), and Sotos Syndrome[a]

	Beckwith-Wiedemann Syndrome[a]	Hemihyperplasia (Hemihypertrophy)[a]	Sotos Syndrome
Tumor frequency[b]	7.5%	5.9%	2.2%
Malignant tumors	Wilms tumor[c]	Wilms tumor[c]	Wilms tumor
	Adrenocortical carcinoma[c]	Adrenocortical carcinoma[c]	Hepatocellular carcinoma
	Hepatoblastoma[c]	Hepatoblastoma[c]	Neuroblastoma
	Hepatocellular carcinoma	Neuroblastoma	Acute lymphocytic leukemia
	Glioblastoma	Pheochromocytoma	Non-Hodgkin lymphoma
	Neuroblastoma	Testicular carcinoma	Epidermoid carcinoma of the vagina
	Rhabdomyosarcoma	Undifferentiated sarcoma	Small cell carcinoma of the lung
	Malignant lymphoma		Sacrococcygeal teratoma
	Pancreatoblastoma		
	Carcinoid tumor		
	Congenital mesoblastic nephroma		
	Renal cell carcinoma		
	Myelodysplasia		
	Yolk sac tumor		
	Intratubular germ cell neoplasm		
Benign tumors	Adrenal adenoma	Adrenal adenoma	Multiple hemangiomas
	Teratoma		Osteochondroma
	Fibroadenoma		Large hairy nevus
	Ganglioneuroma		Giant cell granuloma of mandible
	Myxoma		
	Cardiac hamartoma		
	Bladder hamartoma		
	Chest wall hamartoma		
	Fibrous hamartoma		
	Chorangioma		
	Digital fibroma		
	Hepatic hemangioma		
	Bladder neck polyp		

[a]Not all cases of hemihyperplasia are part of the Beckwith-Wiedemann spectrum.
[b]Could be overestimates because of ascertainment bias.
[c]Most common neoplasms in descending order of frequency.
Source: Adapted from Cole et al. (23), Sayedabadi et al. (70), Nance et al. (60), Cohen (14,22), Wiedemann (82), Hoyme et al. (43), Hersh et al. (41a), and Jonas and Kimonis (45a). See Chapters 2, 3, and 6.

Table 1–6 Mulliken Classification[a]

	Hemangioma	Vascular Malformation
Presentation	Usually not present at birth	Always present at birth, but may not be apparent in some cases
Female/Male Ratio	3:1 (higher in some series)	1:1
Cellular	Endothelial hyperplasia	Flat endothelium
Hematologic	Primary platelet trapping with profound thrombocytopenia (Kasabach-Merritt phenomenon) found only with Kaposiform hemangioendothelioma and tufted angioma but *not* with common infantile hemangioma[b]	Localized intravascular coagulopathy (chronic consumptive coagulopathy in which platelet count is minimally depressed[b]
Course	Rapid postnatal growth followed by slow involution	Growth is commensurate with child's growth

[a]Adapted from Mulliken and Glowacki (58).
[b]Adapted from Sarkar et al. (69).

Table 1–7 Biological Classification of Vascular Malformations

Single channel
  Arterial (AM)
  Capillary (CM)
  Lymphatic (LM)
  Venous (VM)
Complex/combined
  CLM
  CVM
  CLVM
  LVM

Source: Adapted from Mulliken (59).

normal infants by 1 year of age and macular stains are found in about 40% of normal newborns, they queried whether either of these are pathogenetically related in the syndromes in which they have been described. True hemangiomas only occur rarely in malformation syndromes, but vascular malformations are common. Overgrowth syndromes with vascular malformations include Klippel-Trenaunay syndrome, Maffucci syndrome, Proteus syndrome, Bannayan-Riley-Ruvalcaba syndrome, and macrocephaly–cutis marmorata syndrome. Macular stain is found with Beckwith-Wiedemann syndrome.

SYNDROME DESIGNATIONS

There are many different ways of naming syndromes in general and there are advantages and disadvantages of each method (20). When possible, I prefer familiar nomenclature of any kind for known syndrome designations in preference to introducing new names to avoid unnecessary learning hurdles and also to avoid confusion in a field already encumbered by too many names to remember. In some cases, valid "lumping" or "splitting" does require a name change. An example is the Bannayan-Riley-Ruvalcaba syndrome (BRRS). Originally thought to be three separate entities, the name BRRS was an attempt to preserve the earlier used nomenclature by combining the names of the first authors of the three previously known syndromes to keep learning hurdles to a minimum (15). BRRS was adopted by Gorlin et al. (36,37) and others (1,31). Other terms have been suggested, such as HAM syndrome (26) and PTEN-MATCHS (27). *PTEN* mutations have been found in both BRRS and Cowden syndrome and phenotypic overlap has been observed. Marsh et al. (55) demonstrated that the *PTEN* mutational spectrum also involves overlap, suggesting a single entity they called the "PTEN hamartoma-tumor syndrome."

REFERENCES

1. Arch EM, Goodman BK, Van Wesep RA: Deletion of PTEN in a patient with the Bannayan-Riley-Ruvalcaba syndrome suggests allelism with Cowden disease. Am J Med Genet 71:489–493, 1997.
2. Ballantyne JW: *Manual of Antenatal Pathology and Hygiene*. William Green and Sons, Edinburgh, 1904.

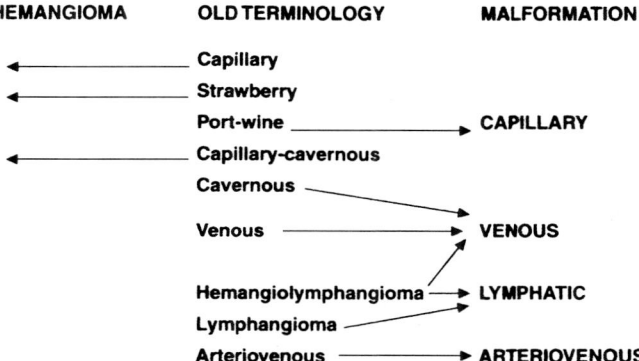

Figure 1–3 Confusion resulting from "standard" terminology of vascular lesions. Adapted from Mulliken (59).

3. Beach AP: A giant birth, the child weighing twenty-three and three quarters pounds. Med Rec 15:271, 1879.
4. Beckwith JB: Nephrogenic rests and the pathogenesis of Wilms tumor: Developmental and clinical considerations. Am J Med Genet 79: 268–273, 1998.
5. Beckwith JB: Precursor lesions of Wilms tumor: Clinical and biological implications. Med Pediatr Oncol 21:158–168, 1993.
6. Beighton P: *Inherited Disorders of the Skeleton.* Churchill Livingstone, New York, pp. 454–473, 1988.
7. Biesecker LG, Happle R, Mulliken JE, Weksberg R, Graham JM Jr, Viljoen DL, Cohen MM Jr: Proteus syndrome: Diagnostic criteria, differential diagnosis, and patient evaluation. Am J Med Genet 84:389–395, 1999.
8. Biesecker LG, Peters KF, Darling TN, Choyke P, Hill S, Schimke N, Cunningham M, Meltzer P, Cohen MM Jr: Clinical differentiation between Proteus syndrome from hemihyperplasia: Description of a distinct form of hemihyperplasia. Am J Med Genet 79:311–318, 1998.
9. Boyd ME, Usher RH, McLean FH: Fetal macrosomia: Prediction, risks, proposed management. Obstet Gynecol 61:715–722, 1983.
10. Brown LM, Pottern LM, Hoover RN: Prenatal and perinatal risk factors for testicular cancer. Cancer Res 46:4812–4816, 1986.
11. Brzustowicz LM, Farrell S, Khan ME, Weksberg R: Mapping of a new SGBS locus to chromosome Xp22 in a family with a severe form of Simpson-Golabi-Behmel syndrome. Am J Hum Genet, in press.
12. Burns AJ, Kaplan LC, Mulliken JB: Is there an association between hemangioma and syndromes with dysmorphic features? Pediatrics 88:1257–1267, 1991.
13. Cohen MM Jr (ed.): The Gorlin Symposium on Overgrowth. Am J Med Genet 79:233–305, 1998.
14. Cohen MM Jr: A comprehensive and critical assessment of overgrowth and overgrowth syndromes, in Harris H and Hirschhorn K (eds) Advances in Human Genetics. New York, Plenum Press, vol 18, Ch 4, pp 181–303; Addendum, 1989, pp 373–376.
15. Cohen MM Jr: Letter to the editor: Bannayan-Riley-Ruvalcaba syndrome: Renaming three formerly recognized syndromes as one etiologic entity. Am J Med Genet 35:291, 1990.
16. Cohen MM Jr: Overgrowth syndromes. In: *Associated Congenital Malformations.* M El-Shafie and CH Klippel, eds. Williams & Wilkins, Baltimore, pp. 71–104, 1981.
17. Cohen MM Jr: Overgrowth syndromes: An update. Adv Pediatr 46:441–491, 1999.
18. Cohen MM Jr: Perspectives on overgrowth syndromes. Am J Med Genet 79:234–237 1998.
19. Cohen MM Jr: Proteus syndrome: Clinical evidence for somatic mosaicism and selective review. Am J Med Genet 47:645–652, 1993.
20. Cohen MM Jr: Syndrome designations. J Med Genet 13:266–270, 1976.
21. Cohen MM Jr: The large-for-gestational age infant in dysmorphic perspective. In: *Clinical Genetics: Problems in Diagnosis and Counseling.* AM Wiley, TP Carter, S Kelly, and IH Porter eds. Academic Press, New York, pp. 153–169, 1982.
22. Cohen MM Jr: Tumors and non-tumors in Sotos syndrome. Am J Med Genet 84:173–175, 1999.
23. Cole TRP, Hughes HE, Jeffreys MJ, Williams GT, Arnold MM: Small cell lung carcinoma in a patient with Sotos syndrome: Are genes at 3p21 involved in both conditions? J Med Genet 29:338–341, 1992.
24. Daling JR, Starzyk, P, Pishan AF, Weiss NS: Birth weight and the incidence of childhood cancer. J Natl Cancer Inst 72:1039–1041, 1984.
25. Deng C, Wynshaw-Boris A, Zhou F, Kuo A, Leder P: Fibroblast growth factor receptor 3 is a negative regulator of bone growth. Cell 84: 911–921, 1996.
26. DiLiberti JH: Comments on Dr. Cohen's letter. Am J Med Genet 35:292, 1990.
27. DiLiberti JH: Inherited macrocephaly—hamartoma syndromes. Am J Med Genet 79:284–290, 1998.
28. Elejalde BR, Giraldo C, Jimenez R, Gilbert EF: Acrocephalopolydactylous dysplasia. Birth Defects 13(3B):53–67, 1977.
29. Elliott JP, Freeman RK, McQuown DS, Patel JM: Ultrasonic prediction of fetal macrosomia in diabetic patients. Obstet Gynecol 60:159–162, 1982.
30. Emerson JC, Malone KE, Daling JR, Starzyk P: Childhood brain tumor risk in relation to birth characteristics. J Clin Epidemiol 44:1159–1166, 1991.
31. Fargnoli MC, Orlow SJ, Semel-Concepcion J, Bolognia JL: Clinicopathologic findings in the Bannayan-Riley-Ruvalcaba syndrome. Arch Dermatol 132:1214–1218, 1996.
32. Fasal E, Jackson EW, Lauber MR. Birth characteristics and leukemia in childhood. J Natl Cancer Inst 47:501–509, 1971.
33. Fraumeni JF Jr: Stature and malignant tumors of bone in childhood and adolescence. Cancer 20:967–973, 1967.
34. Gabbe SG, Mestman JH, Freeman RK: Management and outcome of class A diabetes mellitus. Am J Obstet Gynecol 127:465–469, 1977.
35. Gordon PL, Wilroy RS, Lasater OE, Cohen MM Jr: Neoplasms in Proteus syndrome. Am J Med Genet 57:74–78, 1995.
36. Gorlin RJ, Cohen MM Jr, Condon LM, Burke BA: Bannayan-Riley-Ruvalcaba syndrome. Am J Med Genet 44:307–314, 1992.
37. Gorlin RJ, Cohen MM Jr, Levin LS: *Syndromes*

38. Gould GM, Pyle WL. *Anomalies and Curiosities of Medicine.* W.B. Saunders, Philadelphia, 1896.
39. Gruenwald P: Growth of the human fetus. 1. Normal growth and its variation. Am J Obstet Gynecol 94:1112–1119, 1966.
40. Hatada I, Ohashi H, Fukushima Y, Kaneko Y, Inoue M, Komoto Y, Okada A, Ohishi S, Nabetani A, Morisaki H, Nakayama M, Niikawa N, Mukai T: An imprinted gene $p57^{KIP2}$ is mutated in Beckwith-Wiedemann syndrome. Nat Genet 14:171–173, 1996.
41. Hellman LM, Pritchard JA, eds: *Williams Obstetrics*, 14th ed. Appleton-Century-Crofts, New York, 1971.
41a. Hersh JH, Cole TRP, Bloom AS, Bertolone SJ, Hughes HE: Risk of malignancy in Sotos syndrome. J Pediatr 120:572–574, 1992.
42. Horger EO, Facog M, Miller C, Conner ED: Relation of large birth weight to maternal diabetes mellitus. Obstet Gynecol 45:150–154, 1975.
43. Hoyme HE, Seaver LH, Jones KL, Procopia F, Crooks W, Feingold M: Isolated hemihyperplasia (hemihypertrophy): Report of a prospective multicenter study of the incidence of neoplasia and review. Am J Med Genet 79:274–278, 1998.
44. Ikeda H, Matsuyama S, Tanimura M: Association between hepatoblastoma and very low birth weight: a trend or a chance? J Pediatr 130:557–560, 1997.
45. Irving I: The EMG syndrome (exomphalos, macroglossia, gigantism). In *Progress in Pediatrics*, Vol. 1. RP Rickham, WC Hacker, and J Prevolt, eds. Urban and Schwarzenberg, Munich, pp. 1–61, 1970.
45a. Jonas RE, Kimonis VE. Brief clinical report. Chest wall hamartoma with Wiedemann-Beckwith syndrome: Clinical report and brief review of chromosome 11p15.5-related tumors. Am J Med Genet 101:221–225, 2001.
46. Kaltreider DF: *Effects of Height and Weight on Pregnancy and the Newborn.* Charles C. Thomas, Springfield, IL, 1963.
47. Kessner DM: Infant death: An analysis by maternal risk and health care. Proc Natl Acad Sci USA 70:90–125, 1973.
48. Kitzmiller JL, Cloherty JP, Younger MD, Tobatabaii A, Rothchild SB, Sosenko I, Epstein MF, Singh S, Neff RK: Diabetic pregnancy and perinatal morbidity. Am J Obstet Gynecol 131:560–588, 1978.
49. Leisenring WM, Breslow NE, Evans IE, Beckwith JB, Coppes MJ, Grundy P: Increased birth weight of national Wilms tumor study patients suggest a growth factor excess. Cancer Res 54:4680–4683, 1994.
50. Leonard CO: Prenatal diagnosis of the large for gestational age fetus. 9th Annual David W. Smith Workshop on Malformations and Morphogenesis, Oakland, California, August 3–7, 1988.
51. Li M, Squire JA, Weksberg R: Molecular genetics of Wiedemann-Beckwith syndrome. Am J Med Genet 79:253–259, 1998.
52. Li M, Squire JA, Weksberg R: Overgrowth syndromes and genomic imprinting: From mouse to man. Clin Genet 53:165–170, 1998.
53. Lindblad P, Zack M, Adami H-O, Erickson A: Maternal and perinatal risk factors for Wilms tumor: A nationwide nested case control study in Sweden. Int J Cancer 51:38–41, 1992.
54. Lubchenco LO, Hansman C, Dressler M: Intrauterine growth as estimated from liveborn birth weight data at 24 to 42 weeks of gestation. Pediatrics 32:793–800, 1963.
55. Marsh DJ, Kum JB, Lunetta KL, Bennett MJ, Gorlin RJ, Ahmed SF, Bodurtha J, Crowe C, Curtis MA, Dasouki M, Dunn T, Feit H, Geraghty MT, Graham JM Jr, Hodgson SV, Hunter A, Korf BR, Manchester D, Miesfeldt S, Murday VA, Nathanson KL, Parisi M, Pober B, Romano C, Tolmie JL, Trembath R, Winter RM, Zackai EH, Zori RT, Weng L-P, Dahia PLM, Eng C: *PTEN* mutation spectrum and genotype–phenotype correlations in Bannayan-Riley-Ruvalcaba syndrome suggest a single entity with Cowden syndrome. Hum Mol Genet 8:1461–1472, 1999.
56. Marsh DJ, Dahia PLM, Zheng Z, Liaw D, Parsons R, Gorlin RJ, Eng C: Germline mutations in *PTEN* are present in Bannayan-Zonana syndrome. Nat Genet 16:333–334, 1997.
57. Moss JM, Mulholland HB: Diabetes and pregnancy prediabetic state. Ann Intern Med 34:678–692, 1951.
58. Mulliken JB, Glowacki J: Hemangiomas and vascular malformations in infants and children: A classification based on endothelial characteristics. Plast Reconstr Surg 69:412–420, 1982.
59. Mulliken JB: Cutaneous vascular anomalies. Semin Vasc Surg 6:204–218, 1993.
60. Nance MA, Neglia JP, Talwar D, Berry SA: Neuroblastoma in a patient with Sotos syndrome. J Med Genet 27:130–132, 1990.
61. Naski MC, Wang Q, Xu J, Ornitz DM: Graded activation of fibroblast growth factor receptor 3 by mutations causing achondroplasia and thana-tophoric dysplasia. Nat Genet 13:233–237, 1996.
62. Neri G, Martini-Neri ME, Opitz JM, Freed JJ: The Perlman syndrome: Clinical and biological aspects. In: *Endocrine and Genetics of Growth.* Alan R. Liss, New York, pp. 269–276, 1985.
63. Niswander JR, Singer J, Westphal M: Weight gain during pregnancy and prepregnancy weight. Obstet Gynecol 33:482–491, 1969.
64. Olshan AF: Letter to the editor: Wiedemann-Beckwith syndrome, Wilms tumor, birth weight, and insulin-like growth factor 2. Am J Med Genet 57:640, 1995.

65. Pilia G, Hughes-Benzie RM, MacKenzie A, Baybayan P, Chen EY, Huber R, Neri G, Cao A, Forabosco A, Schlessinger D: Mutations in *GPC3*, a glypican gene, cause the Simpson–Golabi–Behmel overgrowth syndrome. Nat Genet 12: 241–247, 1996.
66. Rabelais F: *Gargantua and Pantagruel*. Portable Viking Edition, New York, 1976.
67. Ross JA, Perentesis JP, Robison LL, Davies SM: Big babies and infant leukemia: A role for insulin-like growth factor-1? Cancer Causes Control 7:553–559, 1996.
68. Ross JA: Hepatoblastoma and birth weight: Too little, too big, or just right? J Pediatr 130:516–517, 1997.
69. Sarkar M, Mulliken JB, Kozakewich HPW, Robertson RL, Burrows PE: Thrombocytopenic coagulopathy (Kasabach-Merritt phenomenon) is associated with kaposiform hemangioendothelioma and not with common infantile hemangioma. Plast Reconstr Surg 100:1377–1386, 1997.
70. Seyedabadi S, Bard DS, Zuna RE: Epidermoid carcinoma of the vagina in a patient with cerebral gigantism. J Ark Med Soc 78:123–127, 1981.
71. Smeets E, Fryns J-P, Cohen MM Jr: Regional Proteus syndrome and somatic mosaicism. Am J Med Genet 51:29–31, 1994.
72. Spellacy WN, Miller S, Winegar A, Peterson PQ: Macrosomia—maternal characteristics and infant complications. Obstet Gynecol 66:158–161, 1985.
73. Stallone LA, Ziel HK: Management of gestational diabetes. Am J Obstet Gynecol 119:1091–1094, 1974.
74. Stevenson DK, Hopper AO, Cohen RS, Bucalo LR, Kerner JA, Sunshine P: Medical progress: Macrosomia: Causes and consequences. J Pediatr 100:515–520, 1982.
75. Tjalma RA: Canine bone sarcoma: Estimation of relative risk as a function of body size. J Natl Cancer Inst 36:1137–1150, 1966.
76. Van Allen MI, Brown ZA, Plovie B, Hanson ML, Knopp RH: Deformation in infants of diabetic and control pregnancies. Am J Med Genet 53:210–215, 1994.
77. Weaver DD: Overgrowth syndromes and disorders: Definition, classification, and discussion. Growth Genet Horm 10:1–4, 1994.
78. Webster MK, Donoghue DJ: Constitutive activation of fibroblast growth factor receptor 3 by the transmembrane domain point mutation found in achondroplasia. EMBO J 15:520–527, 1996.
79. Weksberg R, Squire J: Molecular genetics of Beckwith-Wiedemann syndrome. In: *Studies in Stomatology and Craniofacial Biology*. MM Cohen, Jr and BJ Baum eds. IOS Press, Amsterdam, 1997, pp. 273–287.
80. Weksberg R, Squire JA, Templeton DM: Glypicans: A growing trend. Nat Genet 12:225–227, 1996.
81. Wertelecki W, Mantel N: Increased birth weight in leukemia. Pediatr Res 7:132–138, 1973.
82. Wiedemann H-R: Tumors and hemihyperplasia associated with Wiedemann-Beckwith syndrome. Eur J Pediatr 141:129, 1983.

Beckwith-Wiedemann Syndrome

Beckwith-Wiedemann syndrome (BWS) (OMIM 130650)[a] is a relatively common genetic overgrowth disorder, defined classically by omphalocele, macroglossia, and macrosomia. Other common features include hemihyperplasia, ear anomalies (anterior linear lobe creases, posterior helical pits), umbilical hernia, visceromegaly, adrenocortical cytomegaly, renal abnormalities, and neonatal hypoglycemia. Children with BWS are at increased risk for developing embryonal tumors.

The population incidence has been estimated as 1 in 13,700 (96) with equal numbers of affected males and females (81). The true incidence may be significantly higher as mild cases may be undiagnosed.

HISTORICAL PERSPECTIVE

Beckwith (6) was the first to present the syndromic association between omphalocele, hyperplastic kidneys and pancreas, and adrenal cytomegaly (Fig. 2–1). The following year, Wiedemann (108) published a case report describing three siblings. One child was born with umbilical hernia and macrosomia, the other two with exomphalos, macroglossia, and gigantism. This characteristic triad led to the designation EMG syndrome. However, none of the three cardinal features is a diagnostic requisite. In fact, the eponyms Beckwith-Wiedemann syndrome (BWS) or Wiedemann-Beckwith syndrome (WBS) are now favored.

[a]On-Line Mendelian Inheritance in Man number.

PHENOTYPE AND DIAGNOSTIC CRITERIA

The BWS phenotype can be extremely variable. Many geneticists have proposed a traditional approach to developing diagnostic criteria for BWS—that is, the utilization of at least two major criteria and one minor criterion (Table 2–1). Although this is useful in some situations, a high index of suspicion must be maintained for those children presenting with fewer findings (e.g., macroglossia and ear creases) in order to identify children at risk for tumor development and to address recurrence risk estimation for family members.

MOLECULAR GENETICS OF BECKWITH-WIEDEMANN SYNDROME

Beckwith-Wiedemann syndrome is a complex, multigenic disorder caused by modifications of growth regulatory genes on chromosome 11p15 (Fig. 2–2) (58,59). To explain the current molecular data for BWS, one must invoke not only the involvement of multiple genes but also genomic imprinting.

GENOMIC IMPRINTING

Genomic imprinting is a process by which one copy of a gene is preferentially silenced according to its parental origin (2). Although imprinted autosomal genes are inherited in a Mendelian manner, the expression of each allele is parent-of-origin specific. The molecular basis of im-

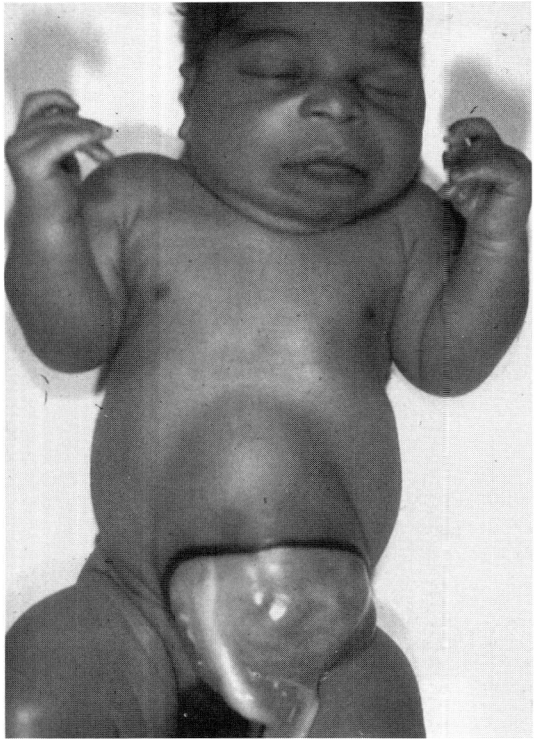

Figure 2–1 Beckwith-Wiedemann syndrome. Note omphalocele and macroglossia. Courtesy of R. Spencer, Los Angeles, California, and J.B. Beckwith, Missoula, Montana.

printing involves epigenetic modification—that is, two alleles, identical in nucleotide sequence, but of opposite parental origin, are regulated differently in the same nucleus. Epigenetic modifications involve DNA methylation and probably also chromatin structure/function; these modifications define the transcriptional activity of imprinted alleles. Genomic imprinting is reversible; the silent, imprinted allele can be reactivated when passed through the germline of the opposite parental sex and the active allele silenced.

Although only approximately 30 imprinted genes have been identified to date, 100–200 are estimated to exist in the human genome. Imprinting is recognized to be an important factor in several inherited human diseases and many tumors (60,82,93,98). It is important to understand the mechanisms underlying the establishment and maintenance of imprinting in order to know how such mechanisms are disrupted in pathological states. Imprinted genes tend to occur in clusters or domains. The concept of an imprinting center regulating expression of multiple genes within an "imprinted domain" was first defined for the Prader-Willi (PWS) and Angelman (AS) syndromes, two neurobehavioral diseases mapping to chromosome 15q11–q13 (75,76). Imprinting centers are thought to regulate imprint switching by determining parent of origin-specific chromatin structures and methylation patterns that are propagated along the chromosome (75). These DNA modifications define parent of origin-specific epigenotypes. Mutations in imprinting centers result in the failure to reset imprints in the germline, leading to inheritance of an inappropriate epigenotype across the entire interval; e.g., deletion of the PWS/AS imprinting center leads to altered methylation and transcription over the entire 1 Mb domain (14). Structural and functional characteristics of imprinting centers are beginning to emerge and it appears that differentially methylated regions (DMRs) and chromatin boundary elements that deny access to transcriptional machinery are features of imprinting centers. The downstream targets of imprinting centers are only partially understood, but likely include many factors that regulate gene-specific imprinting, i.e., promoters, enhancers and antisense transcripts. Oppositely imprinted antisense transcripts are proposed to regulate transcription of overlapping genes (1,46,47,70, 86,87,113).

BECKWITH-WIEDEMANN SYNDROME AND EPIGENETICS

Beckwith-Wiedemann syndrome is genetically extremely complex (59,60,104). Imprinted genes implicated in the etiology of BWS map to the 11p15 imprinted region (Fig. 2–2) and include the paternally expressed (maternally silenced) genes *IGF2* (insulin-like growth factor 2) and *KvLQT1-AS*, and the maternally expressed (paternally silenced) genes *H19*, $p57^{KIP2}$, and *KvLQT1*.

Only 10% of BWS cases have a demonstrable DNA sequence alteration. Most of these occur as mutations in the $p57^{KIP2}$ gene (44,53,57). Chromosome 11p15 abnormalities (paternal duplications and maternal translocation/inversions) account for another 1%–2% (67,88,102,106).

Table 2–1 Diagnostic Criteria for Beckwith-Wiedemann Syndrome[a]

MAJOR FINDINGS

Positive family history (one or more family members with a clinical diagnosis of BWS or a history of features suggestive of BWS)
Macrosomia (traditionally defined as height and weight ≥97%)
Anterior linear ear lobe creases/posterior helical ear pits
Macroglossia
Omphalocele (also called exomphalos)/umbilical hernia
Visceromegaly involving one or more intraabdominal organs including liver, spleen, kidneys, adrenals, and pancreas
Embryonal tumor (e.g., Wilms tumor, hepatoblastoma, rhabdomyosarcoma) in childhood
Hemihyperplasia defined as asymmetric overgrowth of region(s) of the body
Adrenocortical cytomegaly
Renal abnormalities including structural abnormalities, nephromegaly, nephrocalcinosis
Cleft palate (rare)

MINOR FINDINGS

Polyhydramnios
Prematurity
Neonatal hypoglycemia
Facial nevus flammeus
Capillary malformation
Characteristic facies, including midfacial hypoplasia and infraorbital creases
Cardiomegaly/structural cardiac anomalies/rarely cardiomyopathy
Diastasis recti
Advanced bone age
Monozygotic twining. Monozygotic twins with BWS are usually female and discordant; however, both male and female monozygotic twins concordant for BWS have been reported, as well as monozygotic male twins discordant for BWS.

[a]No consensus diagnostic criteria for BWS exist, although it is generally accepted that a diagnosis requires the presence of at least three findings (two major and one minor). Since children with milder phenotypes have developed tumors, special diagnostic consideration must be given to such children. That is, individuals presenting with fewer than three features, e.g. macroglossia and umbilical hernia or just hemihyperplasia, should be considered candidates for tumor surveillance.

Thus, in 90% of cases, the primary molecular change is either epigenetic or unknown. Furthermore, multiple BWS-associated epigenetic alterations may occur in the same individual (Table 2–2). Paternal 11p15 uniparental disomy (two paternal copies of a chromosomal region with no maternal copies, i.e., two paternal epigenotypes) occurs in approximately 20% of BWS cases (59) (Fig. 2–3). The most common epigenetic alterations associated with BWS are expression of the normally silent maternal allele of *IGF2* (25%–50%) (103) and/or loss of methylation of *KvDMR1* (50%) (91). Loss of methylation at *KvDMR1* is associated with loss of imprint of KvLQT1-AS, the antisense transcript in intron 10 of *KvLQT1* (55,77). Many questions remain about how such lesions lead to BWS and its associated tumor predisposition.

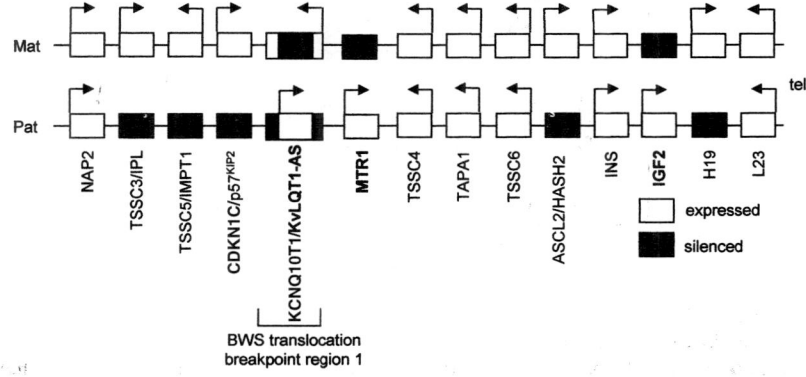

Figure 2–2 Genes and their imprinting status on human chromosome 11p15. When different nomenclature is used, both terms are shown. Mat refers to the maternally derived chromosome; Pat refers to the paternally derived chromosome.

Table 2–2 Beckwith-Wiedemann Syndrome Genetic and Epigenetic Subgroups[a]

Group	Inheritance	Frequency (%)	Karyotype	DNA	RNA
A	Sporadic	50	Normal	KvDMR1 LOM	KvLQT1-AS LOI
B	Sporadic	25–50	Normal	Normal H19 methylation	IGF2 LOI
C	Sporadic	10–20	Normal	Paternal UPD	
D	Sporadic	10–20	Normal	Unknown	Unknown
E	Sporadic	5–10	Normal	$p57^{KIP2}$	
F	Autosomal dominant	5	Normal	$p57^{KIP2}$	
G	Autosomal dominant	5	Normal	Unknown	
H	Sporadic	2	Normal	H19 methylation	IGF2 LOI
I	Sporadic[b]	1	11p15 duplication		
J	Sporadic[b]	1	11p15 translocation/inversion	Disruption of KvLQT1	
K	Monozygotic twins	Rare	Normal	Unknown	Unknown

LOI, loss of imprint; LOM, loss of methylation; UPD, uniparental disomy.
[a]The molecular abnormalities presented here are not always mutually exclusive.
[b]May present as sporadic or recurrent cases in families.

BECKWITH-WIEDEMANN SYNDROME GENETIC AND EPIGENETIC SUBGROUPS

Table 2–2 shows estimated frequencies of known genetic/epigenetic BWS subgroups. These data indicate that BWS is a multigenic disorder with clear parent-of-origin effects, and that BWS and its related tumors result from dysregulation of several imprinted growth regulatory genes on chromosome 11p15. BWS can presently be categorized into eleven genetic/epigenetic groups. The majority of BWS cases (about 90%) are sporadic and without chromosomal abnormalities (Groups A–E and H–J). The other 10% of BWS cases exhibit an autosomal dominant inheritance pattern, with demonstrated linkage to chromosome 11p15 in some families (Groups F and G). Chromosomal rearrangements of 11p15 associated with the BWS phenotype have also been

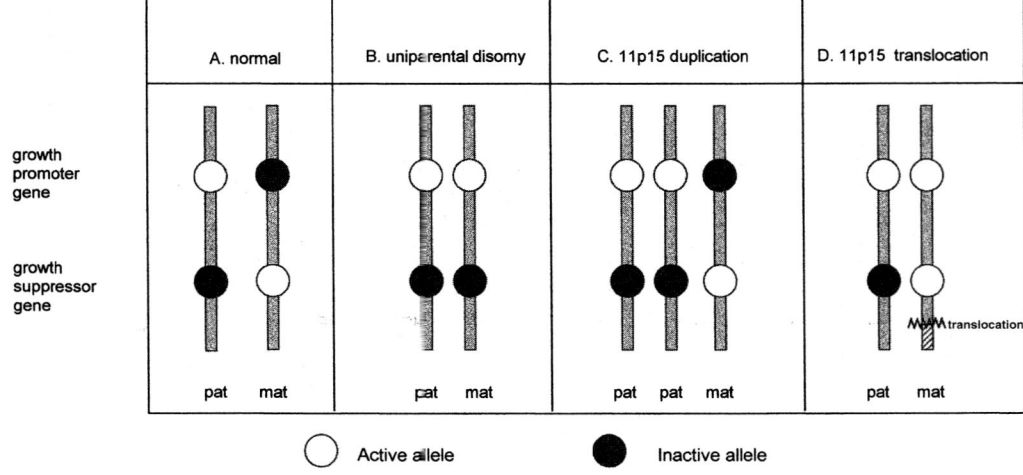

Figure 2–3 Gene dosage models for 11p15 uniparental disomy, chromosomal duplication, and chromosomal translocation. The paternal duplications and paternal uniparental disomy are associated with increased gene dosage of paternally expressed growth promoter genes. The maternal rearrangements are associated with cis-activation of normally suppressed growth promoting genes.

observed in 1%–2% of cases (Groups I and J). Translocations and inversions of the 11p15 region typically show maternal inheritance (Group J), while duplications are usually paternally inherited (Group I). This parent of origin–specific segregation, combined with observations of uniparental disomy (UPD) and preferential maternal transmission in autosomal dominant pedigrees, provide compelling evidence that the 11p15 region houses genes subject to genomic imprinting.

Genetic alterations in BWS can affect both maternally expressed growth suppressor genes and paternally expressed growth promoter genes. Approximately 10%–20% of patients with BWS have paternal UPD (Group C). All patients with 11p15 UPD exhibit somatic mosaicism (45a). This implies that both parental contributions of 11p15 are required in early development and that 11p15 UPD arises postzygotically and may be found in only some tissues. In paternal 11p15 UPD, the BWS phenotype with its tumor predisposition is likely caused by a combination of increased expression of paternally expressed growth promoter genes (e.g., *IGF2*) and diminished expression of maternally expressed growth suppressor genes (e.g., *H19*). Figure 2–3 illustrates this situation in schematic form, depicting the relative gene dosages for 11p15 UPD, 11p15 duplication, and 11p15 translocation/inversion.

IMPRINTED GENES IMPLICATED IN BECKWITH-WIEDEMANN SYNDROME

Recently, many 11p15 imprinted genes have been identified. Figure 2–2 shows all known imprinted and nonimprinted 11p15 loci. Imprinted genes implicated in the pathogenesis of overgrowth and tumorigenesis in BWS are discussed below.

IGF2

IGF2, a paternally expressed embryonic growth factor, exhibits a pattern of tissue-specific expression closely paralleling the organs exhibiting overgrowth in BWS. Transgenic mice that overexpress *IGF2* exhibit many BWS features (overgrowth, visceromegaly, macroglossia) (94b). Therefore, *IGF2* is thought to play a significant role in the pathogenesis of BWS. Disruption of *IGF2* imprinting occurs in some BWS patients (Group B) (103) and in multiple tumors (61), including Wilms tumor (98). Interestingly, *IGF2* expression may be increased by several mechanisms, including transcriptional control by promoter/enhancer elements (see *H19*, below); gene dosage effects (11p15 paternal duplications and UPD); and imprint regulation by imprinting centers and/or changes in chromatin structure/function. The role of such mechanisms in *IGF2* dysregulation remains a rich area for investigation.

H19

The maternally expressed *H19* gene encodes a biologically active, untranslated mRNA that may function as a tumor suppressor (42). *H19* and *IGF2* are coordinately regulated in some normal tissues and tumors. The two genes compete for a common set of downstream enhancers, ensuring monoallelic expression of the maternal H19 allele coincident with monoallelic expression of paternal *IGF2* (3,15). In most cases of sporadic Wilms tumor, 11p15 biallelic expression of *IGF2* is accompanied by silencing of *H19* and by methylation of both *H19* alleles, suggesting epigenetic alteration of an imprinting center (see model in Fig. 2–4). This occurs only rarely in BWS (Group H). In most cases of BWS with biallelic *IGF2* expression, there is disruption of the coordinate regulation of *H19* and *IGF2*; that is, normal monoallelic maternal *H19* expression is maintained (94). This *H19*-independent loss of *IGF2* imprint is seen in up to 50% of BWS cases (Group B). Recently, a DMR that regulates *H19*-independent *IGF2* imprinting was identified upstream of the murine *IGF2* gene (22). However, the syntenic region in humans is not differentially methylated (70), and mice carrying a deletion of this element do not exhibit overgrowth (22). Therefore, the molecular basis of the asymmetric change in *H19/IGF2* expression in BWS remains unknown.

p57^{KIP2}

A member of the cyclin-dependent kinase inhibitor family, *p57^{KIP2}* (also known as *CDKN1C*) is a maternally expressed growth inhibitory gene that plays a role in the pathogenesis of BWS and

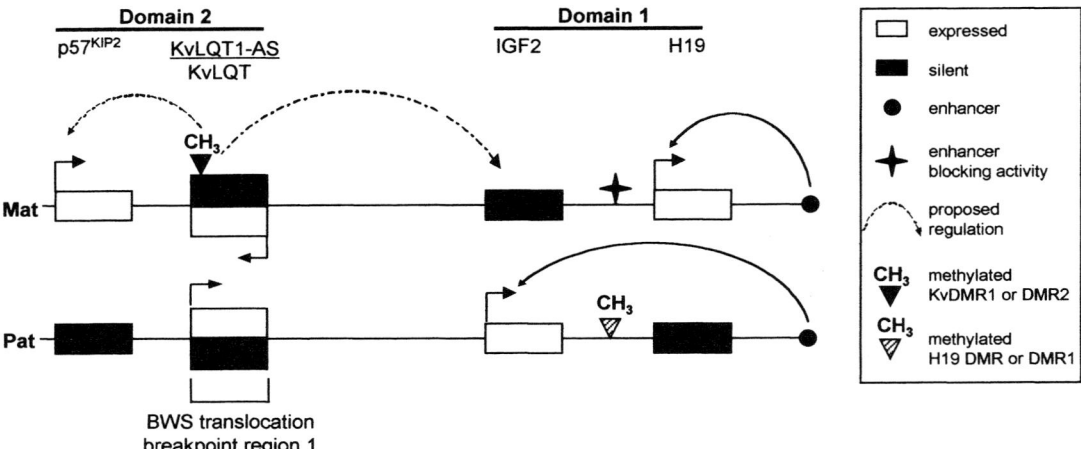

Figure 2–4 Model for imprinted gene and imprinting center function on 11p15.

related tumors. $p57^{KIP2}$ negatively regulates cell proliferation (69). A variety of $p57^{KIP2}$ mutations occur in BWS patients who can exhibit cleft palate, omphalocele, overgrowth, macroglossia, and ear creases; there is only one case of neuroblastoma (44,53,57). Mice with targeted disruption of the $p57^{KIP2}$ gene (115,117) exhibit a spectrum of abnormalities similar to BWS but distinct from the IGF2-overexpressing mouse model. These features include omphalocele, renal medullary dysplasia, adrenal cortical hyperplasia, and cytomegaly, but overgrowth is absent. Notably, $p57^{KIP2}$ mutations occur in only 5%–10% of sporadic BWS (Group E) but in 25% of autosomal dominant pedigrees (44,53,57,78, 115,117) (Group F). In the other 75% of autosomal dominant cases, either cryptic mutations alter p57KIP2 expression, or another 11p15 gene may be involved. It has recently been shown that loss of imprint for *IGF2* occurs in BWS cases with $p57^{KIP2}$ mutations (57) (Group G). The mechanism is unknown but is independent of the putative imprinting center *KvDMR1* (see next section and Fig. 2–4).

KvLQT1/KvLQT1-AS

The maternally expressed *KvLQT1* gene product forms part of a potassium channel and is related to at least two cardiac arrhythmia syndromes (74,100). There are six known translocation sites associated with BWS and tumors, spanning the length of this gene (67,88). These data imply that the *KvLQT1* locus harbors an imprinting center for the 11p15 region. A putative imprinting center, KvDMR1, has been identified in intron 10 of the *KvLQT1* gene. This differentially methylated region, *KvDMR1*, is associated with an imprinted paternally expressed antisense transcript of *KvLQT1* called KvLQT1-AS or KCNQ1OT1 (55,91). The normal functions of KvLQT1-AS and KvDMR1 are not well understood. Approximately 50% of BWS cases show loss of methylation on the maternal allele at KvDMR1; this correlates with biallelic expression or loss of imprint of KvLQT1-AS (55,91) (Group A). In BWS cases with loss of methylation at KvDMR1 and loss of imprint for KvLQT1-AS, only some show *IGF2* loss of imprint (55,91). It is unknown whether KvDMR1 acts as a regional imprinting center to regulate *p57^{KIP2}* and/or *IGF2* imprinting in BWS.

TSSC3/IPL

The *TSSC3* gene (72) is paternally imprinted in placenta, most fetal tissues, and in adult liver and lung. It shows homology to *TDAG51*, a gene involved in apoptosis. Loss of apoptosis is a well-recognized mechanism leading to cancer (72). Intriguingly, a recent study identified biallelic expression for *TSSC3* in normal adult brain but "gain of imprinting" in human neuroblastoma and brain tumors (72), constituting a novel imprinting mechanism for decreasing expression of a potential growth inhibitory gene. Aberrant imprinting of this gene has not been demonstrated in BWS to date.

TSSC5/IMPT1

The *TSSC5* gene (also known as *ORCTL2* or *BWRIA*) is a recently identified imprinted gene in the 11p15 region (27). This gene shows preferential maternal expression in the fetus and is centromeric to $p57^{KIP2}$. Although this gene is known to have negative growth regulatory functions, it has not been directly implicated in BWS.

BECKWITH-WIEDEMANN SYNDROME WITH UNKNOWN ETIOLOGIES

In many instances, the molecular etiology of BWS remains unknown (Group D). An especially enigmatic group is the collection of monozygous (MZ) twin pairs (Group K). Fewer than 20 such twin pairs have been reported; typically they are female and discordant for BWS (9,10,13,20,38,63,65,79). Three pairs of male MZ twins discordant for BWS have been reported (16,56), and three other pairs are unpublished. One concordant (35) male twin pair and one concordant female pair have also been reported (20). Asymmetric expression of BWS in these MZ twins could result from abnormalities in temporally related developmental processes such as imprinting, X-inactivation, and twinning (65,80).

A MODEL FOR REGULATION OF IMPRINTED GENES IN THE 11P15 REGION

A possible mechanism explaining how an imprinting center regulates imprinting has recently emerged (43). A differentially methylated region 2 kb upstream of the mouse *H19* gene (H19DMR) regulates imprinted expression of *H19* and *IGF2* (Domain 1) by functioning as a chromatin boundary element (Fig. 2–4). An analogous human H19DMR has been identified (43). Figure 2–4 depicts a hypothetical model for imprint regulation within the BWS region. The model describes at least two imprinted domains on 11p15, but the limits of each domain have yet to be precisely defined. Domain 1 would be telomeric and includes *IGF2* and *H19*, while the more centromeric domain 2 involves *KvLQT1/KvLQT1-AS* and possibly $p57^{KIP2}$ (48). The Domain 1 imprinting center is H19DMR, while KvDMR1 is the postulated imprinting center for Domain 2 (37a,66). On the maternal chromosome, H19DMR is unmethylated, permitting the binding of boundary proteins such as CTCF, and blocking access of the *IGF2* promoter to downstream enhancers. Thus, the maternal copy of *H19* uses these enhancers and is transcribed. Methylation of the H19DMR on the paternal chromosome prevents binding of proteins associated with development of a chromatin boundary, so that the *IGF2* promoter has access to the downstream enhancers and *H19* is silenced (43). Far less is known about the mechanism for imprint regulation in Domain 2. No common enhancers or boundary elements have been identified in the region. It is possible that the mechanism for imprint regulation in Domain 2 is not the same as for Domain 1. In fact, homozygous deletion of the *Dnmt1* cytosine DNA methyltransferase gene results in erasure of the *H19* imprint in Domain 1, while the $p57^{KIP2}$ imprint remains intact in Domain 2 (82). The fact that translocations through *KvLQT1* do not affect *KvDMR1/KvLQT1-AS* but do result in altered *IGF2* imprinting indicate that there may be molecular interactions between the two hypothesized imprinted domains.

BECKWITH-WIEDEMANN SYNDROME, IMPRINTING, AND CANCER

In recent years, it has become apparent that abnormal genomic imprinting plays a role in the inactivation of tumor suppressor genes and in the development of certain types of cancers (93,98). Since imprinted genes are functionally haploid, somatic mutation of the expressed allele will reduce the number of "hits" required for the development of a tumor. Thus, for a single imprinted gene, the "two-hit" model for carcinogenesis (49) can be modified to "one-hit". Since imprinted genes cluster within large imprinted domains, one hit (e.g., loss of heterozygosity, imprinting center mutation) can alter the function of multiple imprinted growth regulatory genes, generating many hits in a tumorigenic pathway. Over the last 10 years, the BWS/11p15.5 region has been strongly associated with tumorigenesis (97,98), including not only childhood embryonal tumors (94a) and brain tumors (72), but also a variety of common adult malignancies such as breast, testicular and lung cancer (51,52,84,97,98,111,112,116).

DIAGNOSTIC TESTING AND RECURRENCE RISK

Elucidation of the molecular etiology of each BWS clinical group is important for the determination of recurrence risks. In general, the recurrence risk in future pregnancies is assumed to be low if neither parent manifests signs of the condition.

Currently, chromosome testing and molecular testing are useful for diagnostic confirmation and recurrence risk estimation. Not enough is known yet about the relationship between genotype and phenotype for testing to have medical management implications. An exception to this involves the identification of a chromosome abnormality such as a duplication of 11p15, as this is associated with developmental delay (90). All children with BWS should be karyotyped with high-resolution banding for the 11p15 region.

Paternal UPD for 11p15 can be ascertained by RFLP analysis of multiple loci or by methylation studies of imprinted genes on 11p15. Since all cases of UPD associated with BWS involve somatic mosaicism, a negative result for UPD in one tissue (e.g., blood) is not conclusive. Obtaining other tissues (e.g., skin), especially in the event of surgery, should be considered. In fact, UPD for 11p15 can be limited to just normal kidney tissue surrounding a Wilms tumor in a phenotypically normal child. For BWS, the finding of 11p15 UPD confers a low recurrence risk since it usually arises from a postzygotic somatic recombination event.

Testing for $p57^{KIP2}$ is currently available through research laboratories. If a $p57^{KIP2}$ mutation is found in a child with BWS, the parents should be offered testing since parental mutations carry a 50% risk of transmission. Although mutations in $p57^{KIP2}$ are usually maternally transmitted, both parents should be tested, as there have been two cases of paternal transmission of a $p57^{KIP2}$ mutation associated with BWS (54,57). If no mutation is found in either parent, prenatal testing might still be considered because of the theoretical possibility of gonadal mosaicism; such a case has not yet been reported.

The validity of using epigenetic changes in the 11p15 region for BWS diagnosis remains to be established. Although *KvDMR1* loss of methylation and *KvLQT1-AS* loss of imprint have been demonstrated in approximately 50% of BWS cases, the proposal that this should form the basis for BWS diagnostic testing should be viewed with caution. In 1993, *IGF2* loss of imprint in association with BWS was a parallel finding. However, over the last 8 years, it has been shown that loss of *IGF2* imprint occurs not only in BWS cases but also in non-BWS cases with overgrowth and tumors (71). *IGF2* loss of imprint can also be seen in normal individuals, where it has been postulated to represent a marker for tumor predisposition (26). Therefore, we still do not recommend *IGF2* expression analysis as a diagnostic test for BWS. Similarly, *KvDMR1* methylation status will need to be examined more carefully before it can be used as a diagnostic test for BWS. The usefulness of *H19* methylation studies to identify Group H (Table 2–2) BWS cases also remains to be established in the clinical arena.

With respect to recurrence risk, in general, epigenetic changes such as loss of *IGF2* imprint are not associated with significant recurrence risks. However, such epigenetic lesions may occur in conjunction with other 11p15 molecular alterations (for example, translocations of 11p15), which may have a significant recurrence risk.

NATURAL HISTORY

Up to 20% of infants with BWS die in the perinatal period of complications from prematurity, macroglossia, and rarely cardiomyopathy (81,107). Most individuals with BWS have a good prognosis for physical health and mental development. However, individuals with BWS and 11p15 duplications are developmentally delayed and have other congenital malformations outside the BWS spectrum. In addition, although many embryonal tumors seen in children with BWS have a good prognosis, some of them are associated with significant morbidity and mortality.

Growth

Growth excess can be manifested in BWS as whole body overgrowth or regional overgrowth affecting areas of the body or specific organs. This overgrowth has been demonstrated in a variety of tissues to represent cellular hyperplasia (see Figs. 2–6, 2–10, 2–11, 2–13, 2–14, 2–15).

Even though macrosomia is not a diagnostic requisite for BWS, most individuals with BWS have birth weights and lengths at or above the 97th centile for gestational age (107). Nevertheless, the onset of overgrowth can vary from the prenatal period to as late as 1 year of age (101a). Head circumference may be proportional to other growth parameters or closer to the normal range. If the head circumference is within the normal range, relative microcephaly does not correlate with poor developmental outcome.

Growth typically continues at an increased rate through the first few years of life, with bone age often at the upper limit of normal. Several studies have shown a decreased growth rate from mid-childhood through puberty (107) with adult heights typically clustering between the 50th and 90th centiles (81,107).

Hemihyperplasia (asymmetric overgrowth restricted to one or more regions of the body) occurs in about 25% of BWS cases (33), but may not be apparent at birth (Fig. 2–9).

Development

Contrary to early reports, mental development is generally normal in BWS. Development may be delayed if there is a chromosomal duplication involving 11p15, if there are complications of prematurity, or a period of uncontrolled or undetected hypoglycemia.

Chest/Cardiovascular

Information regarding cardiovascular problems in BWS is generally anecdotal. Cardiac malformations have an incidence ranging from 9% to 34% (33,81); cardiomegaly is the diagnosis in about half of these. Cardiomyopathy, though reported, is very rare. A dome-shaped defect of the diaphragm has been reported (Fig. 2–5). In addition, diaphragmatic eventration has been found during ultrasound screening for embryonal tumors, but is uncommon.

Pregnancy/Perinatal

Beckwith-Wiedemann syndrome is associated with an increased incidence of prematurity, perhaps as high as 50% (107). Polyhydramnios and fetal macrosomia are also common (33). In pregnancies with an identified BWS fetus, findings frequently include a long umbilical cord and an enlarged placenta, averaging almost twice the normal weight for gestational age (107).

Endocrine/Metabolic

Hypoglycemia, due to hyperplastic changes in the pancreas (Fig. 2–6) and consequent hyperinsulinemia, affects about 30%–50% of infants with BWS (34,81). Mosaicism for 11p15 UPD has been shown to be the underlying pathogenetic mechanism in focal nesidioblastosis of the pancreas in individuals who do not have BWS (28); similarly, 11p15 UPD in the pancreas of BWS cases would play an analogous role in the hypoglycemia in BWS. Other genetic modifications within the BWS locus must cause hypoglycemia for other BWS subgroups.

Polycythemia, hypocalcemia, hypercholesterolemia, hyperlipidemia, and hypothyroidism have been documented in some BWS cases.

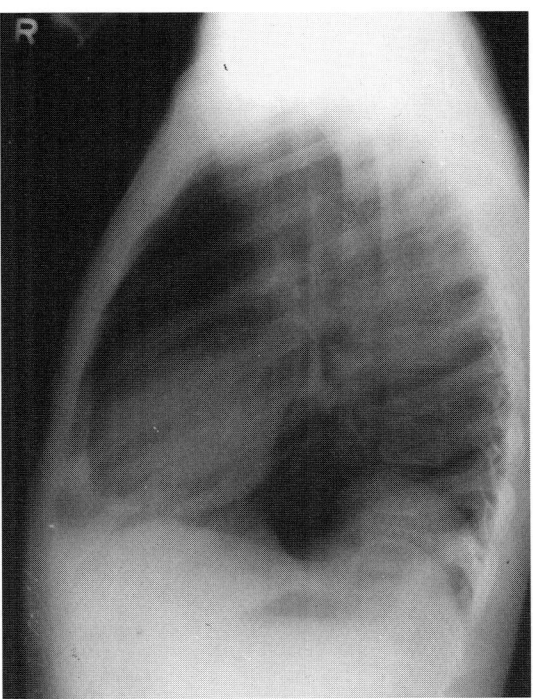

Figure 2–5 Beckwith-Wiedemann syndrome. Dome-shaped defect of diaphragm. From Cohen (21a).

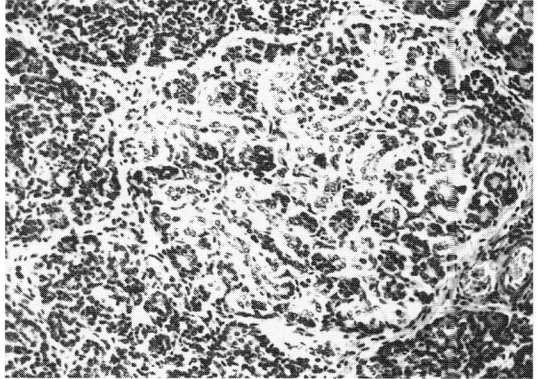

Figure 2–6 Beckwith-Wiedemann syndrome. Pancreas. Nodular mass of hyperplastic ductular elements surrounded by hyperplastic acinar tissue. From Beckwith (6a).

Craniofacial

Characteristic facial features in BWS include macroglossia, anterior earlobe creases (Fig. 2–7) and posterior helical pits (Fig. 2–8), nevus flammeus, and prominent eyes with infraorbital creases. Although biopsies of the tongue have usually been normal, Borstlap and de Wilde (12a) reported three cases with angiomatous vascular anomalies. Mild to moderate macroglossia often resolves spontaneously as the jaw grows to accommodate the tongue. However, macroglossia can occasionally lead to serious feeding or respiratory complications, and sometimes to speech articulation problems. As jaw growth accelerates to accommodate the tongue, malocclusion requiring intervention may also occur. Hemihyperplasia affecting one side of the face and/or tongue can also produce an unusual appearance. These facial features often show improvement over time (Fig. 2–9).

Abdomen

Omphalocele, umbilical hernia, and diastasis recti are very common findings in children with BWS. Less common findings include inguinal hernia, prune belly sequence, and gastrointestinal malformations such as atresia, stenosis, and malrotation.

Visceromegaly is common and may involve any or all of the following: liver, spleen, pancreas, kidneys, and adrenal glands. Adrenocortical cytomegaly (Fig. 2–10) is considered a hallmark of BWS; other renal findings are discussed below. Hyperplastic changes in the pancreas may be associated with neonatal hypoglycemia, but functional problems due to splenomegaly or hepatomegaly have generally not been reported.

Genitourinary

Renal anomalies, including unilateral or bilateral nephromegaly (Fig. 2–11), are quite common. The following have also been noted: renal medullary dysplasia (Fig. 2–12), persistent nephrogenic activity zones (Fig. 2–13), duplicated collecting system, nephrocalcinosis, medullary sponge kidney, cystic changes, hydronephrosis, neprolithiasis, and diverticulae (12,19).

Enlargement of the bladder, uterus, phallus, clitoris, ovaries (Fig. 2–14), and testes (Fig. 2–15) has also been reported.

Neoplasia

Approximately 7.5% of children with BWS develop tumors (109). In comparison, the popula-

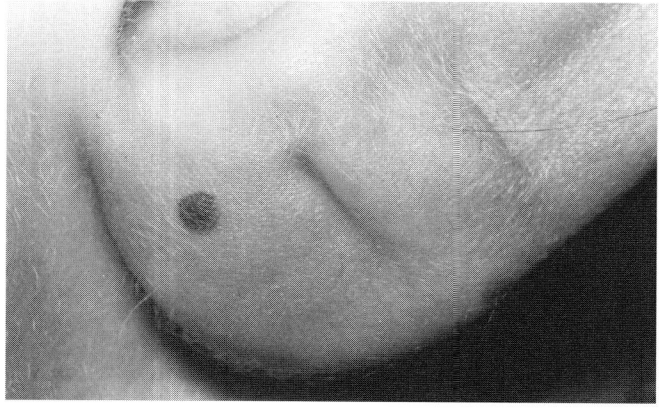

Figure 2–7 Beckwith-Wiedemann syndrome. Earlobe groove. From Cohen (21a).

Figure 2–8 Beckwith-Wiedemann syndrome. Circular indentation, posterior rim of helix. From Cohen (21a).

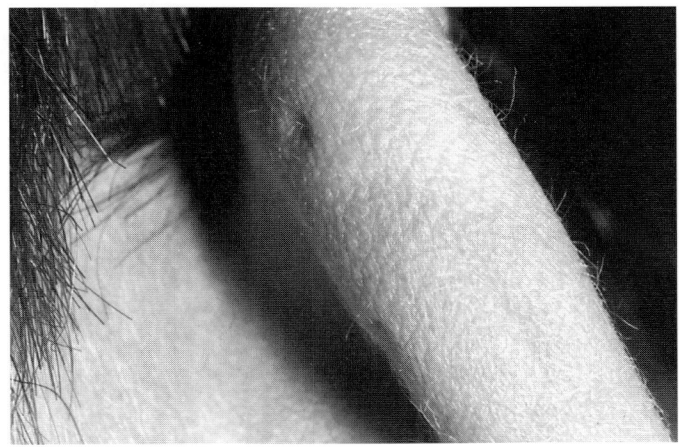

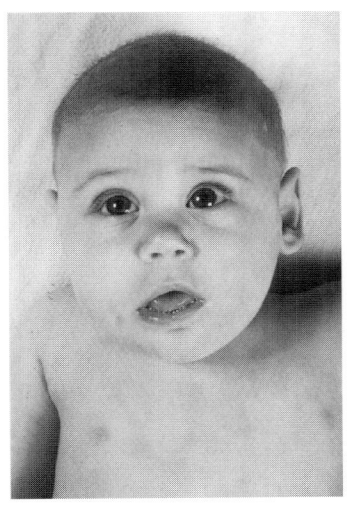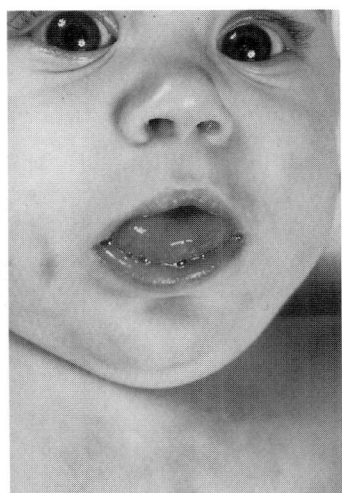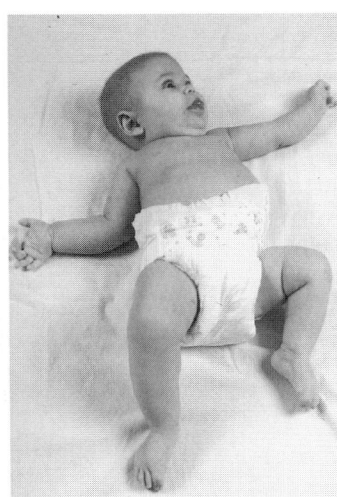

A

Figure 2–9 Beckwith-Wiedemann syndrome patient with uniparental disomy of chromosome 11p15. **A–E**: Evolution of facial features. Macroglossia from 5 months to 8.5 years. This patient did not have a tongue reduction or any orthodontic intervention. Panel **C** (right) shows hemihyperplasia of her leg.

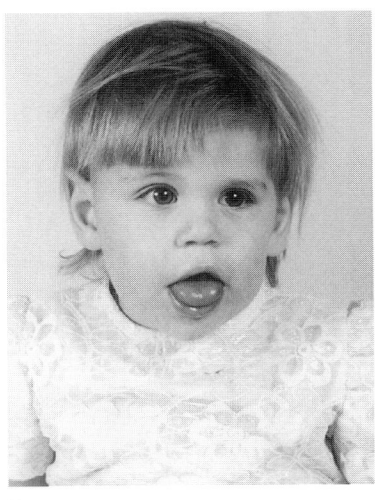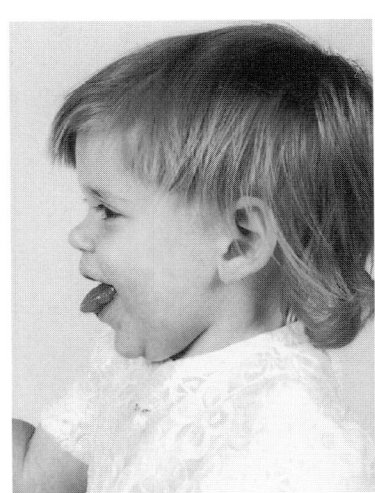

B

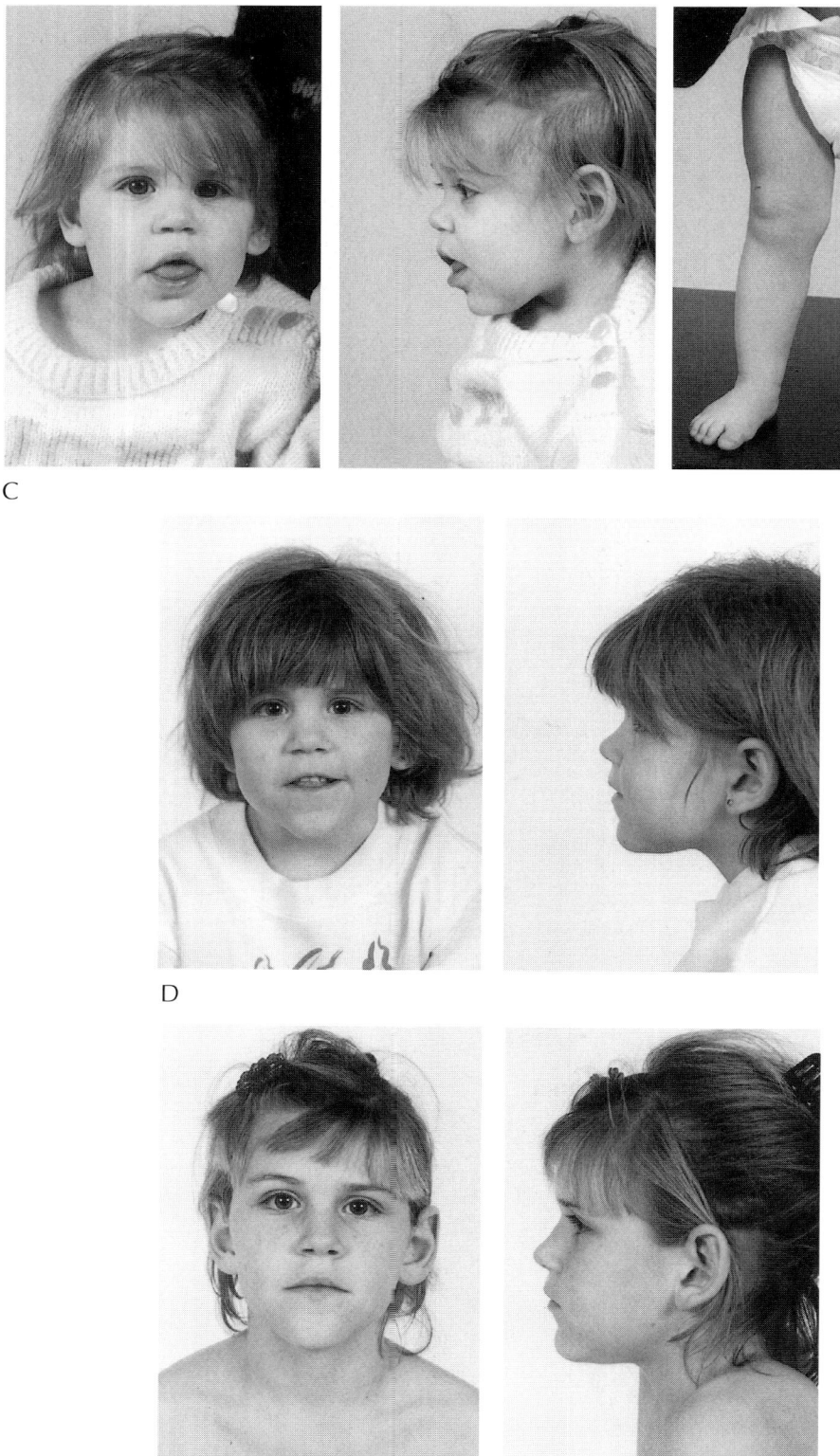

C

D

E

Figure 2–9 (continued).

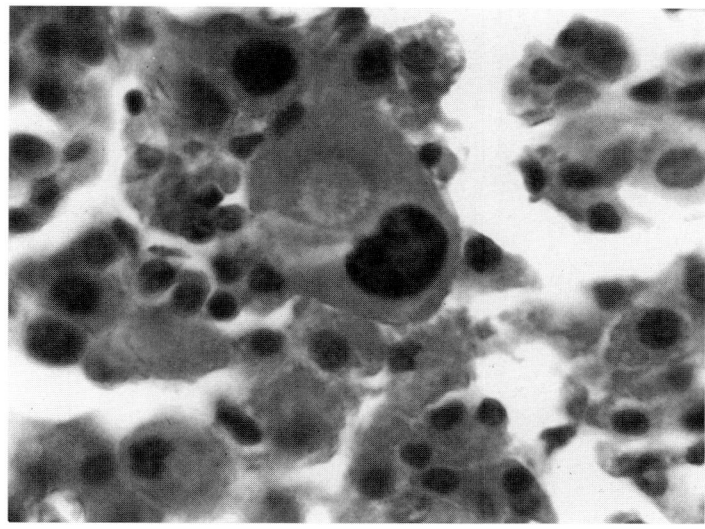

Figure 2–10 Beckwith-Wiedemann syndrome. Extreme cytomegaly of the adrenal cortex. Courtesy of J.B. Beckwith, Missoula, Montana.

tion risks for the two most common tumors, Wilms tumor and hepatoblastoma, are 1 in 10,000 and 1 in 100,000, respectively.

A comprehensive list of neoplasms reported in association with BWS is shown in Table 2–3. The most common malignancies reported in association with BWS are embryonal tumors such as Wilms tumor, hepatoblastoma, rhabdomyosarcoma, and neuroblastoma. The treatment outcomes for Wilms tumor are almost identical for children with or without BWS (82a).

Reports are only beginning to emerge on tumor risk and BWS molecular subgroups (10a,33a). BWS associated with hemihyperplasia confers an increased cancer risk, but the tumor site does not always correlate with the side of the overgrowth (45). Several other factors also appear to be associated with tumor development in BWS. These include nephromegaly (29) and nephrogenic rests or nephroblastomatosis (23). Nephrogenic rests, which represent abnormally persistent nephrogenic cells, are thought to be

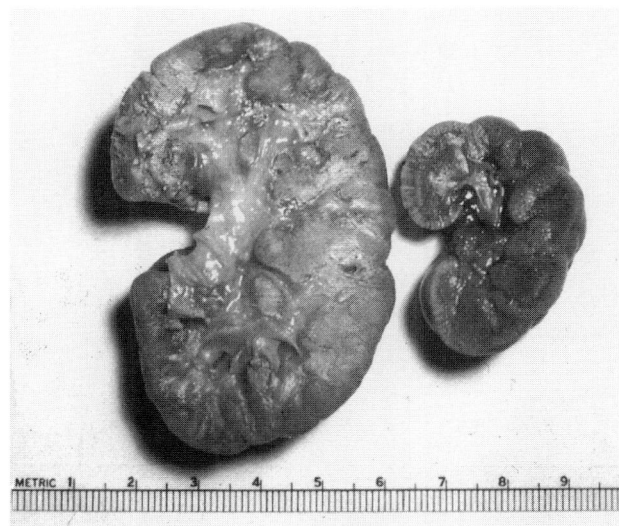

Figure 2–11 Beckwith-Wiedemann syndrome kidney compared with normal term newborn control. Courtesy of J.B. Beckwith, Missoula, Montana.

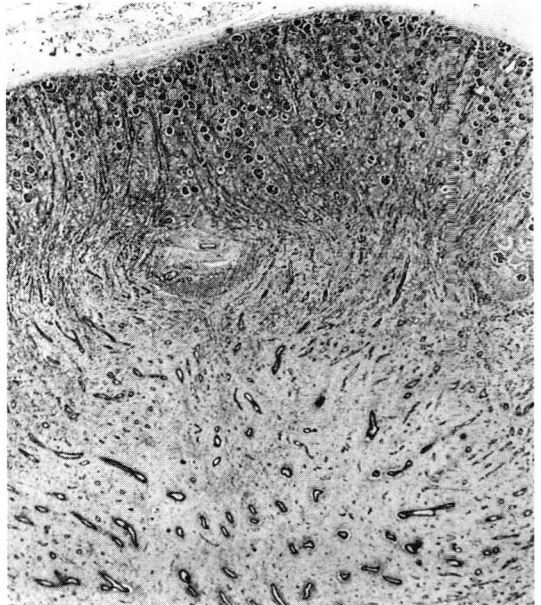

Figure 2–12 Beckwith-Wiedemann syndrome. Renal medullary dysplasia. From Beckwith (6a).

precursors of Wilms tumor. In BWS, nephrogenic rests occur in a perilobar distribution (7).

By mid-childhood (age 8), the risk of tumor development for individuals with BWS falls significantly and is thought to approximate the tumor risk for the general population.

PRENATAL PATIENT EVALUATION

Level II ultrasound at 19–20 weeks and again at 32 weeks gestation, as well as serum AFP (at 16 weeks gestation) should be offered to individuals with BWS undertaking a pregnancy and to parents who have had a previous child with BWS. Ultrasound screening, in conjunction with AFP screening, should be used to look for an abdominal wall defect. Ultrasound can also be used to assess growth parameters advanced for gestational age (likely not detectable until late in the second trimester), and to detect organomegaly, renal anomalies, cleft palate, cardiac abnormality, and macroglossia. In addition, there has been one report of an early ultrasound, between 10 and 14 weeks gestation, revealing increased nuchal translucency thickness and exomphalos in a fetus later found to have BWS (92).

Some families may wish to undertake prenatal testing for pregnancy and delivery management, and others, possibly to decide whether or not to continue with the pregnancy. If a molecular lesion has been identified, (e.g., $p57^{KIP2}$ mutation), the possibility of prenatal diagnosis by CVS or amniocentesis may be considered.

If BWS is suspected or diagnosed during pregnancy, delivery at a high-risk unit should be considered because of the increased risk of fetal macrosomia and maternal preeclampsia and eclampsia and for delivery management of omphalocele and/or macroglossia.

POSTNATAL PATIENT EVALUATION

It is recommended that neonates with BWS be screened for hypoglycemia. Parents should be advised of typical hypoglycemic manifestations and

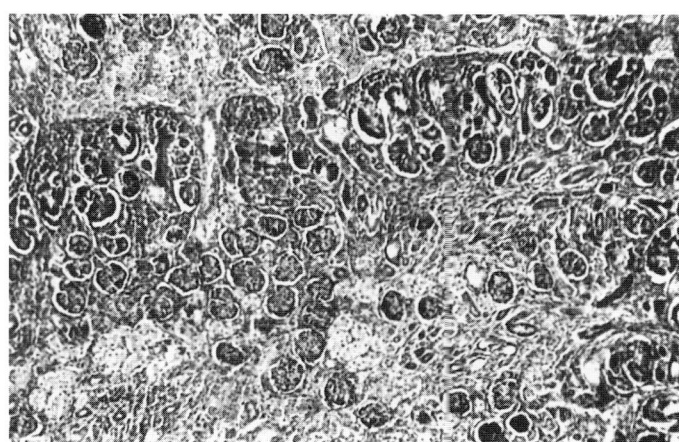

Figure 2–13 Beckwith-Wiedemann syndrome. Persistent nephrogenic activity zones. Courtesy of J.B. Beckwith, Missoula, Montana.

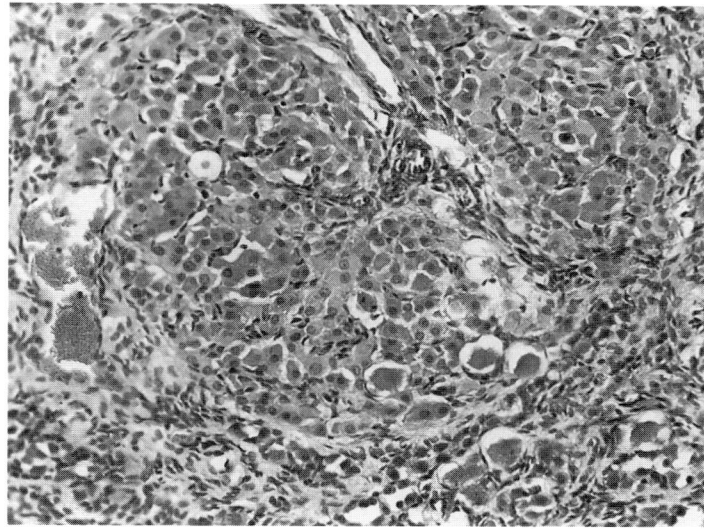

Figure 2–14 Beckwith-Wiedemann syndrome. Ovarian section. Adenomatous hyperplasia, hilus. Courtesy of J.B. Beckwith, Missoula, Montana.

the need for rapid intervention. In rare cases, hypoglycemia may be severe or prolonged. In such cases, evaluation by a pediatric endocrinologist is suggested.

Abdominal imaging for tumor surveillance (see below) is also useful for detecting renal malformations that may require referral to a nephrologist. Also, if there is evidence of calcium deposition in the kidney, periodic evaluation of urinary calcium excretion is indicated.

Developmental evaluation should be part of routine follow-up, and growth parameters should be measured at all clinic visits. Familial heights are helpful in the assessment of growth parameters. A bone age may assist in predicting adult height. In cases of hemihyperplasia, leg length discrepancies >1 cm and/or scoliosis should be referred for orthopedic evaluation.

Macroglossia may necessitate feeding adjustments or even partial tongue resection in the first few years of life. Some craniofacial surgeons opt for tongue reduction later if orthodontic and/or cosmetic concerns have not resolved, e.g., by preschool age. Early evaluation by a craniofacial team is helpful in determining the necessity and timing of intervention.

A high index of suspicion for cardiac problems should be maintained; also, a standard cardiac evaluation should precede any surgical procedure.

Tumor development has been associated with several BWS molecular groups. To date, tumors have been seen most frequently in BWS cases

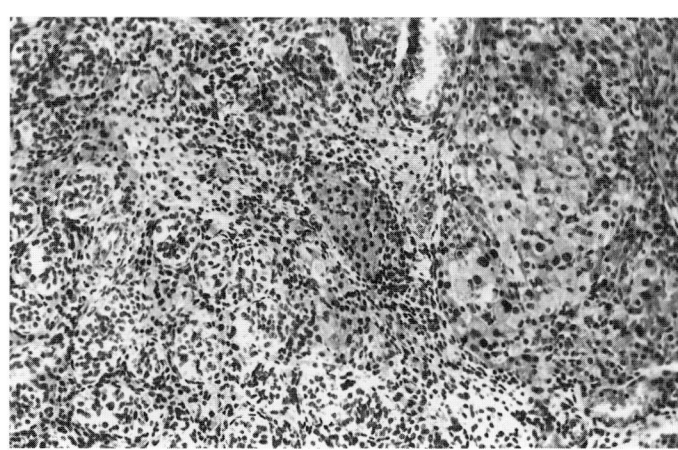

Figure 2–15 Beckwith-Wiedemann syndrome. Section of testis showing extreme hyperplasia of Leydig cells, with cytomegaly near upper right corner of field. From Beckwith (6a).

Table 2–3 Malignant/Premalignant and Benign Tumors in Beckwith-Wiedemann Syndrome[a]

Malignant/Premalignant Tumors	Benign Tumors
Wilms tumor	Adrenal adenoma
Adrenal cortical carcinoma	Fibroadenoma
Hepatoblastoma	Fibrous hamartoma
Hepatocellular carcinoma	Ganglioneuroma
Glioblastoma	Myxoma
Neuroblastoma	Teratoma
Carcinoid tumor	ACTH-independent testosterone-secreting adrenal adenoma
Rhabdomyosarcoma	Cardiac hamartoma
Malignant lymphoma	Chorangioma
Pancreatoblastoma	Digital fibroma
Congenital mesoblastic nephroma	Hepatic hemangioendothelioma
Myelodysplasia	Congenital gastric teratoma
Yolk sac tumor	Ganglioneuroma
Renal cell carcinoma	Benign bladder neck polyp
Intratubular germ cell neoplasia	Hamartoma of the urinary bladder
	Breast fibroadenoma

[a]This table is based on reports and reviews from Benirschke (8), Bockrath et al. (11), Crankson and Ahmed (24), Craver and Heinrich (25), Drut et al. (30–32), Falik-Borenstein et al. (37), Gorlin et al. (39), Koishi et al. (50), Matsumoto et al. (68), Raine et al. (83), Reddy et al. (85), Sirinelli et al. (89), Sutherland et al. (95), Weinstein et al. (101), Wiedemann (109), Williams et al. (110), Yamaguchi et al. (114).

with 11p15 UPD (Group C) or H19 maternal methylation (Group H) (10a,33a) and less frequently in BWS cases with imprinting defects of KvDMR1/KvLQT1-AS (101a) and mutations of $p57^{KIP2}$ (54). Because of the increased tumor risk, it is currently recommended that *all* children with suspected or confirmed BWS be screened every 3 months with abdominal ultrasounds until age 8. One of the potential benefits of a regular screening protocol is earlier diagnosis (18) and higher salvage of normal renal parenchyma (4). A baseline MRI or CT is suggested at the time of entry into a tumor surveillance program (5,21). Evaluation for elevated or rising alpha-fetoprotein levels in the first few years of life can be used for early detection of hepatoblastoma. In the first year of life, children with BWS tend to have higher levels of alpha-fetoprotein than the normal population (36). Although generally not incorporated into tumor screening protocols, screening for neuroblastoma has been previously suggested (17).

DIFFERENTIAL DIAGNOSIS

Several other overgrowth syndromes, as well as maternal diabetes mellitus, should be considered in the differential diagnosis of children presenting with macrosomia or other features characteristic of BWS. Features not commonly associated with BWS (such as developmental delay in the absence of 11p15 duplication) point to other diagnoses. Some children with hypotonia appear to have enlarged tongues. Also, large children can have other independent diagnoses. Isolated hemihyperplasia (see Chapter 3) should be considered when asymmetric overgrowth is the only finding. Several syndromes with phenotypes overlapping BWS are discussed below.

Simpson-Golabi-Behmel syndrome (SGBS) (see Chapter 4) has the following features in common with BWS: macrosomia, visceromegaly, macroglossia, and renal cysts. Findings that are more specific for SGBS include a characteristic facial coarseness, cleft lip, cardiac defects (62), supernumerary nipples, polydactyly or other skeletal anomalies, and an X-linked pattern of inheritance. The SGBS is caused by mutations in *GPC3*, a gene on the X-chromosome that encodes an extracellular proteoglycan (glypican-3) thought to act as a growth regulator during development (73,105).

Perlman syndrome (see Chapter 5) is characterized by macrosomia, increased risk of neonatal mortality, mental retardation, nephroblastomatosis, and a high incidence of bilateral Wilms tumor, usually occurring in the first year of life. The face is round with an upsweep of the anterior scalp hair, depressed nasal bridge, and micrognathia. The molecular etiology of Perlman syndrome is unknown but its autosomal recessive inheritance implies a distinct genetic basis (40,41).

In the neonatal period, Costello syndrome (see Chapter 15) can be confused with BWS. Infants with Costello syndrome typically present with overgrowth, cardiac defects, and edema. Over time, these patients are clearly distinguishable from BWS patients by their distinctive features and failure to thrive (99).

REFERENCES

1. Barlow DP: Competition—A common motif for the imprinting mechanism? EMBO J 16:6899–6905, 1997.
2. Barlow DP: Gametic imprinting in mammals. Science 270:1610–1613, 1995.
3. Bartolomei MS, Tilghman SM: Genomic imprinting in mammals. Annu Rev Genet 31:493–525, 1997.
4. Beckwith JB: personal communication, 2000.
5. Beckwith JB: Children at increased risk for Wilms tumor: monitoring issues [editorial; comment]. J Pediatr 132:377–379, 1998.
6. Beckwith JB: Extreme cytomegaly of the adrenal fetal cortex, omphalocele, hyperplasia of kidneys and pancreas and Leydig-cell hyperplasia: Another syndrome? Western Society for Pediatric Research, Los Angeles, California, 1963.
6a. Beckwith JB: Macroglossia, omphalocele, adrenal cytomegaly, gigantism, and hyperplastic visceromegaly. Birth Defects 5(2):188–196, 1969.
7. Beckwith JB, Kiviat NB, Bonadio JF: Nephrogenic rests, nephroblastomatosis, and the pathogenesis of Wilms' tumor. Pediatr Pathol 10:1–36, 1990.
8. Benirschke K: Recent trends in chorangiomas, especially those of multiple and recurrent chorangiomas. Pediatr Dev Pathol 2:264–269, 1999.
9. Benke PJ: Familial Beckwith-Wiedemann syndrome. Annual Birth Defects Conference, San Francisco, California, 1978.
10. Berry AC, Belton EM, Chantler C: Monozygotic twins discordant for Wiedemann-Beckwith syndrome and the implications for genetic counselling. J Med Genet 17:136–138, 1980.
10a. Bliek J, Maas SM, Ruijten JM, Hennekam RCM, Alders M, Westerveld A, Mannens MMAM: Increased tumor risk for BWS patients correlates with aberrant $H19$ and not $KCNQ1OT1$ methylation: Occurrence of $KCNQ1OT1$ hypomethylation in familial cases of BWS. Hum Mol Genet 10:467–476, 2001.
11. Bockrath JM, Maizels M, Firlit CF: Benign bladder neck polyp causing tandem obstruction of the urinary tract in a patient with Beckwith-Wiedemann syndrome. J Urol 128:1309–1312, 1982.
12. Borer JG, Kaefer M, Barnewolt CE, Elias ER, Hobbs N, Retik AB, Peters CA: Renal findings on radiological follow-up of patients with Beckwith-Wiedemann syndrome. J Urol 161:235–239, 1999.
12a. Borstlap WA, de Wilde PCM. Macroglossia in Beckwith-Wiedemann syndrome. J Craniomaxillofac Surg (Suppl 1) 28:9, 2000.
13. Bose B, Wilkie RA, Madlom M, Forsyth JS, Faed MJ: Wiedemann-Beckwith syndrome in one of monozygotic twins. Arch Dis Child 60:1191–1192, 1985.
14. Buiting K, Saitoh S, Gross S, Dittrich B, Schwartz S, Nicholls RD, Horsthemke B: Inherited microdeletions in the Angelman and Prader-Willi syndromes define an imprinting centre on human chromosome 15 [published erratum appears in Nat Genet 1995;10:249]. Nat Genet 9:395–400, 1995.
15. Caspary T, Cleary MA, Baker CC, Guan XJ, Tilghman SM: Multiple mechanisms regulate imprinting of the mouse distal chromosome 7 gene cluster. Mol Cell Biol 18:3466–3474, 1998.
16. Chien CH, Lee JS, Tsai WY, Wang TR: Wiedemann-Beckwith syndrome with congenital central hypothyroidism in one of monozygotic twins. J Formos Med Assoc 89:132–136, 1990.
17. Chitayat D, Friedman JM, Dimmick JE: Neuroblastoma in a child with Wiedemann-Beckwith syndrome. Am J Med Genet 35:433–436, 1990.
18. Choyke PL, Siegel MJ, Craft AW, Green DM, DeBaun MR: Screening for Wilms tumor in children with Beckwith-Wiedemann syndrome or idiopathic hemihypertrophy. Med Pediatr Oncol 32:196–200, 1999.
19. Choyke PL, Siegel MJ, Oz O, Sotelo-Avila C, DeBaun MR: Nonmalignant renal disease in pediatric patients with Beckwith-Wiedemann syndrome. Am J Roentgenol 171:733–737, 1998.
20. Clayton-Smith J, Read AP, Donnai D: Monozygotic twinning and Wiedemann-Beckwith syndrome. Am J Med Genet 42:633–637, 1992.
21. Clericuzio CL, D'Angio GJ, Duncan M, Green DM, Knudson AG Jr: Summary and recommendations of the workshop held at the First International Conference on Molecular and Clinical Genetics of Childhood Renal Tumors, Albuquerque, New Mexico. Med Pediatr Oncol 1992.
21a. Cohen MM Jr: Overgrowth syndromes. In: *Associated Congenital Malformations*. M. El-Shafie and CH Klippel, eds. Williams & Wilkins, Baltimore, 1981, pp. 71–104.

22. Constancia M, Pickard B, Kelsey G, Reik W: Imprinting mechanisms. Genome Res 8:881–900, 1998.
23. Coppes MJ, Arnold M, Beckwith JB, Ritchey ML, D'Angio GJ, Green DM, Breslow NE: Factors affecting the risk of contralateral Wilms tumor development: A report from the National Wilms Tumor Study Group. Cancer 85:1616–1625, 1999.
24. Crankson S, Ahmed S: Benign bladder neck polyp and ureteropelvic obstruction in Beckwith-Wiedemann syndrome. Aust N Z J Surg 61:955–957, 1991.
25. Craver RD, Heinrich S: Bone invasion by a recurrent digital fibroma of infancy in a child with Beckwith-Wiedemann syndrome. Pediatr Pathol Lab Med 15:147–151, 1995.
26. Cui H, Horon IL, Ohlsson R, Hamilton SR, Feinberg AP: Loss of imprinting in normal tissue of colorectal cancer patients with microsatellite instability [see comments]. Nat Med 4:1276–1280, 1998.
27. Dao D, Frank D, Qian N, O'Keefe D, Vosatka RJ, Walsh CP, Tycko B: IMPT1, an imprinted gene similar to polyspecific transporter and multi-drug resistance genes. Hum Mol Genet 7:597–608, 1998.
28. de Lonlay P, Fournet JC, Rahier J Gross-Morand MS, Poggi-Travert F, Foussier V, Bonnefont JP, Brusset MC, Brunelle F, Robert JJ, Nihoul-Fekete C, Saudubray JM, Junien C: Somatic deletion of the imprinted 11p15 region in sporadic persistent hyperinsulinemic hypoglycemia of infancy is specific of focal adenomatous hyperplasia and endorses partial pancreatectomy. J Clin Invest 100:802–807, 1997.
29. DeBaun MR, Siegel MJ, Choyke PL: Nephromegaly in infancy and early childhood: A risk factor for Wilms tumor in Beckwith-Wiedemann syndrome [see comments]. J Pediatr 132:401–404, 1998.
30. Drut R, Drut RM, Toulouse JC: Hepatic hemangioendotheliomas, placental chorioangiomas, and dysmorphic kidneys in Beckwith-Wiedemann syndrome. Pediatr Pathol 12:197–203, 1992.
31. Drut R, Jones MC: Congenital pancreatoblastoma in Beckwith-Wiedemann syndrome: an emerging association. Pediatr Pathol 8:331–339, 1988.
32. Drut R, Mortera M, Drut RM: Yolk sac tumor of the placenta in Wiedemann-Beckwith syndrome. Pediatr Dev Pathol 1:534–537, 1998.
33. Elliott M, Maher ER: Beckwith-Wiedemann syndrome. J Med Genet 31:560–564, 1994.
33a. Engel JR, Smallwood A, Harper A, Higgins MJ, Oshimura M, Reik W, Schofield PN, Maher ER: Epigenotype-phenotype correlations in Beckwith-Wiedemann syndrome. J Med Genet 37:921–926, 2000.
34. Engstrom W, Lindham S, Schofield P: Wiedemann-Beckwith syndrome. Eur J Pediatr 147:450–457, 1988.
35. Estabrooks LL, Lamb AN, Kirkman HN, Boyer S, Wiley JE, Callanan ND, Rao KW: Beckwith-Wiedemann syndrome in twins with a duplication of chromosome [15q11.2–q13] mat. Am J Hum Genet 45(Suppl):A75, 1989.
36. Everman DB, Shuman C, Dzolganovski B, O'Riordan MA, Weksberg R, Robin NH: Serum alpha-fetoprotein levels in Beckwith-Wiedemann syndrome. J Pediatr 137:123–127, 2000.
37. Falik-Borenstein TC, Korenberg JR, Davos I, Platt LD, Gans S, Goodman B, Schreck R, Graham JM Jr: Congenital gastric teratoma in Wiedemann-Beckwith syndrome. Am J Med Genet 38:52–57, 1991.
37a. Feinberg AP: The two-domain hypothesis in Beckwith-Wiedemann syndrome. J Clin Invest 106:739–740, 2000.
38. Franceschini P, Guala A, Vardeu MP, Franceschini D: Monozygotic twinning and Wiedemann-Beckwith syndrome [letter]. Am J Med Genet 46:353–354, 1993.
39. Gorlin RJ, Cohen MM Jr, Levin LS, eds. Syndromes of the Head and Neck, 3rd ed. Oxford University Press, New York, 1990.
40. Greenberg F, Stein F, Gresik MV, Finegold MJ, Carpenter RJ, Riccardi VM, Beaudet AL: The Perlman familial nephroblastomatosis syndrome. Am J Med Genet 24:101–110, 1986.
41. Grundy RG, Pritchard J, Baraitser M, Risdon A, Robards M: Perlman and Wiedemann-Beckwith syndromes: Two distinct conditions associated with Wilms' tumour. Eur J Pediatr 151:895–898, 1992.
42. Hao Y, Crenshaw T, Moulton T, Newcomb E, Tycko B: Tumour-suppressor activity of H19 RNA. Nature 365:764–767, 1993.
43. Hark AT, Schoenherr CJ, Katz DJ, Ingram RS, Levorse JM, Tilghman SM: CTCF mediates methylation-sensitive enhancer-blocking activity at the H19/Igf2 locus [see comments]. Nature 405:486–489, 2000.
44. Hatada I, Ohashi H, Fukushima Y, Kaneko Y, Inoue M, Komoto Y, Okada A, Ohishi S, Nabetani A, Morisaki H, Nakayama M, Niikawa N, Mukai T: An imprinted gene $p57^{KIP2}$ is mutated in Beckwith-Wiedemann syndrome [see comments]. Nat Genet 14:171–173, 1996.
45. Hoyme HE, Seaver LH, Jones KL, Procopio F, Crooks W, Feingold M: Isolated hemihyperplasia (hemihypertrophy): Report of a prospective multicenter study of the incidence of neoplasia and review. Am J Med Genet 79:274–278, 1998.
45a. Itoh N, Becroft DMO, Reeve AE, Morison IM: Proportion of cells with paternal 11p15 uniparental disomy correlated with organ enlargement in Wiedemann-Beckwith syndrome. Am J Med Genet 92:111–116, 2000.

46. Jong MT, Carey AH, Caldwell KA, Lau MH, Handel MA, Driscoll DJ, Stewart CL, Rinchik EM, Nicholls RD: Imprinting of a RING zinc-finger encoding gene in the mouse chromosome region homologous to the Prader-Willi syndrome genetic region. Hum Mol Genet 8:795–803, 1999.
47. Jong MT, Gray TA, Ji Y, Glenn CC, Saitoh S, Driscoll DJ, Nicholls RD: A novel imprinted gene, encoding a RING zinc-finger protein, and overlapping antisense transcript in the Prader-Willi syndrome critical region. Hum Mol Genet 8:783–793, 1999.
48. Kawame H, Gartler SM, Hansen RS: Allele-specific replication timing in imprinted domains: Absence of asynchrony at several loci. Hum Mol Genet 4:2287–2293, 1995.
49. Knudson AG Jr, Strong LC: Mutation and cancer: A model for Wilms' tumor of the kidney. J Natl Cancer Inst 48:313–324, 1972.
50. Koishi S, Kubota M, Taniguchi Y, Takei N, Mamada M, Akiyama Y, Furusho K, Hayashidera T: Myelodysplasia in a child with Beckwith-Wiedemann syndrome previously treated for hepatoblastoma with multi-agent chemotherapy [letter]. J Pediatr Hematol Oncol 18:419–420, 1996.
51. Kondo M, Matsuoka S, Uchida K, Osada H, Nagatake M, Takagi K, Harper JW, Takahashi T, Elledge SJ: Selective maternal-allele loss in human lung cancers of the maternally expressed $p57^{KIP2}$ gene at 11p15.5. Oncogene 12:1365–1368, 1996.
52. Lai S, Goepfert H, Gillenwater AM, Luna MA, El-Naggar AK: Loss of imprinting and genetic alterations of the cyclin-dependent kinase inhibitor $p57^{KIP2}$ gene in head and neck squamous cell carcinoma [in process citation]. Clin Cancer Res 6:3172–3176, 2000.
53. Lam WW, Hatada I, Ohishi S, Mukai T, Joyce JA, Cole TR, Donnai D, Reik W, Schofield PN, Maher ER: Analysis of germline *CDKN1C* (*$p57^{KIP2}$*) mutations in familial and sporadic Beckwith-Wiedemann syndrome (BWS) provides a novel genotype–phenotype correlation. J Med Genet 36:518–523, 1999.
54. Lee MP, DeBaun M, Randhawa G, Reichard BA, Elledge SJ, Feinberg AP: Low frequency of $p57^{KIP2}$ mutation in Beckwith-Wiedemann syndrome. Am J Hum Genet 61:304–309, 1997.
55. Lee MP, DeBaun MR, Mitsuya K, Galonek HL, Brandenburg S, Oshimura M, Feinberg AP: Loss of imprinting of a paternally expressed transcript, with antisense orientation to KVLQT1, occurs frequently in Beckwith-Wiedemann syndrome and is independent of insulin-like growth factor II imprinting. Proc Natl Acad Sci USA 96:5203–5208, 1999.
56. Leonard NJ, Bernier FP, Rudd N, Machin GA, Bamforth F, Bamforth S, Grundy P, Johnson C: Two pairs of male monozygotic twins discordant for Wiedemann-Beckwith syndrome. Am J Med Genet 61:253–257, 1996.
57. Li M, Squire J, Shuman C, Smith AC, Chitayat D, Weksberg R: Imprinting status of 11p15 genes in Beckwith-Wiedemann syndrome with $p57^{KIP2}$. Genomics 74:370–376, 2001.
58. Li M, Squire JA, Weksberg R: Molecular genetics of Beckwith-Wiedemann syndrome. Curr Opin Pediatr 9:623–629, 1997.
59. Li M, Squire JA, Weksberg R: Molecular genetics of Wiedemann-Beckwith syndrome. Am J Med Genet 79:253–259, 1998.
60. Li M, Squire JA, Weksberg R: Overgrowth syndromes and genomic imprinting: from mouse to man. Clin Genet 53:165–170, 1998.
61. Li X, Adam G, Cui H, Sandstedt B, Ohlsson R, Ekstrom TJ: Expression, promoter usage and parental imprinting status of insulin-like growth factor II (IGF2) in human hepatoblastoma: Uncoupling of IGF2 and H19 imprinting. Oncogene 11:221–229, 1995.
62. Lin AE, Neri G, Hughes-Benzie R, Weksberg R: Cardiac anomalies in the Simpson-Golabi-Behmel syndrome. Am J Med Genet 83:378–381, 1999.
63. Litz CE, Taylor KA, Qiu JS, Pescovitz OH, de Martinville B: Absence of detectable chromosomal and molecular abnormalities in monozygotic twins discordant for the Wiedemann-Beckwith syndrome. Am J Med Genet 30:821–833, 1988.
64. Lubinsky M, Herrmann J, Kosseff AL, Opitz JM: Letter: Autosomal-dominant sex-dependent transmission of the Wiedemann-Beckwith syndrome. Lancet 1:932, 1974.
65. Lubinsky MS, Hall JG: Genomic imprinting, monozygous twinning, and X inactivation [letter] [see comments]. Lancet 337:1288, 1991.
66. Maher ER, Reik W: Beckwith-Wiedemann syndrome: Imprinting in clusters revisited [see comments]. J Clin Invest 105:247–252, 2000.
67. Mannens M, Hoovers JM, Redeker E, Verjaal M, Feinberg AP, Little P, Boavida M, Coad N, Steenman M, Bliek J: Parental imprinting of human chromosome region 11p15.3-pter involved in the Beckwith-Wiedemann syndrome and various human neoplasia. Eur J Hum Genet 2:3–23, 1994.
68. Matsumoto T, Kinoshita E, Maeda H, Niikawa N, Kurosaki N, Harada N, Yun K, Sawai T, Aoki S, Kondoh T, et al.: Molecular analysis of a patient with Beckwith-Wiedemann syndrome, rhabdomyosarcoma and renal cell carcinoma. Jpn J Hum Genet 39:225–234, 1994.
69. Matsuoka S, Edwards MC, Bai C, Parker S, Zhang P, Baldini A, Harper JW, Elledge SJ: $p57^{KIP2}$, a structurally distinct member of the p21CIP1 Cdk inhibitor family, is a candidate tumor suppressor gene. Genes Dev 9:650–662, 1995.

70. Moore T, Constancia M, Zubair M, Bailleul B, Feil R, Sasaki H, Reik W: Multiple imprinted sense and antisense transcripts, differential methylation and tandem repeats in a putative imprinting control region upstream of mouse Igf2. Proc Natl Acad Sci USA 94:12509–12514, 1997.
71. Morison IM, Becroft DM, Taniguchi T, Woods CG, Reeve AE: Somatic overgrowth associated with overexpression of insulin-like growth factor II. Nat Med 2:311–316, 1996.
72. Muller S, van den Boom D, Zirkel D, Koster H, Berthold F, Schwab M, Westphal M, Zumkeller W: Retention of imprinting of the human apoptosis-related gene *TSSC3* in human brain tumors. Hum Mol Genet 9:757–763, 2000.
73. Neri G, Gurrieri F, Zanni G, Lin A: Clinical and molecular aspects of the Simpson-Golabi-Behmel syndrome. Am J Med Genet 79:279–283, 1998.
74. Neyroud N, Tesson F, Denjoy I, Leibovici M, Donger C, Barhanin J, Faure S, Gary F, Coumel P, Petit C, Schwartz K, Guicheney P: A novel mutation in the potassium channel gene *KVLQT1* causes the Jervell and Lange-Nielsen cardioauditory syndrome [see comments]. Nat Genet 15:186–189, 1997.
75. Nicholls RD: The impact of genomic imprinting for neurobehavioral and developmental disorders. J Clin Invest 105:413–418, 2000.
76. Nicholls RD, Saitoh S, Horsthemke B: Imprinting in Prader-Willi and Angelman syndromes. Trends Genet 14:194–200, 1998.
77. Neumann R, Kubicka P, Barlow DP: Characteristics of imprinted genes. Nat Genet 9:12–13, 1995.
78. Okamoto K, Morison IM, Reeve AE, Tommerup N, Wiedemann H-R, Friedrich U: Is *p57KIP2* mutation a common mechanism for Beckwith-Wiedemann syndrome or somatic overgrowth? J Med Genet 35:86, 1998.
79. Olney AH, Buehler BA, Waziri M: Wiedemann-Beckwith syndrome in apparently discordant monozygotic twins. Am J Med Genet 29:491–499, 1988.
80. Orstavik RE, Tommerup N, Eiklid K, Orstavik KH: Non-random X chromosome inactivation in an affected twin in a monozygotic twin pair discordant for Wiedemann-Beckwith syndrome. Am J Med Genet 56:210–214, 1995.
81. Pettenati MJ, Haines JL, Higgins RR, Wappner RS, Palmer CG, Weaver DD: Wiedemann-Beckwith syndrome: Presentation of clinical and cytogenetic data on 22 new cases and review of the literature. Hum Genet 74:143–154 1986.
82. Pfeifer K. Mechanisms of genomic imprinting. Am J Hum Genet 67:777–787, 2000.
82a. Porteus MH, Narkool P, Nemberg D, Guthrie K, Breslow N, Green DM, Diller L: Characteristics and outcome of children with Beckwith-Wiedemann syndrome and Wilms' tumor: A report from the National Wilms Tumor Study Group. J Clin Oncol 18:2026–2031, 2000.
83. Raine PA, Noblett HR, Houghton-Allen BW, Campbell PE: Breast fibroadenoma and cardiac anomaly associated with EMG (Beckwith-Wiedemann) syndrome. J Pediatr 94:633–634, 1979.
84. Rainier S, Johnson LA, Dobry CJ, Ping AJ, Grundy PE, Feinberg AP: Relaxation of imprinted genes in human cancer. Nature 362:747–749, 1993.
85. Reddy JK, Schimke RN, Chang CH, Svoboda DJ, Slaven J, Therou L: Beckwith-Wiedemann syndrome. Wilms' tumor, cardiac hamartoma, persistent visceromegaly, and glomeruloneogenesis in a 2-year-old boy. Arch Pathol 94:523–532, 1972.
86. Reik W, Constancia M: Genomic imprinting. Making sense or antisense? [news; comment]. Nature 389:669–671, 1997.
87. Rougeulle C, Cardoso C, Fontes M, Colleaux L, Lalande M: An imprinted antisense RNA overlaps UBE3A and a second maternally expressed transcript [letter]. Nat Genet 19:15–16, 1998.
88. Sait SN, Nowak NJ, Singh-Kahlon P, Weksberg R, Squire J, Shows TB, Higgins MJ: Localization of Beckwith-Wiedemann and rhabdoid tumor chromosome rearrangements to a defined interval in chromosome band 11p15.5. Genes Chromosomes Cancer 11:97–105, 1994.
89. Sirinelli D, Silberman B, Baudon JJ, Sinnassamy P, Gruner M, Montagne JP: Beckwith-Wiedemann syndrome and neural crest tumors. A report of two cases. Pediatr Radiol 19:242–245, 1989.
90. Slavotinek A, Gaunt L, Donnai D: Paternally inherited duplications of 11p15.5 and Beckwith-Wiedemann syndrome. J Med Genet 34:819–826, 1997.
91. Smilinich NJ, Day CD, Fitzpatrick GV, Caldwell GM, Lossie AC, Cooper PR, Smallwood AC, Joyce JA, Schofield PN, Reik W, Nicholls RD, Weksberg R, Driscoll DJ, Maher ER, Shows TB, Higgins MJ: A maternally methylated CpG island in KvLQT1 is associated with an antisense paternal transcript and loss of imprinting in Beckwith-Wiedemann syndrome. Proc Natl Acad Sci USA 96:8064–8069, 1999.
92. Souka AP, Snijders RJ, Novakov A, Soares W, Nicolaides KH: Defects and syndromes in chromosomally normal fetuses with increased nuchal translucency thickness at 10–14 weeks of gestation [see comments]. Ultrasound Obstet Gynecol 11:391–400, 1998.
93. Squire J, Weksberg R: Genomic imprinting in tumours. Semin Cancer Biol 7:41–47, 1996.
94. Squire JA, Li M, Perlikowski S, Fei YL, Bayani J, Zhang ZM, Weksberg R: Alterations of *H19* imprinting and *IGF2* replication timing are infrequent in Beckwith-Wiedemann syndrome. Genomics 65:234–242, 2000.
94a. Steenman M, Westerveld A, Mannens M: Ge-

netics of Beckwith-Wiedemann syndrome-associated tumors: Common genetic pathways. Genes Chromosomes Cancer 28:1–13, 2000.
94b. Sun FL, Dean WL, Kelsey G, Allen ND, Reik W: Transactivation of igf2 in a mouse model of Beckwith-Wiedemann syndrome. Nature 389: 809–815, 1997.
95. Sutherland RW, Wiener JS, Hicks MJ, Hawkins EP, Chintagumpala M: Congenital mesoblastic nephroma in a child with the Beckwith-Wiedemann syndrome. J Urol 158:1532–1533, 1997.
96. Thorburn MJ, Wright ES, Miller CG, Smith-Read EH: Exomphalos-macroglossia-gigantism syndrome in Jamaican infants. Am J Dis Child 119:316–321, 1970.
97. Tycko B: Genomic imprinting and cancer. In *Genomic Imprinting: An Interdisciplinary Approach*. R. Ohlsson, ed. Springer-Verlag, Berlin and Heidelberg, pp. 133–169, 1999.
98. Tycko B: Genomic imprinting and human neoplasia. In: *DNA Alterations in Cancer*. M. Ehrlich, ed. Eaton Publishing: Natwick, MA, pp. 333–349, 1999.
99. van Eeghen AM, van Gelderen I, Hennekam RC: Costello syndrome: Report and review. Am J Med Genet 82:187–193, 1999.
100. Wang Q, Curran ME, Splawski I, Burn TC, Millholland JM, VanRaay TJ, Shen J, Timothy KW, Vincent GM, de Jager T, Schwartz PJ, Toubin JA, Moss AJ, Atkinson DL, Landes GM, Connors TD, Keating MT: Positional cloning of a novel potassium channel gene: *KVLQT1* mutations cause cardiac arrhythmias. Nat Genet 12:17–23, 1996.
101. Weinstein JM, Backonja M, Houston LW, Gilbert EE, Finlay JL, Duff TA, Chun RW: Optic glioma associated with Beckwith-Wiedemann syndrome. Pediatr Neurol 2:308–310, 1986.
101a. Weksberg R: Unpublished data, 2001.
102. Weksberg R, Glaves M, Teshima I, Waziri M, Patil S, Williams BR: Molecular characterization of Beckwith-Wiedemann syndrome (BWS) patients with partial duplication of chromosome 11p excludes the gene *MYOD1* from the BWS region. Genomics 8:693–698, 1990.
103. Weksberg R, Shen DR, Fei YL, Song QL, Squire J: Disruption of insulin-like growth factor 2 imprinting in Beckwith-Wiedemann syndrome. Nat Genet 5:143–150, 1993.
104. Weksberg R, Squire JA: Molecular biology of Beckwith-Wiedemann syndrome. Med Pediatr Oncol 27:462–469, 1996.
105. Weksberg R, Squire JA, Templeton DM: Glypicans: a growing trend [news; comment]. Nat Genet 12:225–227, 1996.
106. Weksberg R, Teshima I, Williams BR, Greenberg CR, Pueschel SM, Chernos JE, Fowlow SB, Hoyme E, Anderson IJ, Whiteman DA: Molecular characterization of cytogenetic alterations associated with the Beckwith-Wiedemann syndrome (BWS) phenotype refines the localization and suggests the gene for BWS is imprinted. Hum Mol Genet 2: 549–556, 1993.
107. Weng EY, Moeschler JB, Graham JM Jr: Longitudinal observations on 15 children with Wiedemann-Beckwith syndrome. Am J Med Genet 56:366–373, 1995.
108. Wiedemann H-R: Complexe malformatif familial avec hernie ombilicale et macroglossie, un "syndrome nouveau". J Génét Hum 13:223–232, 1964.
109. Wiedemann H-R: Tumours and hemihypertrophy associated with Wiedemann-Beckwith syndrome. Eur J Pediatr 141:129, 1983.
110. Williams MP, Ibrahim SK, Rickwood AM: Hamartoma of the urinary bladder in an infant with Beckwith-Wiedemann syndrome. Br J Urol 65:106–107, 1990.
111. Wu HK, Squire JA, Catzavelos CG, Weksberg R: Relaxation of imprinting of human insulin-like growth factor II gene, *IGF2*, in sporadic breast carcinomas. Biochem Biophys Res Commun 235:123–129, 1997.
112. Wu HK, Weksberg R, Minden MD, Squire JA: Loss of imprinting of human insulin-like growth factor II gene, *IGF2*, in acute myeloid leukemia. Biochem Biophys Res Commun 235:466–472, 1997.
113. Wutz A, Smrzka OW, Schweifer N, Schellander K, Wagner EF, Barlow DP: Imprinted expression of the *Igf2r* gene depends on an intronic CpG island [see comments]. Nature 389:745–749, 1997.
114. Yamaguchi T, Fukuda T, Uetani M, Hayashi K, Kurosaki N, Maeda H, Matsumoto T, Miyake H: Renal cell carcinoma in a patient with Beckwith-Wiedemann syndrome. Pediatr Radiol 26:312–314, 1996.
115. Yan Y, Frisen J, Lee MH, Massague J, Barbacid M: Ablation of the CDK inhibitor p57^{KIP2} results in increased apoptosis and delayed differentiation during mouse development. Genes Dev 11:973–983, 1997.
116. Yballe CM, Vu TH, Hoffman AR: Imprinting and expression of insulin-like growth factor-II and H19 in normal breast tissue and breast tumor. J Clin Endocrinol Metab 81:1607–1612, 1996.
117. Zhang P, Liegeois NJ, Wong C, Finegold M, Hou H, Thompson JC, Silverman A, Harper JW, DePinho RA, Elledge SJ: Altered cell differentiation and proliferation in mice lacking *p57^{KIP2}* indicates a role in Beckwith-Wiedemann syndrome. Nature 387:151–158, 1997.

3

Hemihyperplasia (Hemihypertrophy)

Although the term *hemihypertrophy* has been used conventionally and frequently in the medical literature, it is inappropriate because the condition so obviously refers to hemihyperplasia—an increase in cell number, not an increase in cell size. Differences between asymmetry, hemihyperplasia, hemihypertrophy, hematrophy, and preferential laterality have been discussed by Cohen (2,3).

NOSOLOGY

The most extensive reviews are those of Cohen (1), Ringrose et al. (15), Parker and Skako (14), and Gorlin and Meskin (6). A variety of abnormalities have been observed in association with hemihyperplasia affecting the limbs, teeth, skin, liver, kidneys, and genitalia (1,6,10,14,15) (Table 3–1). The enlarged area may vary from a single digit or limb or unilateral facial enlargement to involvement of half the body (Figs. 3–1 to 3–5). Hemihyperplasia may be segmental, unilateral, or crossed. In some cases, the defect is limited to a single system, e.g., muscular, vascular, skeletal, or nervous system, but it may frequently involve multiple systems (1). Bones have been found to be unilaterally enlarged, and increased bone age on the affected side has been reported (3,14).

Subsets of hemihyperplasia are listed in the Chapter 1 (Table 1–2). One subset overlaps and is continuous with Beckwith-Wiedemann syndrome (1) (Chapter 2). The hemihyperplasia/multiple lipomatosis syndrome is often confused with Proteus syndrome (Chapter 9).

EPIDEMIOLOGY

Almost all cases of hemihyperplasia are sporadic if incomplete forms of the Beckwith-Wiedemann syndrome (Chapter 2) and neurofibromatosis (Chapter 12) are excluded. Tomooka (17) estimated a hemihyperplasia birth prevalence of 1/86,000 livebirths. Increased birth weight has been observed (mean, 3.8 kg) (9). A 2:1 female predominance has been noted (18).

ETIOLOGIC CONSIDERATIONS

The etiology and pathogenesis are poorly understood. A tendency toward dizygotic twinning has been observed in some cases. Chromosomal anomalies, including diploid/triploid mosaicism, trisomy 18 mosaicism, translocation 13q;7p, partial G and B monosomy with B/G translocation, and abnormally large chromosome number 3 have been reported (1). Many other theories have been advanced to explain hemihyperplasia, including anatomical and functional vascular or lymphatic abnormalities; lesions of the central nervous system leading to altered neurotropic action; endocrine abnormalities; asymmetric cell division and deviation of the twinning process; fusion of two eggs following fertilization, leading to unequal reg-

Table 3–1 Abnormalities Associated with Hemihyperplasia (Hemihypertrophy)[a]

SKIN	LIVER
Nevi	Cyst
Pigmentation	Focal nodular hyperplasia
Cutis marmorata	
Telangiectasis	**KIDNEY**
Nevus flammeus	Medullary sponge kidney
Coarse skin on affected side	Unilateral nephromegaly
Ichthyosis on affected side	Abnormal collecting system
Hirsuitism	Polycystic kidneys
Hypertrichosis	
Thicker hair on affected side	**GENITALIA**
Excessive secretions of sebaceous and sweat glands	Hypospadias
Increased skin temperature on affected side	Cryptorchidism
	Macropenis
LIMB	Enlarged testis on affected side
Macrodactyly	Clitoromegaly
Polydactyly	
Syndactyly	**DENTAL, ORAL**
Clubfoot	Enlarged teeth on affected side
	Early eruption of teeth on affected side
SKELETAL	Abnormal tooth roots
Increased bone age on affected side	Enlarged alveolar ridge on affected side
Compensatory scoliosis	Enlarged tongue on affected side
Hip dysplasia	
	OTHER
CENTRAL NERVOUS SYSTEM	Strabismus
Hemimegalencephaly	Tracheoesophageal fistula
Cerebral hemiatrophy	Supernumerary nipples
Macrocephaly	Umbilical hernia
Cyst of septum pellucidum	Inguinal hernia
Mental deficiency	Short stature
Seizures	
CARDIOVASCULAR	
Congenital heart defects	

[a] See reviews by Ringrose et al. (15), Parker and Shalko (14), and Gorlin and Meskin (6).
Source: Adapted from Cohen (1).

ulative ability in the two halves; and mitochondrial damage to an over-ripened egg leading to over-regeneration (13). The range of variability of the clinical abnormalities in hemihyperplasia (1,6,8,14,15) together with the large number of sporadic cases means almost certain etiologic heterogeneity (Table 3–1).

TUMORS

Hoyme et al. (8) reported an associated tumor incidence of 5.9%. A 1.36:1 right-sided predominance and a 1.88:1 female-to-male sex ratio was found in 168 patients. Tumors may occur ipsilateral and sometimes contralateral to the hemihyperplastic side (8). Most common are Wilms tumor, adrenal cortical carcinoma, and hepatoblastoma, in that order (4,5,7,12,14). Other tumors have been noted: adrenal neuroblastoma, adrenal adenoma, pheochromocytoma (16) (Figs. 3–6 to 3–8), testicular carcinoma, undifferentiated sarcoma, and leiomyosarcoma (1). Neoplasms associated with hemihyperplasia are compared with those found in Beckwith-Wiedemann and Sotos syndromes in Chapter 1 (Table 1–5).

Meadows et al. (11) reported an unusual family in which a mother with hemihyperplasia gave birth to three children, each of whom developed Wilms tumor, but each of whom had no evidence of hemihyperplasia. A fourth child had duplication of the renal collecting system but no evidence of hemihyperplasia or Wilms tumor (Fig. 3–9).

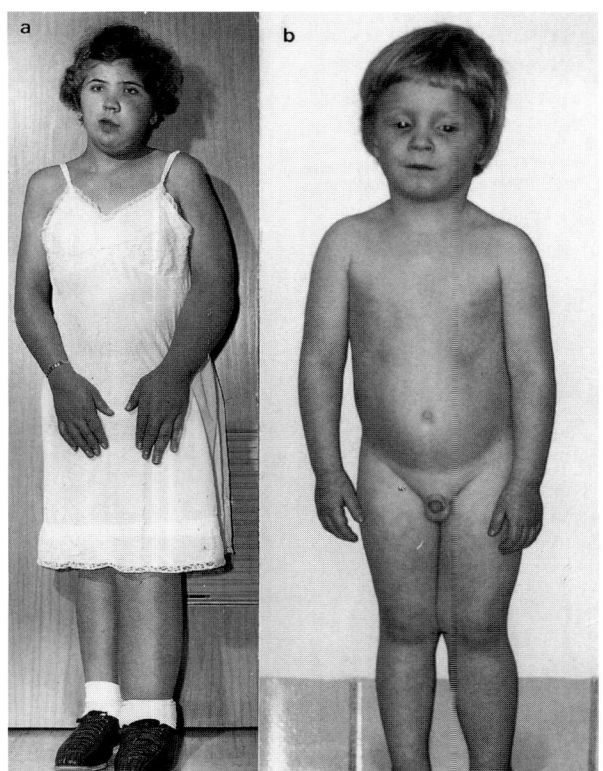

Figure 3–1 Hemihyperplasia. **a:** Involvement of half the body. From Gorlin and Meskin (6). **b:** Milder degree of involvement. From Cohen (1).

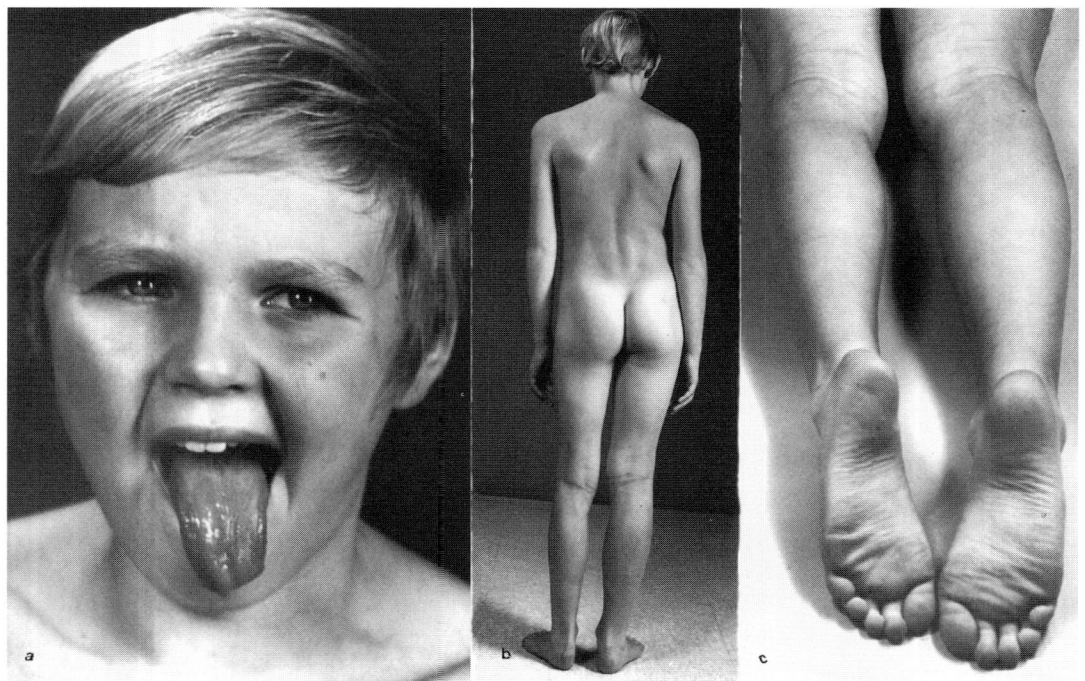

Figure 3–2 Hemihyperplasia. **a–c:** Involvement on right side. From Schnakenburg et al. (16).

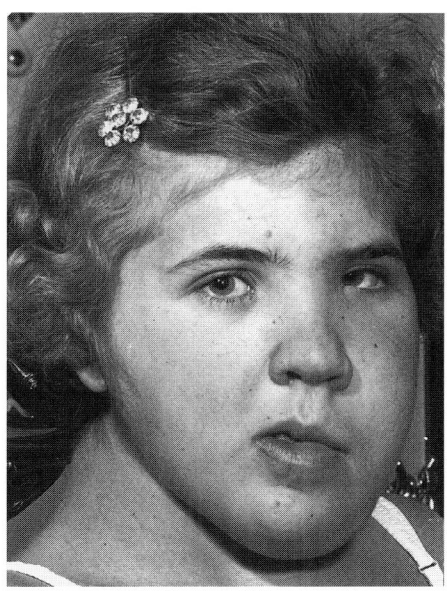

Figure 3–3 Hemihyperplasia. Full face view of patient shown in Figure 3–1a. From Gorlin and Meskin (6).

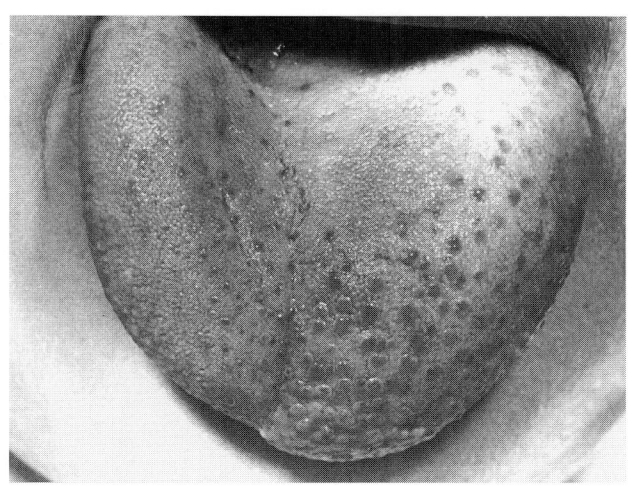

Figure 3–4 Hemihypierplasia. Tongue involvement with enlarged fungiform papillae. Note sharp demarcation line. Same patient as shown in Figure 3–1a. From Gorlin and Meskin (6).

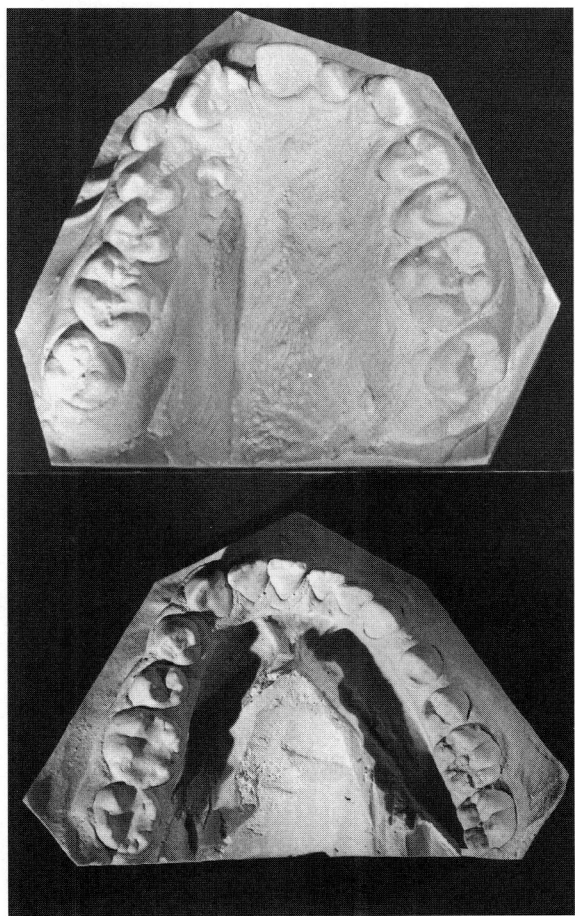

Figure 3–5 Hemihyperplasia. Casts of jaws. Note differences in width of bone and size of teeth on affected and normal sides. Same patient as shown in Figure 3–1a. From Gorlin and Meskin (6).

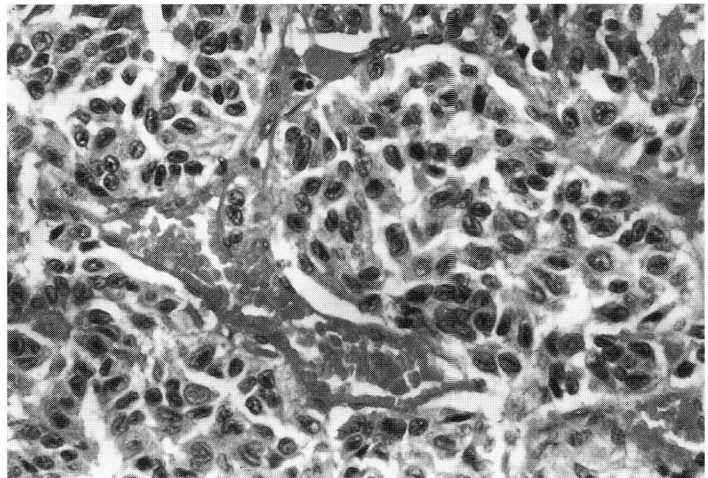

Figure 3–6 Hemihyperplasia. Malignant pheochromocytoma. Alveolar pattern. Note pleomorphism and mitotic activity. Same patient as shown in Figure 3–2. From Schnakenburg et al. (16).

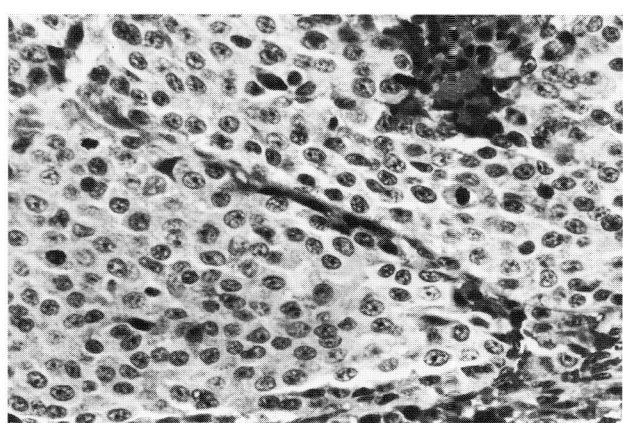

Figure 3–7 Hemihyperplasia. Malignant pheochromocytoma. Solid pattern. Note nuclear pleomorphism and mitotic figures. Same patient as shown in Figure 3–2. From Schnakenburg et al. (16).

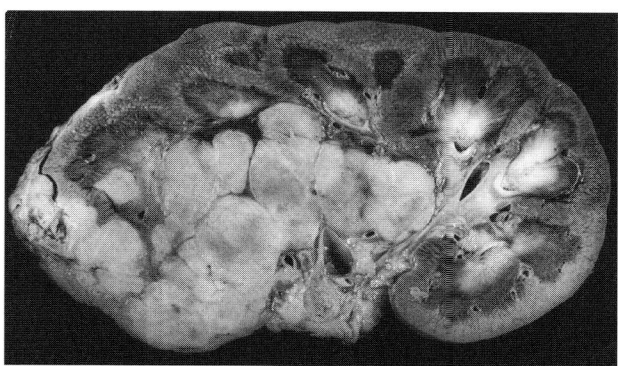

Figure 3–8 Hemihyperplasia. Metastases of malignant pheochromocytoma at hilus of right kidney with invasion into parenchyma. Same patient as shown in Figure 3–2. From Schnakenburg et al. (16).

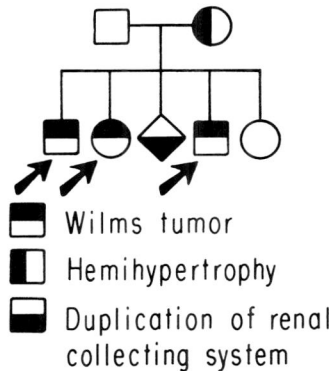

Figure 3–9 Pedigree in which mother has hemihyperplasia. Three children had Wilms tumor but no evidence of hemihyperplasia. From Meadows (11).

REFERENCES

1. Cohen MM Jr: A comprehensive and critical assessment of overgrowth and overgrowth syndromes. In Harris H and Hirschhorn K (eds): *Advances in Human Genetics*, New York: Plenum Press, 1989, Vol 18, Ch 4, pp 181–303; Addendum, pp 373–376.
2. Cohen MM Jr: Perspectives on craniofacial asymmetry IV. Hemi-asymmetries. Int J Oral Maxillofac Surg 24:134–141, 1995.
3. Cohen MM Jr: *The Child With Multiple Birth Defects*, 2nd ed. Oxford University Press, New York, 1997.
4. Fraumeni JF Jr, Geiser CF, Manning MD: Wilms tumor and congenital hemihypertrophy: report of 5 new cases and review of the literature. Pediatrics 40:886–890, 1967.
5. Fraumeni JF Jr, Miller RW: Adrenocortical neoplasms with hemihypertrophy, brain tumors and other disorders. J Pediatr 70:129–138, 1967.
6. Gorlin RJ, Meskin LH: Congenital hemihypertrophy. J Pediatr 61:870–879, 1962.
7. Green DM, Breslow NE, Beckwith JB, Norkool P: Screening of children with hemihypertrophy, aniridia and Wiedemann-Beckwith syndrome in patients with Wilms tumor. Med Pediatr Oncol 21:188–192, 1993.
8. Hoyme HE, Seaver LH, Jones KL, Procopio F, Crooks W, Feingold M: Isolated hemihyperplasia (hemihypertrophy): Report of a prospective multicenter study of the incidence of neoplasia and review. Am J Med Genet 79:274–278, 1998.
9. Leisenring WM, Breslow NE, Evans IE, Beckwith JB, Coppes MJ, Grundy P: Increased birth weights of National Wilms Tumor Study patients suggest a growth factor excess. Cancer Res 54:4680–4683, 1994.
10. Mark S, Clark OH, Kaplan RA: A virilized patient with congenital hemihypertrophy. Postgrad Med J 70:752–755, 1994.
11. Meadows AT: Wilms' tumor in three children of a woman with hemihypertrophy. N Engl J Med 291:23, 1974.
12. Miller RW, Fraumeni JF Jr, Manning MD: Association of Wilms tumor with aniridia, hemihypertrophy and other congenital malformations. N Engl J Med 270:922–927, 1964.
13. Noé O, Berman HH: The etiology of congenital hemihypertrophy and one case report. Arch Pediatr 79:278–288, 1962.
14. Parker DA, Shalko RG: Congenital asymmetry: Report of 10 cases with associated developmental abnormalities. Pediatrics 44:584–589, 1969.
15. Ringrose RE, Jabbour JT, Keele DK: Hemihypertrophy. Pediatrics 36:434–448, 1965.
16. Schnakenburg K, Muller M, Dorner K, Harms D, Schwarze EW, Grosse FR, Wiedemann H-R: Congenital hemihypertrophy and malignant giant pheochromocytoma—a previously undescribed coincidence. Eur J Pediatr 122:263–273, 1976.
17. Tomooka Y: Congenital hemihypertrophy and medullary sponge kidney. Br J Radiol 61:851–853, 1988.
18. Warkany J: *Congenital Malformations: Notes and Comments*. Year Book Medical Publishers, Chicago, 1971, p. 163.

4

Simpson-Golabi-Behmel Syndrome

Simpson-Golabi-Behmel syndrome (OMIM 312870)[a] is an X-linked overgrowth syndrome characterized by prenatal and postnatal overgrowth, dysmorphic facial features, and a spectrum of congenital malformations that overlap with other overgrowth syndromes, particularly Beckwith-Wiedemann syndrome (see Chapter 2).

HISTORICAL PERSPECTIVE

In 1975, Simpson et al. (39) described two maternal male cousins with macrocephaly, coarse face, broad hands, and normal intelligence. In 1984, Behmel et al. (1) reported several males from a large family with additional findings, including congenital heart defects, polydactyly, and frequent infant mortality. They noted X-linked inheritance and mild expression in female carriers. Golabi and Rosen (9), also in 1984, independently observed a family with several affected males with malformations of the internal organs and early death. In the same year, Opitz (31) noted a family with severely affected males. In 1988, Neri et al. (28) recorded a family of three affected males, noting that it was the same disorder described by Simpson et al. (39), Golabi and Rosen (9), and Behmel et al. (1,2). They coined the eponym "Simpson-Golabi-Behmel syndrome."

ETIOLOGY

Molecular Biology of Glypicans

Two major families of cell surface proteoglycans are glypicans and syndecans. Other cell surface proteoglycans are also known, such as CD44 and betaglycan. Syndecans have highly conserved membrane spanning regions and short cytoplasmic tails. Glypicans are anchored to the peripheral membrane by a glycosylphosphatidylinositol linkage (3,5,38). At present, six glypican genes are known: glypican/GPC1 (6), cerebroglypican/GPC2 (41), OCI-5/GPC3 (7,34), k-glypican/GPC4 (51), GPC5 (46), and GPC6 (48). There is also a Drosophila homologue, dally (18,26). Each gene has a tissue-specific developmental pattern of expression.

Molecular Biology of GPC3

GPC3 contains 8 exons spanning over 500 kb of genomic DNA (47). The transcript is widely expressed during development in the same spectrum of tissues affected in Simpson-Golabi-Behmel syndrome. Adult expression is limited to the placenta, lung, ovary, and mammary gland (33). Critical cis-acting promoter elements regulating developmental or tissue-specific GPC3 expression have yet to be identified (15,21).[b]

[b]Gene silencing by CpG methylation has been reported for GPC3 in ovarian cancer cells and in the context of X-inactivation (24). However, restricted tissue-specific expression in human GPC3 makes similar studies in Simpson-Golabi-Behmel patients difficult.

[a]On-Line Mendelian Inheritance in Man number.

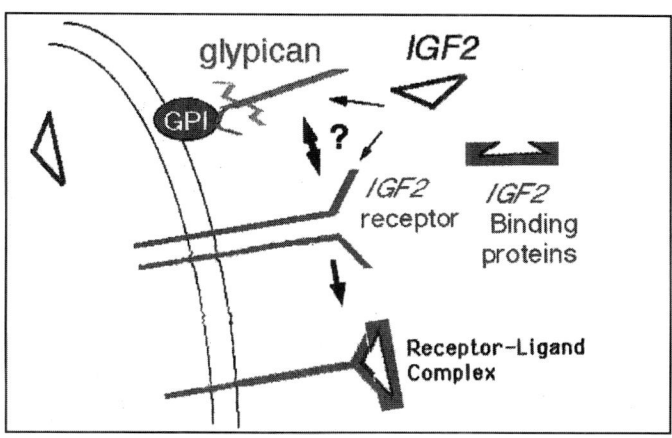

Figure 4–1 Putative role of *GPC3* in modulating *IGF2* interaction with IGF2R. The figure depicts *IGF2* interactions at the cell membrane with homodimeric IGF2R and the potential role of *GPC3* in facilitating ligand association. IGF2 binding proteins are depicted as rectangles that can chaperone *IGF2* (triangles) to dimerized IGF2R. GPC3 is anchored to the peripheral membrane by the GPI linkage shown as an oval. From Weksberg et al. (53).

GPC3 is likely involved in (*a*) regulating cell proliferation and apoptosis and (*b*) modulating cellular responses to growth factors (10,40).

Clinical overlap between Simpson-Golabi-Behmel syndrome and Beckwith-Wiedemann syndrome is known to occur. Beckwith-Wiedemann syndrome is a multigenic disorder involving many growth regulatory molecules such as IGF2 (see Chapter 2). Pilia et al. (34) suggested that GPC3 forms a complex with IGF2 and might modulate IGF2 action. However, this has not been confirmed by Filmus (40). Transgenic mice with a loss-of-function mutation in the Igf2 receptor (Igf2r) are overgrown (50). GPC3-null mice exhibit some of the features of Simpson-Golabi-Behmel syndrome, including overgrowth (4a). The similarity of mouse mutant phenotypes suggests that GPC3 and IGF2R function sequentially or as coreceptors for IGF2 (53) (Fig. 4–1).

Gene Mapping

Simpson-Golabi-Behmel syndrome has been mapped to Xq26 by several investigators (16,17a,32,54). Pilia et al. (34) first identified *GPC3* as the Simpson-Golabi-Behmel locus. *GPC3* and *GPC4* are juxtaposed at Xq26 (13). A second locus has been mapped to Xp22[c] by using a large family with a severe phenotype. Whether this locus is always associated with a severe phenotype or with a spectrum of phenotypes remains to be determined. At present, the Xp22 region contains no known genes that can obviously be implicated in the etiology of the severe form of Simpson-Golabi-Behmel syndrome (4).

GPC3 Mutations

Pilia et al. (34) found deletions and translocations at both ends of the gene in different patients with Simpson-Golabi-Behmel syndrome. Deletions recorded by a number of investigations (17,22, 25,30,47,49,52,55)[d,e] have been identified in all exons with no specific genotype–phenotype correlations. Li et al. (22) reported the largest series of patients screened for *GPC3* deletions. They identified seven deleted patients and reviewed the literature. Combining all cases to date, they noted that *GPC3* deletions had been identified in 40% of cases ($n = 65$) (Table 4–1). Based on the structural changes in the *GPC3* gene, it is likely that the function of its protein is severely curtailed or lost in every case (34).

Veugelers et al. (49) identified six *GPC3* point mutations of the missense, nonsense, frameshift, and splice site types. A single nucleotide dele-

---

[c]This has been called Simpson-Golabi-Behmel syndrome, type 2 (OMIM 300209)[a].

[d]Veugelers et al. (49) identified a deletion that affected *GPC3* and *GPC4*, which flanks the centromeric end of *GPC3* on Xq26. However, it was the *GPC3* deletion that caused Simpson-Golabi-Behmel syndrome.

[e]Xuan et al. (55) identified a *GPC3* deletion in a Dutch-Canadian family; a *normal* daughter of a Simpson-Golabi-Behmel syndrome carrier who had skeletal abnormalities and Wilms tumor raised the possibility of a trans effect from the maternal carrier in Simpson-Golabi-Behmel syndrome kindreds.

Table 4-1 GPC3 Deletion Mutations and Associated Clinical Findings

Patients[a]	Exon Deletion/ Mutation	Prenatal Overgrowth	Postnatal Overgrowth	Coarse Facies	Cleft Lip/ Palate	Macro-glossia	Cardiac Defects	Hernias	Renal Tract Abnormalities	Super-numerary Nipples	Skeletal Abnormalities	Hand Anomalies	Develop-mental Delay	Embryonal Tumors
W1	1	+	NA	+	−	−	−	u	+	NA	+	+	−	−
W2	3–5	NA	+	NA	−	−	+	d	−	−	+	−	NA	+
W3	3–5	+	+	+	−	+	−	−	+	+	+	+	NA	−
W4	4–5	+	+	+	+	+	−	i	+	+	+	−	+	−
W5	36652	+	NA	+	−	−	−	−	−	−	−	+	NA	+
W6	6–7	+	+	+	−	−	−	−	+	+	+	+	+	−
W7	8	+	NA	−	−	−	−	u	−	−	−	+	−	−
L1	1	NA	NA	+	−	+	−	d/u	−	+	+	NA	+	+
L2	1	+	+	+	NA	NA	+	+	−	−	±	+	−	−
L3	1–2	+	+	−	NA	−	−	+	−	−	−	NA	−	+
L4	1–2	+	NA	+	NA	NA	−	+	−	−	−	NA	+	+
L5	2	+	+	−	−	−	−	−	−	−	−	+	+	+
L6	2	+	NA	+	+	+	+	i/u	+	+	+	+	+	+
L7	2	+	NA	+	−	+	−	d/u	+	−	−	−	+	−
L8	2–4	+	NA	+	+	+	−	d/i	−	+	+	NA	+	−
L9	3	+	+	+	−	−	−	−	−	−	−	+	−	−
L10	3	+	+	+	−	−	+	−	+	+	+	+	+	+
L11	3	+	NA	+	−	−	−	−	+	+	+	+	+	−
L12	3	+	+	+	−	−	+	d/u	+	+	+	+	−	−
L13	3–4	+	NA	+	−	−	+	u	+	+	+	+	+	−
L14	3–8	+	NA	+	NA	+	+	u	+	−	+	NA	+	−
L15	4–5	+	+	−	NA	NA	+	−	+	+	+	−	−	−
L16	5	+	+	−	−	−	−	−	−	−	−	+	+	−
L17	6–8	+	NA	+	+	+	+	NA	+	NA	+	+	−	−
L18	6–8	+	NA	+	−	+	−	u	−	−	+	NA	+	−
L19	7	NA	+	+	−	−	−	−	+	+	−	+	−	−
L20	7–8	+	NA	+	NA	NA	−	u	+	NA	+	NA	NA	−
L21	8	+	+	+	NA	NA	−	−	+	−	−	NA	+	−

[a]W, Weksberg's cases; L, Literature cases.

Source: From Li et al. (22).

Table 4–2 Findings in Simpson-Golabi-Behmel Syndrome

Clinical Findings	Relative Frequency[a]
NEONATAL	
Macrosomia	+++
Fetal hydrops	+
CRANIOFACIAL	
Macrocephaly	+++
Coarse face	+++
Downslanting palpebral fissures	++
Macrostomia/macroglossia	++
Dental malocclusion	++
Cleft lip/palate	+
Central groove of lower lip	++
HANDS	
Polydactyly	++
Fingernail hypoplasia	++
Cutaneous syndactyly	+
CHEST/ABDOMEN	
Supernumerary nipples	+++
Pectus excavatum	+++
Rib/vertebral abnormalities	++
Diastasis recti	++
Coccygeal skin tags	+
Umbilical/inguinal hernias	++
GENITALIA	
Hypospadias	+
Cryptorchidism	++
INTERNAL ORGANS	
Congenital heart defects	++
Heart arrythmias	++
Diaphragmatic defect	+
Hepatosplenomegaly	++
Hyperplastic islets of Langerhans	+
Cystic dysplasia of kidneys	++
NEUROLOGICAL	
Hypotonia	+++
Mental retardation	±
OTHER	
Advanced bone age	++
Neonatal death	++

[a]Frequency of clinical findings approximately estimated as nearly constant (+++), frequent (++), occasionally reported (+), or absent (−).

Source: From Neri et al. (29).

CLINICAL PHENOTYPE

The clinical spectrum is broad, ranging from mildly affected female carriers to multiple malformations in males to neonatal death in males (~50%) (28). Overgrowth is of prenatal onset and continues postnatally. Birth length, birth weight, and birth head circumference of affected males are usually well above the 97th centile and adult height attainment can exceed 2.0 m, although height is variable.

Features of Simpson-Golabi-Behmel syndrome are summarized in Tables 4–1 (22) and 4–2 (8,29,42) and illustrated in Figures 4–2 to 4–5. Findings include ocular hypertelorism, downslanting palpebral fissures, epicanthic folds, short nose, macrostomia, macroglossia, central groove of the lower lip, and malocclusion. Cleft lip and palate have been reported on occasion. The hands and feet are relatively short and broad. Other abnormalities may include metatarsus varus, talipes equinovarus, fingernail

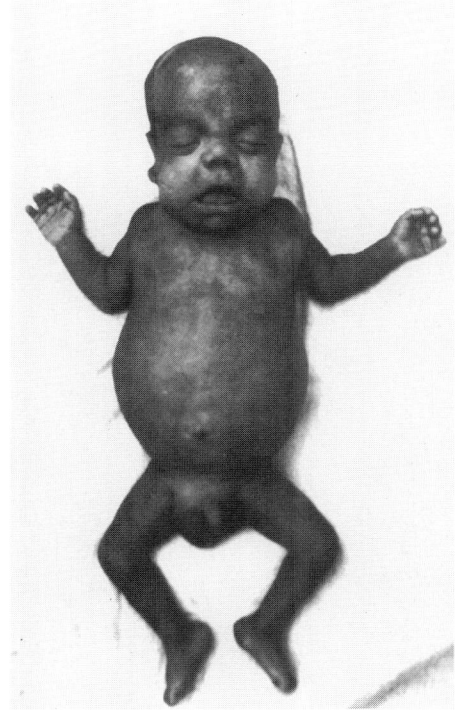

Figure 4–2 Simpson-Golabi-Behmel syndrome. Note ocular hypertelorism, broad flat nose, and large mouth. Weight greater than 90th centile at birth. From Golabi and Rosen (9).

tion was also noted in one case by Okamoto et al. (30). To date, point mutations have not been recorded by other investigators. Alternative gene silencing mechanisms and other genes involved in the pathogenesis of Simpson-Golabi-Behmel syndrome are possibilities to consider.

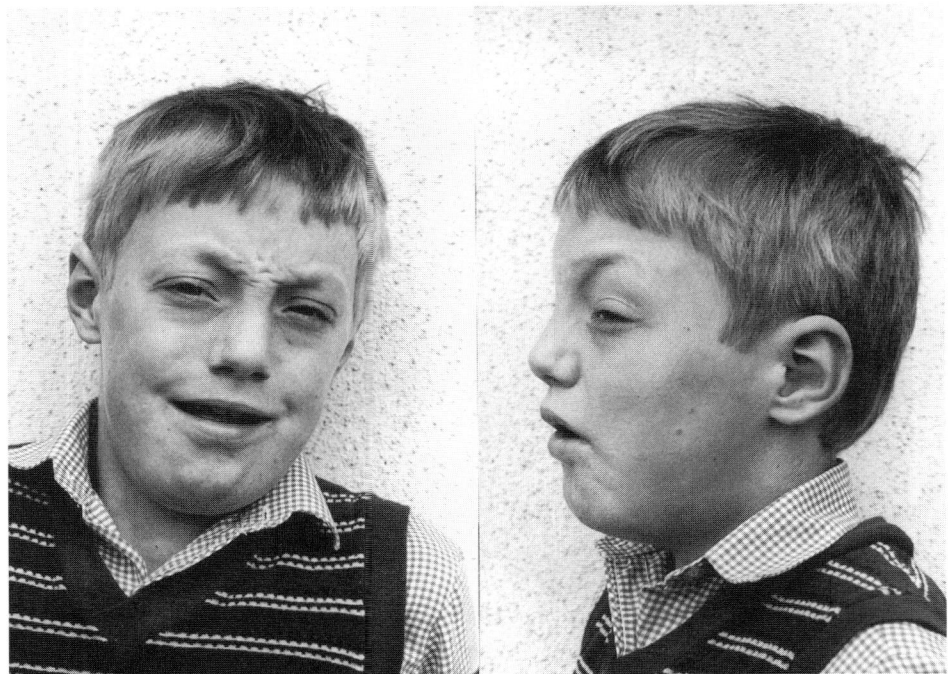

Figure 4–3 Simpson-Golabi-Behmel syndrome. Coarse face, wide nasal bridge, and wide mouth. From Golabi and Rosen (9).

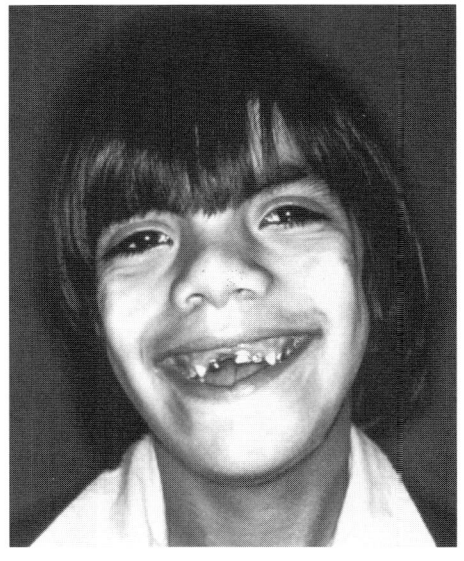

Figure 4–4 Simpson-Golabi-Behmel syndrome. Ocular hypertelorism, short, broad upturned nose, and large mouth. From Golabi and Rosen (9).

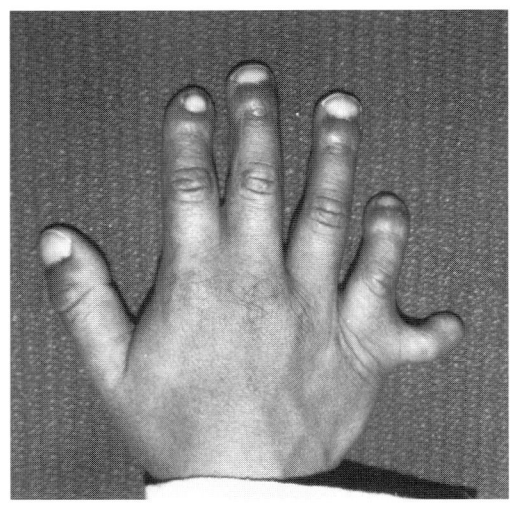

Figure 4–5 Simpson-Golabi-Behmel syndrome. Postaxial polydactyly and mild soft tissue syndactyly between the second and third fingers. From Golabi and Rosen (9).

hypoplasia, cutaneous syndactyly, and polydactyly. Transverse palmar creases are commonly found together with dermatoglyphic features such as an excess of triradii and interdigital loops and an irregular mixture of fingertip arches, loops, and whorls.

Extra nipples are a frequent finding. Genitalia are usually normal, although hypospadias and cryptorchidism have been reported on occasion (36,44). Organomegaly is common, especially affecting the liver, spleen, and the kidneys, which show multicystic dysplasia. Lung segmentation defects have been noted. A diaphragmatic defect has been reported in several patients. Cardiac abnormalities have been found in 36% of patients ($n = 101$) (23). When cardiac analysis was restricted to fully described patients, this figure rose to 47% (23). Findings included ventricular septal defect, patent ductus arteriosus, pulmonic stenosis, cardiac arrhythmias, and cardiomyopathy (12,20,23). Gastrointestinal malrotation, pyloric ring, and Meckel diverticulum have been described and may cause gastrointestinal obstruction. Kim et al. (19a) noted a choledochal cyst.

Radiographic findings consist of advanced bone age, vertebral segmentation defects such as C2–C3 fusion, cervical ribs (usually with 13 pairs of ribs), six lumbar vertebrae, sacrococcygeal defects, and scoliosis.

Hypotonia is a constant finding. Secondary consequences include mouth-breathing facies, highly arched palate, pectus excavatum, downsloping shoulders, diastasis recti, umbilical hernia, inguinal hernias, and cryptorchidism. Mental deficiency has been reported, although most patients have normal intelligence. Because psychological problems are common, counseling and support are essential.

NEOPLASMS

To date, Wilms tumor has been recorded in three patients (16,22,54), nephroblastomatosis in two (22,45), and nephrogenic rests in one (17). Hepatoblastoma was noted by Li et al. (22). Tumor surveillance in Simpson-Golabi-Behmel syndrome should follow the same protocol used for Beckwith-Wiedemann syndrome (see Chapter 2).

DIAGNOSIS

Simpson-Golabi-Behmel syndrome is variably expressed in severely affected males who die during the neonatal period, males with dysmorphic features, and mildly affected female carriers. Males have even been noted *without* typical facial changes and have even been found in a family whose other members had typical facial changes (22,25). Both familial and sporadic cases with *GPC3* mutations have been recorded. Li et al. (22) found *GPC3* mutations in five sporadic cases.

Clinical overlap with Beckwith-Wiedemann syndrome is problematic (see Chapter 2). Certain clinical traits can be useful in distinguishing the two syndromes. The combination of minor facial anomalies, skeletal/hand anomalies, and supernumerary nipples is found only in Simpson-Golabi-Behmel syndrome (22).

Finding a *GPC3* mutation establishes the diagnosis of Simpson-Golabi-Behmel syndrome; this (*a*) rules out Beckwith-Wiedemann syndrome, (*b*) facilitates the screening of carrier mothers, and (*c*) assumes importance in defining recurrence risk for families.

DIFFERENTIAL DIAGNOSIS

A number of patients with other diagnoses have been reassessed and found to have Simpson-Golabi-Behmel syndrome. Neri et al. (28) and Punnett (35) reassessed several patients originally diagnosed with Beckwith-Wiedemann syndrome and reassigned them as examples of Simpson-Golabi-Behmel syndrome. One patient initally diagnosed as having Weaver syndrome (43) was subsequently recognized as having Simpson-Golabi-Behmel syndrome (19).

Verloes et al. (45) pointed out clinical overlap between Simpson-Golabi-Behmel syndrome and Perlman syndrome. However, the two syndromes are easily distinguishable on a clinical basis (27) (see Chapter 5). One patient originally described as having Perlman syndrome but who had some features at variance with that diagnosis (11) was later found to have Simpson-Golabi-Behmel syndrome; Li et al. (22) found a *GPC3* mutation in an affected relative. Another patient initially diagnosed with Sotos syndrome (37) was found to have Simpson-Golabi-Behmel syndrome by Li et al. (22), who noted a *GPC3* mutation in an affected relative in that family also.

Wilms tumor is also found with Beckwith-Wiedemann syndrome (see Chapter 2), hemihyperplasia (see Chapter 3), Perlman syndrome (see Chapter 5), Sotos syndrome (see Chapter 6), and Weaver syndrome (see Chapter 7).

REFERENCES

1. Behmel A, Plöchl E, Rosenkranz W: A new X-linked dysplasia gigantism syndrome: Identical with the Simpson dysplasia syndrome? Hum Genet 67:409–413, 1984.
2. Behmel A, Plöchl E, Rosenkranz W: A new X-linked dysplasia gigantism syndrome: Follow-up in the first family and report on a second Austrian family. Am J Genet 30:275–285, 1988.
3. Bernfield M, Kokenyesi R, Kato M, Hinkes MT, Spring J, Gallo RL, Lose EJ: Biology of the syndecans: A family of transmembrane heparan sulfate proteoglycans. Annu Rev Cell Biol 8:365–393, 1992.
4. Brzustowicz LM, Farrell S, Kahn MB, Weksberg R: Mapping of a new SGB locus to chromosome Xq22 in a family with a severe form of Simpson-Golabi-Behmel syndrome. Am J Hum Genet 65:779–783, 1999.
4a. Cano-Gauci DF, Song H, Yang H, McKerlie C, Choo B, Shi W, Pullano R, Piscione TD, Grisaru S, Soon S, Sedlackova L, Tanswell AK, Lockwood GA, Mak TW, Yeger H, Rosenblum ND, Filmus J: Glypican-3-deficient mice exhibit developmental overgrowth and some of the abnormalities typical of the Simpson-Golabi-Behmel syndrome. J Cell Biol 146 255–264, 1999.
5. David G: Integral membrane heparan sulphate proteoglycans. FASEB J 7:1023–1030, 1993.
6. David G, Lories V, Decock B, Marynen P, Cassiman JJ, Van den Berghe H: Molecular cloning of a phosphatidylinositol-anchored membrane heparan sulfate proteoglycan from human lung fibroblasts. J Cell Biol 111:3165–3176 1990.
7. Filmus J, Shi W, Wong ZM, Wong MJ: Identification of a new membrane-bound heparan sulphate proteoglycan. Biochem J 311 561–565, 1995.
8. Garganta CL, Bodurtha JN: Report of another family with Simpson-Golabi-Behmel syndrome and a review of the literature. Am J Med Genet 44:129–135, 1992.
9. Golabi M, Rosen L: A new X-linked mental retardation-overgrowth syndrome. Am J Med Genet 17:345–358, 1984.
10. Gonzales AD, Kaya M, Shi W, Song H, Testa JR, Penn LZ, Filmus J: OCI-5/GPC3, a glypican encoded by a gene that is mutated in the Simpson-Golabi-Behmel overgrowth syndrome, induces apoptosis in a cell line-specific manner. J Cell Biol 141:1407–1414, 1998.
11. Greenberg F, Copeland K, Gresik MV: Expanding the spectrum of the Perlan syndrome. Am J Med Genet 29:773–776, 1988.
12. Gurrieri F, Cappa M, Neri G: Further delineation of the Simpson-Golabi-Behmel (SGB) syndrome. Am J Med Genet 44:136–137, 1992.
13. Huber R, Mazzarella R, Chen C-N, Chen E, Ireland M, Lindsay S, Pilia G: Glypican 3 and glypican 4 are juxtaposed in Xq26.1. Gene 225:9–16, 1998.
14. Huber R, Crisponi L, Mazzarella R, Chen C-N, Su Y, Shizuya H, Chen EY, Cao A, Pilia G: Analysis of exon/intron structure and 400 kb of genomic sequence surrounding the 5′-promoter and 3′-terminal ends of the human glypican 3 (GPC3) gene. Genomics 45:48–58, 1997.
15. Huber R, Schlessinger D, Pilia G: Multiple Sp1 sites efficiently drive transcription of the TATA-less promoter of the human glypican 3 (*GPC3*) gene. Gene 214:35–44, 1998.
16. Hughes-Benzie RM, Hunter AGW, Allanson JE, Mackenzie AE: Simpson-Golabi-Behmel syndrome associated with renal dysplasia and embryonal tumor: Localization of the gene to Xqcen–q21. Am J Med Genet 43:428–435, 1992.
17. Hughes-Benzie RM, Pilia G, Xuan JY, Hunter AGW, Chen E, Golabi M, Hurst JA, Kobari J, Marymee K, Pagon RA, Punnett HH, Schelley S, Tolmie JL, Wohlferd MM, Grossman T, Schlessinger D, McKenzie AE: Simpson-Golabi-Behmel syndrome genotype/phenotype analysis of 18 affected males from 7 unrelated families. Am J Med Genet 66:227–234, 1996.
17a. Ireland M, Hughes-Benzie R, Allanson J, Besner A, MacKenzie A, Burn J: Simpson-Golabi-Behmel syndrome in a 5 generation family: A clinical and molecular study. Proc Greenwood Genet Ctr 12:41–44, 1993.
18. Jackson SM, Nakato H, Sugiura M, Jannuzi A, Oakes R, Kaluza V, Golden C, Sellect SB: *dally*, a *Drosophila* glypican, controls cellular responses to the TGFβ-related morphogen, *Dpp*. Development 124:4113–4120, 1997.
19. Kajii T, Tsukahara M: Letter to the editor: The Golabi-Rosen syndrome. Am J Med Genet 19:819, 1984.
19a. Kim S, Idowu O, Chen E: Letter to the editor: Choledochal cyst in Simpson-Golabi-Behmel syndrome. Am J Med Genet 87:267–270, 1999.
20. König R, Fuchs S, Kern C, Langenbeck U: Simpson-Golabi-Behmel syndrome with severe cardiac arrhythmias. Am J Med Genet 38:244–247, 1991.
21. Li M, Pulliano R, Yang HL, Lee HK, Miyamoto NG, Filmus J, Buick RN: Transcriptional regulation of OCI-5/glypican 3: Elongation control of confluence-dependent induction. Oncogene 15:1535–1544, 1997.

22. Li M, Shuman C, Cutiongco E, Bender HA, Stevens C, Wilkins-Haug L, Day-Salvatore D, Yong SL, Geraghty MT, Squire J, Weksberg R: *GPC3* mutation analysis in a spectrum of patients with overgrowth expands the phenotype of Simpson-Golabi-Behmel syndrome. Am J Med Genet 102:161–168, 2001.
23. Lin AE, Neri G, Hughes-Benzie R, Weksberg R: Cardiac anomalies in the Simpson-Golabi-Behmel syndrome. Am J Med Genet 83:378–381, 1999.
24. Lin H, Huber R, Schlessinger D, Morin PJ: Frequent silencing of the *GPC3* gene in ovarian cancer cell lines. Cancer Res 59:807–810, 1999.
25. Lindsay S, Ireland M, O'Brien O, Clayton-Smith J, Hurst JA, Mann J, Cole T, Sampson J, Slaney S, Schlessinger D, Burn J, Pilia GT: Large scale deletions in the *GPC3* gene may account for a minority of cases of Simpson-Golabi-Behmel syndrome. J Med Genet 34:480–483, 1997.
26. Nakato H, Futch TA, Selleck SB: The division abnormally delayed (*dally*) gene: A putative integral membrane proteoglycan required for cell division patterning during postembryonic development of the nervous system in *Drosophila*. Development 121:3687–3702, 1995.
27. Neri G, Martini-Neri ME, Katz BE, Opitz JM: The Perlman syndrome: Familial renal dysplasia with Wilms tumor, fetal gigantism and multiple congenital anomalies. Am J Med Genet 19:195–207, 1984.
28. Neri G, Marini R, Cappa M, Borrelli P, Opitz JM: Simpson-Golabi-Behmel syndrome: An X-linked encephalo-tropho-schisis syndrome. Am J Med Genet 30:287–299, 1988.
29. Neri G, Gurrieri F, Zanni G, Lin A: Clinical and molecular aspects of the Simpson-Golabi-Behmel syndrome. Am J Med Genet 79:279–283, 1998.
30. Okamoto N, Yagi M, Imura K, Wada Y: A clinical and molecular study of a patient with Simpson-Golabi-Behmel syndrome. J Hum Genet 44:327–329, 1999.
31. Opitz JM: The Golabi-Rosen syndrome—Report of a second family. Am J Med Genet 17:359–366, 1984.
32. Orth U, Gurrieri F, Behmel A, Genuardi M, Cremer M, Gal A, Neri G: Gene for Simpson-Golabi-Behmel syndrome is linked to HPRT in Xq26 in two European families. Am J Med Genet 50:388–390, 1994.
33. Pellegrini M, Pilia G, Pantano S, Lucchini F, Uda M, Fumi M, Cao A, Schlessinger D, Forabosco A: *GPC3* expression correlates with the phenotype of the Simpson-Golabi-Behmel syndrome. Dev Dynam 213:431–439, 1998.
34. Pilia G, Hughes-Benzie RM, Mackenzie A, Baybayan P, Chen EV, Huber R, Neri G, Cao A, Forabosco A, Schlessinger D: Mutations in *GPC3*, a glypican gene, cause the Simpson-Golabi-Behmel overgrowth syndrome. Nat Genet 12:241–247, 1996.
35. Punnett HH: Simpson-Golabi-Behmel syndrome (SGBS) in a female with an X-autosome translocation. Am J Med Genet 50:391–393, 1994.
36. Saul RA, Phelan MC, Schwartz CE: Sex chromosome aneuploidy and ambiguous genitalia in the Simpson-Golabi-Behmel syndrome. Proc Greenwood Genet Ctr 13:129, 1994.
37. Scott CI: Cerebral gigantism. Birth Defects 11(2):418–422, 1975.
38. Selleck SB: Overgrowth syndromes and the regulation of signaling complex by proteoglycans. Am J Hum Genet 64:372–377, 1999.
39. Simpson JL, Landey S, New M, German J: A previously unrecognized X-linked syndrome of dysmorphia. Birth Defects 11(2):18–24, 1975.
40. Song HH, Shi W, Filmus J: OCI-5/rat glypican-3 binds to fibroblast growth factor-2 but not to insulin-like growth factor-2. J Biol Chem 272:7574–7577, 1997.
41. Stipp CS, Litwack ED, Lander AD: Cerebroglycan: An integral membrane heparan sulfate proteoglycan that is unique to the developing nervous system and expressed specifically during neuronal differentiation. J Cell Biol 124:149–160, 1994.
42. Terespolsky D, Farrell SA, Siegel-Bartelt J, Weksberg R: Infantile lethal variant of Simpson-Golabi-Behmel syndrome associated with hydrops fetalis. Am J Med Genet 59:329–333, 1995.
43. Tsukahara M, Tanaka S, Kajii T: A Weaver-like syndrome in a Japanese boy. Clin Genet 25:73–78, 1984.
44. Vance GN, Probert RC: Simpson-Golabi-Behmel syndrome and genital abnormalities. Proc Greenwood Genet Ctr 14:116, 1995.
45. Verloes A, Massart B, Dehalleux L, Langhendries J-P, Koulischer L: Clinical overlap of Beckwith-Wiedemann, Perlman and Simpson-Golabi-Behmel syndromes: a diagnostic pitfall. Clin Genet 47:257–262, 1995.
46. Veugelers M, Vermeesch J, Reekmans G, Steinfeld R, Marynen P, David G: Characterization of glypican-5 and chromosomal localization of human *GPC5*, a new member of the glypican gene family. Genomics 40:24–30, 1997.
47. Veugelers M, Vermeesch J, Watanabe K, Yamaguchi Y, Marynen P, David G: *GPC4*, the gene for human k-glypican, flanks *GPC3* on Xq26: Deletion of the GPC3–GPC4 gene cluster in one family with Simpson-Golabi-Behmel syndrome. Genomics 53:1–11, 1998.
48. Veugelers M, De Cat B, Ceulemans H, Bruystens A-M, Coomans C, Durr J, Vermeesch J, Marynen P, David G: Glypican-6, a new member of the glypican family of cell surface heparan sulfate proteoglycans. J Biol Chem 274:26968–26977, 1999.
49. Veugelers M, De Cat B, Muyldermans SY, Reekmans G, Delande N, Frints S, Legius E, Fryns J-P, Schrander-Stumpel C, Weidle B,

Magdalena N, David G: Mutational analysis of the *GPC3/GPC4* glypican gene cluster on Xq26 in patients with Simpson-Golabi-Behmel syndrome: Identification of loss-of-function mutations in the *GPC3* gene. Hum Mol Genet 9: 1321–1328, 2000.
50. Wang Z-Q, Fung MR, Barlow DP, Wagner EF: Regulation of embryonic growth and lysosomal targeting by the imprinted *Igf2/Mpr* gene. Nature 372:464–467, 1994.
51. Watanabe K, Yamada H, Yamaguchi Y: K-glypican: A novel GPI-anchored heparan sulfate proteoglycan that is highly expressed in developing brain and kidney. J Cell Biol 130:1207–1218, 1995.
52. Weksberg R, Li M, Shuman C, Cutiongeo E, Bender HA, Stevens C, Wilkins-Haug L, Wong SL, Squire J: Glypican3 (*GPC3*) deletions: The phenotypic spectrum in overgrowth syndromes. Am J Hum Genet 65(Suppl):A114, 1999.
53. Weksberg R, Squire AJ, Templeton DM: Glypicans: a growing trend. Nat Genet 12:225–227, 1996.
54. Xuan JY, Besner A, Ireland M, Hughes-Benzie RM, Mackenzie AE: Mapping of Simpson-Golabi-Behmel syndrome to Xq25–q27. Hum Mol Genet 3:133–137, 1994.
55. Xuan JY, Hughes-Benzie RM, Mackenzie AE: A small interstitial deletion in the *GPC3* gene causes Simpson-Golabi-Behmel syndrome in a Dutch-Canadian family. J Med Genet 36:57–58, 1999.

5

Perlman Syndrome

Perlman syndrome (OMIM 267000)[a] is characterized by neonatal macrosomia, macrocephaly, full round face, deeply set eyes, nephroblastomatosis, and a predisposition for Wilms tumor.

HISTORICAL PERSPECTIVE

The first report was published by Liban and Kozenitsky (10) in 1970; metanephric hamartomas and nephroblastomatosis were described in two sibs of a consanguineous Yemenite Jewish family. In 1973 and 1975 in follow-up studies of the same family, Perlman et al. (14,15) noted six affected offspring of both sexes. Delineation of the syndrome included fetal gigantism, unusual face, renal hamartomas with or without nephroblastomatosis, and hyperplasia of the islets of Langerhans. In 1984, Greenberg et al. (5) noted a case with fetal ascites, prune belly, hepatomegaly, nephromegaly, and Wilms tumor. In the same year, Neri et al. (11) reported two sibs with fetal gigantism, characteristic face, nephroblastomatosis, Wilms tumor and, in the sole survivor, developmental delay; they proposed the eponym "Perlman syndrome." In 1986, Perlman (13) reported the facial changes in two of his original patients.

ETIOLOGY

To date, 15 cases from six different families have been recorded (2,5,6,8,10–15,15a). The sex ratio is 2M:1F ($n = 15$). Inheritance is autosomal recessive. Cell lines from skin biopsies were established from one patient and her heterozygous mother, but no evidence was found that the patient's cells were larger, grew faster, or produced growth factors when compared to her mother and to a normal control (12). Chromosomes have been normal in all patients studied, except for the case of Chernos et al. (2) with a de novo extra G-positive band at the end of the short arm chromosome 11. Similarly, duplications at the 11p15 region, but of paternal origin, have been reported in patients with Beckwith-Wiedemann syndrome (9,16) (see Chapter 2).

CLINICAL PHENOTYPE

Clinical and pathological features are listed in Table 5–1. Pregnancy and delivery were complicated by polyhydramnios, fetal ascites, breech presentation, and abdominal dystocia and were caused by visceromegaly. Neonatal macrosomia was evident in all cases. Thirteen of the 15 patients died during the neonatal period. In surviving patients, growth parameters fell rapidly to the lower limits of normal. Hypotonia was constant. A 12-year-old girl was reported as moderately retarded, perhaps caused, in part, by chemotherapy and radiation for a recurrent Wilms tumor (11). Another 1-year-old patient had a developmental quotient of 50 (6). A third patient was noted with agenesis of the corpus callosum (8).

Phenotypic features included macrosomia at birth (weight > 98th centile), macrocephaly, full

[a]On-Line Mendelian Inheritance in Man number.

Table 5–1 Features of Perlman Syndrome[a]

Features	Frequencies
GROWTH	
Macrosomia	15/15
Macrocephaly	11/15
CENTRAL NERVOUS SYSTEM	
Hypotonia	15/15
Developmental delay	5/?
Seizures	3/?
FACE	
Full round face	7/7
Deep-set eyes	8/10
Broad low nasal bridge	11/12
Everted upper lip	11/15
Micrognathia	6/6
Low-set ears	9/11
VISCEROMEGALY	
Nephromegaly	13/13
Nephroblastomatosis	10/13
Renal hamartomas	6/10
Wilms tumor	5/15
Hydronephrosis	8/12
Hepatomegaly	10/13
Pancreatic islet cell hyperplasia	8/12
Hypoglycemia	7/10
Cardiomegaly	5/?
Polysplenia/splenomegaly	2/?
OTHER	
Polyhydramnios	8/11
Cryptorchidism	10/10
Neonatal death	13/15

[a]Based on references 2,5,6,10–15,15a.

round face, frontal hairline upsweep, deeply-set eyes, epicanthic folds, broad flat nasal bridge, anteverted nares, inverted V-shaped upper lip, highly arched palate (cleft palate in one patient), micrognathia, and low-set ears (Fig. 5–1). The chest was often broad with pectus excavatum and other anomalies such as prominent, broad, and/or bifid xiphisternum. The abdomen was usually distended with a prune belly–like appearance, resulting from hepatomegaly and nephromegaly. Cryptorchidism and inguinal hernias have been recorded and an excess of fingertip whorls has also been noted (5,6,11–15).

Prenatal diagnosis is possible in some instances, particularly for families at risk for Perlman syndrome. Nephromegaly, fetal ascites, and polyhydramnios are important clues, although they may not appear until later during pregnancy. Such findings should also be critically assessed during routine screening for any pregnancy.

PATHOLOGY

Visceromegaly involves the heart, liver, spleen, pancreas, and kidneys (Table 5–1). Nephromegaly is associated with fetal lobulation. Nephroblastomatosis is characteristic. Histo-

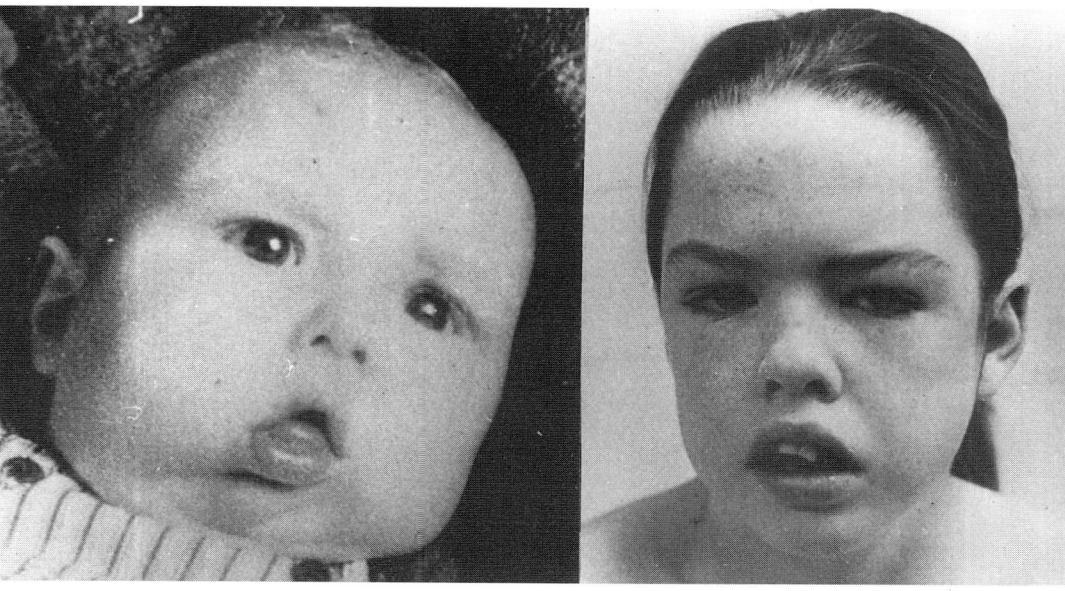

Figure 5–1 Affected brother (6 months) and sister (12 years). From Neri et al. (11).

PERLMAN SYNDROME

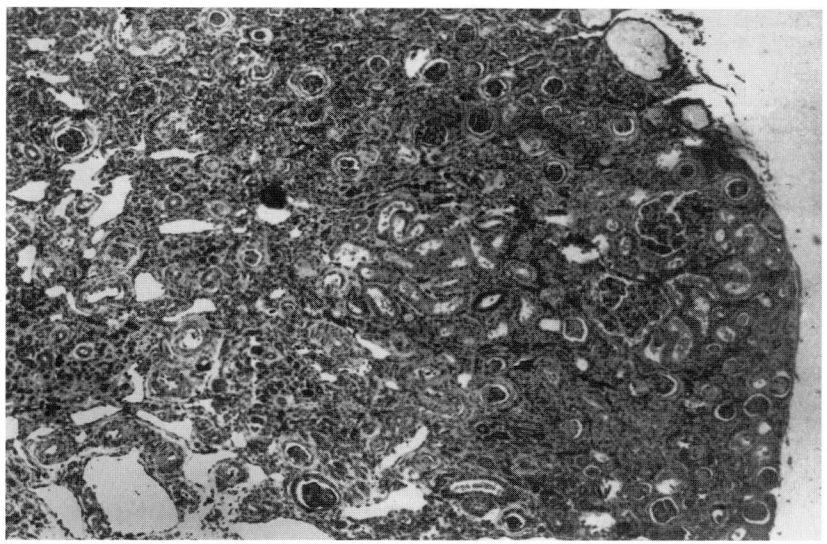

Figure 5–2 Area of cytodifferentiated renal blastema with immature glomeruli and primitive tubular structures. From Neri et al. (11).

pathologic findings include cytodifferentiated nodular renal blastema and nests of immature glomeruli together with sclerotic glomeruli and primitive tubular structures (Fig. 5–2). Foci of hamartomatous tissue can be found in the medulla (5,6,10,11,14,15).

Nephroblastomatosis predisposes to the development of Wilms tumor (1), which has been found in 5 of the 15 reported patients. Dao et al. (3) showed loss of heterozygosity for chromosome 11p markers in a Wilms tumor from the Perlman syndrome patient of Greenberg et al. (6); the opposite result was obtained by Hamel et al. (7) in their patient.

Cytomegaly of the adrenal cortex was found in one case. Hyperplasia of the islets of Langerhans has been noted in several instances (5,6,10,11,14,15) and may be related to macrosomia at birth, apneic episodes, and sudden infant death, possibly from hypoglycemic coma. Atelectasis and volvulus were reported in one case each (8,11).

DIFFERENTIAL DIAGNOSIS

Wilms tumor may also be found in Beckwith-Wiedemann syndrome (Chapter 2), Simpson-Golabi-Behmel syndrome (Chapter 4), hemihyperplasia (Chapter 3), Sotos syndrome (Chapter 6), and Weaver syndrome (Chapter 7). Beckwith-Wiedemann syndrome can be differentiated from Perlman syndrome because the former has capillary stain, macroglossia, omphalocele or umbilical hernia and, in some cases, asymmetry.

The patient reported by Greenberg et al. in 1984 (5) and more fully in 1986 (6) was an example of Perlman syndrome. Greenberg et al. (4) reported a second patient in 1988 with additional features at variance with the diagnosis of Perlman syndrome: diaphragmatic hernia, interrupted aortic arch, anomalous coronary vessels, polysplenia, and hypospadias. Weksberg (17) reclassified this patient as having Simpson-Golabi-Behmel syndrome after another birth in the family was found to have a *GPC3* mutation.

REFERENCES

1. Bove KE, MacAdams AJ: The nephroblastomatosis complex and its relationship to Wilms' tumor: A clinicopathologic treatise. Perspect Pediatr Pathol 7:158–223, 1976.
2. Chernos JR, Fowlow SB, Cox DM: A case of Perlman syndrome associated with a cytogenetic abnormality of chromosome 11. Am J Hum Genet 47(Suppl):A28, 1990.
3. Dao DD, Schroeder WT, Chao L-Y, Kikuchi H,

3. Strong LC, Riccardi VM, Pathak S Nichols WW, Lewis WH, Saunders GF: Genetic mechanisms of tumor-specific loss of 11p DNA sequences in Wilms tumor. Am J Hum Genet 41:202–217, 1987.
4. Greenberg F, Copeland K, Gresik MV: Expanding the spectrum of the Perlman syndrome. Am J Med Genet 29:773–776, 1988.
5. Greenberg F, Stein F, Gresik MV, Finegold MJ, Carpenter RJ, Riccardi VM, Beaudet A: Fetal ascites, prune belly sequence, hepatomegaly, and nephromegaly associated with Wilms tumor. Proc Greenwood Genet Ctr 3:133, 1984.
6. Greenberg F, Stein F, Gresik MV, Finegold MJ, Carpenter RJ, Riccardi VM, Beaudet AL: The Perlman familial nephroblastomatosis syndrome. Am J Med Genet 24:101–110, 1986.
7. Hamel BCJ, Mannens M, Bokkerink JPM: Perlman syndrome: Report of a case and results of molecular studies. Am J Hum Genet 45(Suppl): A48, 1989.
8. Henneveld HT, van Lingen RA, Hamel BCJ, Stolte-Dijkstra I, van Essen AJ: Perlman syndrome: Four additional cases. Am J Med Genet 86:439–446, 1999.
9. Kubota T, Saitoh S, Matsumoto T, Narahara K, Fukushima Y, Jinno YM, Niikawa N: Excess functional copy of allele at chromosomal region 11p15 may cause Wiedemann-Beckwith (EMG) syndrome. Am J Med Genet 49:378–383, 1984.
10. Liban E, Kozenitzky IL: Metanephric hamartomas and nephroblastomatosis in siblings. Cancer 25:885–888, 1970.
11. Neri G, Martini-Neri ME, Katz BE, Opitz JM: The Perlman syndrome: Familial renal dysplasia with Wilms tumor, fetal gigantism and multiple congenital anomalies. Am J Med Genet 19:195–207, 1984.
12. Neri G, Martini-Neri ME, Opitz JM, Freed JJ: The Perlman syndrome: clinical and biological aspects. In: *Endocrine Genetics and Genetics of Growth*. CJ Papadatos and CS Bartsocas, eds. Alan R. Liss, New York, pp. 269–276, 1985.
13. Perlman M: Perlman syndrome: Familial renal dysplasia with Wilms tumor, fetal gigantism, and multiple congenital anomalies. Am J Med Genet 25:793–795, 1986.
14. Perlman M, Goldberg GM, Bar-Ziv J, Danovitch G: Renal hamartomas and nephroblastomatosis with fetal gigantism: A familial syndrome. J Pediatr 83:414–418, 1973.
15. Perlman M, Levin M, Witels B: Syndrome of fetal gigantism, renal hamartomas and nephroblastomatosis with Wilms' tumor. Cancer 35:1212–1217, 1975.
15a. Schilke K, Schaefer F, Waldherr R, Rohrschneider W, John C, Himbert U, Mayatepek E, Tariverdian G: A case of Perlman syndrome: Fetal gigantism, renal dysplasia, and severe neurological deficits. Am J Med Genet 91:29–33, 2000.
16. Waziri M, Patil S, Hanson JW, Bartley JA: Abnormality of chromosome 11 in patients with features of Beckwith-Wiedemann syndrome. J Pediatr 102: 873.876, 1983.
17. Weksberg R: Personal observation, 1999.

6

Sotos Syndrome

Sotos syndrome (OMIM 117550)[a] is an overgrowth syndrome characterized by increased birth length, increased birth weight, excessive growth during the first 4 years of life, advanced bone age, and distinctive facial features including macrodolichocephaly, ocular hypertelorism, and prominent mandible (45). Opitz et al. (38) critically reviewed the syndrome, and Cohen (9) has provided an extensive update. Over 300 cases are found in the literature. Sotos syndrome is relatively common among overgrowth syndromes and appears to occur 10 times more frequently than Weaver syndrome.

ETIOLOGIC CONSIDERATIONS

Most cases are sporadic and increased paternal age has been noted (13). Several reported families have been consistent with autosomal dominant inheritance (38,52). Autosomal recessive inheritance has been proposed (3a,21b,46a), but documentation has been inadequate (21a,46a); the two sibs reported by Boman and Nilson (3a) are convincing, but could be explained by gonadal mosaicism. Brown et al. (4) reported discordant monozygotic twins and suggested that a postconceptual mutation, an epigenetic change, or an environmental factor might be involved.

Lin et al. (30) analyzed seven patients for nerve growth factor (NGF), brain-derived neurotrophic factor (BDNF), and neurotrophin 3 (NT3). Mutations in all three genes were excluded as a cause of Sotos syndrome. Alternatively, mutations may not have been found either because of heterogeneity or because they might have involved the 5' region of each respective neurotrophin gene, which was *not* screened for mutations (30). Faivre et al. (19a) found no evidence of unbalanced growth-related genes from 78 loci of various chromosomal regions in 18 cases of Sotos syndrome.

Chromosomes are almost always normal. Smith et al. (44) found no evidence for uniparental disomy as a common cause of Sotos syndrome ($n = 29$). In a few instances, chromosomal anomalies have been found. Schrander-Stumpel et al. (42) noted a de novo balanced translocation [t(3;6)(p21;p21)]. Cole and Hughes (14) observed a balanced mosaic translocation—46,XY/46XY,t(2;4) (2qter → 2p15::4p14 → 4pter; 4qter → 4p14::2p16.2 → 2pter). Faivre et al. (20) noted a patient with apparent Sotos syndrome and trisomy 20p11.2–p12.1 mosaicism. Cole et al. (15) reported a case with a small cell carcinoma of the lung and queried whether genes at 3p21 could be involved in both Sotos syndrome and the neoplasm. Several cases have involved chromosome 15, suggesting the possibility that a gene or genes on this chromosome may have something to do with Sotos syndrome. Wajntal and Koiffman (49) reported two cases with del(15)(q12) or (q13) and one case with t(15q;15q). Maroun et al. (32) observed a case with de novo t(5;15)(q35;q22).

[a]On-Line Mendelian Inheritance in Man number.

DIAGNOSTIC CONSIDERATIONS

Cole and Hughes (14) evaluated 79 patients with presumed Sotos syndrome and found misdiagnosis in almost 50% of cases. A number of examples of misdiagnosis are found in the literature (see 12,16,17,19,23,24,36). Cohen (8) pointed out that the autosomal recessive condition reported by Nevo et al. (36) was clearly at variance with "cerebral gigantism" and named the condition Nevo syndrome (7,9). Evans (19) reported a patient with Sotos syndrome and peripheral dysostosis and depressed nasal bridge. The most likely diagnosis is pseudohypoparathyroidism with an acrodysostosis phenotype. Several patients with Bannayan-Riley-Ruvalcaba syndrome have been reported as examples of Sotos syndrome (23,24).

Most patients can be diagnosed by craniofacial gestalt accompanied by significant overgrowth. Occasional patients have been confused with Weaver syndrome. Still other patients cannot be confidently diagnosed as having either syndrome. Opitz et al. (38) suggested that the many similarities between Sotos syndrome and Weaver syndrome may possibly indicate allelic rather than locus heterogeneity. Boys with fragile X may overlap phenotypically with Sotos syndrome (3,48).

The clinical findings of Sotos syndrome are listed in Table 6-1, with percentages derived from the combined 102 cases reported by Jaeken et al. (27) and Wit et al. (51).

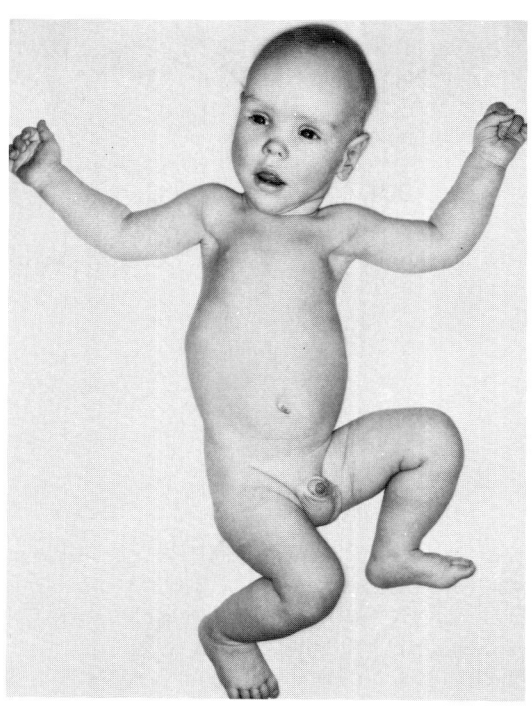

Figure 6-1 Sotos syndrome. Eighteen-month-old male. Large hands and feet. Courtesy of M.M. Steiner, Chicago.

Table 6-1 Clinical Findings in Sotos Syndrome[a,b]

Findings	Total Patients (n)	With Findings (%)
GROWTH		
Large birthweight	19	84
Excessive growth	102	97
Accelerated osseous maturation	102	79
Large hands and feet	80	83
PERFORMANCE		
Developmental retardation	100	84
Lack of fine motor control	92	72
Neonatal adaptation and/or feeding difficulties	80	44
CRANIOFACIAL		
Macrocrania	20	90
Dolichocephaly	100	85
Receding hairline	18	94
Prominent forehead	101	96
Ocular hypertelorism	98	92
Downslanting palpebral fissures	20	65
Pointed chin	101	79
High-arched palate	97	96
Premature eruption of teeth	80	57

[a]Based on 80 cases reviewed by Jaeken et al. (27) and on 22 cases reviewed by Wit et al. (51).
[b]Because the findings are based on sporadic cases, there is an obvious ascertainment bias toward the severe end of the phenotypic spectrum.

GROWTH AND SKELETAL FINDINGS

Overgrowth is commonly evident in the newborn, birthweight averaging 4200 g in males and 4000 g in females (14). Excessive growth is particularly pronounced during the first 4 years of life and bone age is advanced (50) (Figs. 6-1 and 6-2). Agwu et al. (1a) demonstrated that patients are excessively tall at birth, during infancy, and during childhood. Mean birth lengths are 55.6 cm (SD 2.8) in boys and 57.3 cm (SD 3.5) in girls. Disproportionately long limbs cause much

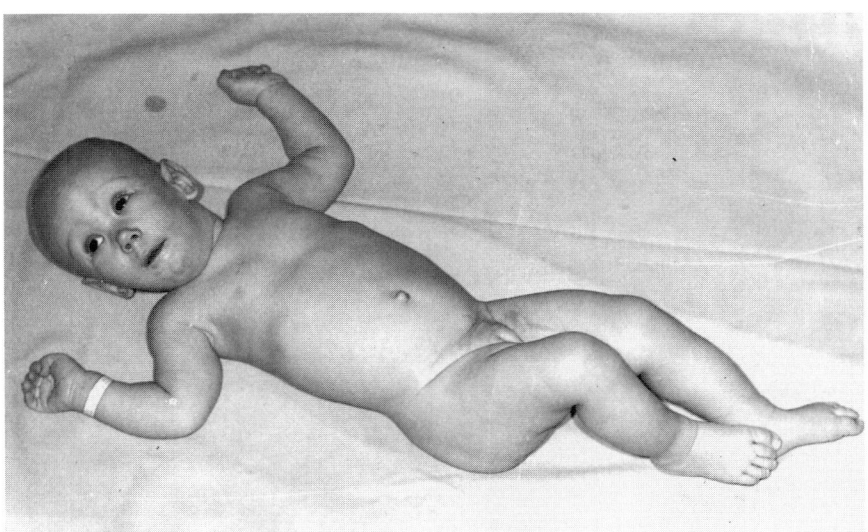

Figure 6–2 Sotos syndrome. Characteristic facial appearance. Large hands and feet. Courtesy of R.J. Gorlin, Minneapolis.

of the increased stature. The onset of menarche appears to occur earlier than usual compared with the average age of onset in British girls. Mean final height attainments are 184.3 cm (SD 6.0) in men and 172.9 cm (SD 5.7) in women. Both are within the normal range for the population, although exceptions are more likely in men than in women.

The hands and feet are large (Figs. 6–1 and 6–2). Dysharmonic maturation and abnormal sequences in the appearance of carpal bones occur in some affected individuals (7). A characteristic metacarpophalangeal profile pattern has been reported (5,6,18). Dijkstra et al. (18) showed that from age 3–7 1/2 years, metacarpophalangeal profile pattern analysis could discriminate between Sotos syndrome and Marfan syndrome. Although these two disorders are commonly differentiated by clinical examination, metacarpophalangeal profile analysis may be a useful adjunct in young children.

PERFORMANCE AND CENTRAL NERVOUS SYSTEM ABNORMALITIES

Neonatal hypotonia and early feeding difficulties are common (14). Most patients have nonprogressive neurologic dysfunction manifested by clumsiness and poor coordination. Cole and Hughes (14) reported a mean DQ/IQ of 78 with a range of 40–129 ($n = 23$), but indicated that their figures probably underestimated ability in Sotos syndrome because some children from regular schools could not be formally assessed. Delay in expressive language and motor development during infancy is particularly common and in some instances may be followed by attainment of normal or near-normal intelligence. Delay in walking until after 15 months of age and speech delay until after 2.5 years are usual. Seizures are found in about 50% of patients, but in about half the cases, they are febrile. Often drooling is observed. Attention deficit may also be a component in some instances. There is a tendency for tone to improve with age, although many children have persistent hypotonic posture and gait (7,9,13,14).

Dilatation of the cerebral ventricles is common. Other abnormalities include absent corpus callosum, prominent cortical sulci, cavum septum pellucidum, and cavum velum interpositi (33,40,41). In a neuroimaging study of 40 patients, Schaefer et al. (41) found prominence of the trigone in 90%, prominence of the occipital horns in 75%, and ventriculomegaly in 63% (Table 6–2).

Table 6–2 Neuroimaging Findings in Sotos Syndrome

Categories	Neuroimaging Abnormalities	Percentage ($n = 40$)
Ventricles	Large	63
	Prominent trigone	90
	Prominent occipital horn	75
Extracerebral fluid	Supratentorial	70
	Posterior fossa	70
Midline anomalies	Cavum septum pellucidum	40
	Cavum vergae	37.5
	Cavum velum interpositum	17.5
	Macrocisterna magna	16.7[a]
	Agenesis of the corpus callosum	2.5
	Hypoplasia of the corpus callosum	97.5[a]
Migration abnormalities	Heterotopias	8.3[a]
Other abnormalities	Periventricular leukomalacia	13.8[a]
	Macrocerebellum	5.5[a]
	Open operculum	2.5

[a]$n = 36$ for these entries.
Source: Adapted from Schaefer et al. (41).

CRANIOFACIAL FEATURES

Dolichocephaly and marked frontal bossing are accentuated by frontoparietal balding. The head circumference is usually well above the 97th centile. Narrow temples make the eyes appear wide-set, but true ocular hypertelorism is not found. The cheeks are full. Although the mandible is long and narrow inferiorly, squared, or pointed, true prognathism is rare (Figs. 6–3 and 6–4). The palate is highly arched, and prematurely erupted deciduous teeth are observed in more than 50% of cases (7,9).

OTHER FINDINGS

Upper respiratory infections are common, particularly otitis media. Constipation is also a problem. About 20% have urinary tract infections. Strabismus is found in about 41% of patients (13).

Congenital heart defects have been discussed by several authors (14,28,33a,35,37,47). Cole and Hughes (14) found congenital heart defects in 12% of Sotos syndrome patients ($n = 41$). Of five cases, four had PDA and one had ASD. Another patient had neonatal supraventricular tachycardia that required digoxin treatment. A high incidence of congenital heart defects and urogenital anomalies have been reported in Japanese reviews (28,33a), suggesting the possibility of heterogeneity.

Mild scoliosis has been reported on occasion and two cases with severe scoliosis have been noted (21a). Other low-frequency abnormalities have been found, including, among others, nys-

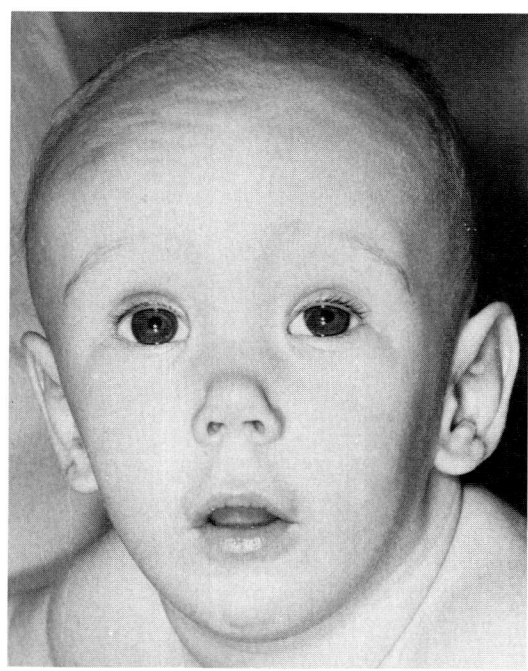

Figure 6–3 Sotos syndrome. Macrocrania, receding hairline, prominent forehead, and pointed chin. Courtesy of R.J. Gorlin, Minneapolis.

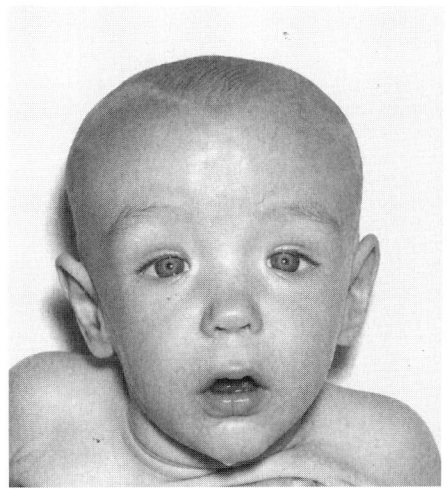 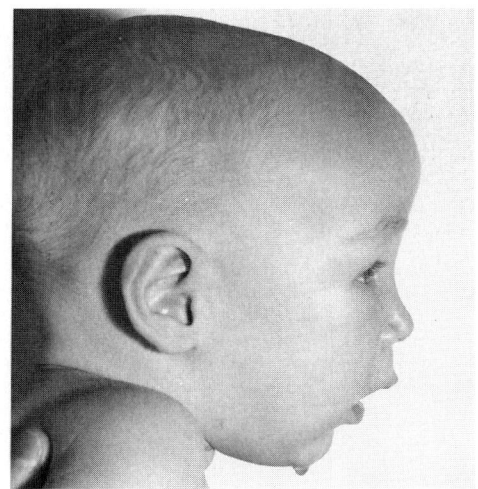

Figure 6–4 Sotos syndrome. Macrodolichocephaly, frontal bossing, ocular hypertelorism, downslanting palpebral fissures, and pointed chin. From Cohen (7).

tagmus, cataracts, juvenile macular degeneration, bones in the anterior fontanelle, vertebra plana, brittle nails, syndactyly, functional megacolon, and autonomic failure with persistent fever (7,9).

NEOPLASMS

Cohen (11) critically reviewed neoplasms reported to occur with Sotos syndrome (Tables 6–3 and 6–4). Tumors have included Wilms tumor,

Table 6–3 Tumors and Nontumors in Sotos Syndrome

Tumor	Age at Diagnosis	Sex	Reference
Wilms tumor	5 years	F	Maldonado et al. (31)
	4.5 years	M	
Neuroblastoma	15 months	F	Nance et al. (34)
	9 years	M	Hersh et al. (25)
Acute lymphocytic leukemia	25 months	M	Hersh et al. (25)
	6 years	M	
Non-Hodgkin lymphoma	8 years	M	Hersh et al. (25)
Hepatocellular carcinoma	14 years	M	Sugarman et al. (46)
Epidermoid carcinoma of the vagina	20 years	F	Seyedabadi et al. (43)
Small cell carcinoma of the lung	22 years	F	Cole et al. (15)
Sacrococcygeal teratoma	Prenatal (38 weeks)	F	Leonard et al. (29)
	Prenatal (27 weeks)	F	
Multiple hemangiomas[a]	2–14 months	F	Abraham and Snodgrass (1) (case 1)
Osteochondroma	7 years	M	Hook and Reynolds (26) (patient C)
Large hairy nevus[b]	Presumed since birth	F	Hook and Reynolds (26) (patient B)
Giant cell granuloma of mandible[c]	13 years	F	Flaggert et al. (21)

[a]Multiple hemangiomas originally listed by the authors as "cavernous haemangiomata." By today's standards hemangiomas cannot be cavernous. See Cohen (10).
[b]Large hairy nevus is not a tumor although it may have an increased risk of malignant transformation.
[c]Giant cell granuloma of the jawbones cannot be considered a tumor. It is different histologically from true giant cell tumors of the long bones. The histologic appearance of giant cell granuloma is identical to lesions found in hyperparathyroidism. In fact, oral and maxillofacial pathologists sign out such biopsies as "consistent with giant cell granuloma; rule out hyperparathyroidism."
Source: From Cohen (11).

Table 6–4 Tumors and Hamartomas in Misdiagnosed Sotos Syndrome Cases

Reported Lesion	Reported Diagnosis	Actual Diagnosis	Reference
Pleomorphic adenoma[a]	Sotos syndrome	Pseudohypoparathyroidism with acrodysostosis phenotype?	Evans (19)
Intestinal polyposis	Sotos syndrome	Bannayan-Riley-Ruvalcaba syndrome	Ruvalcaba et al. (39)
Intestinal polyposis	Sotos syndrome	Bannayan-Riley-Ruvalcaba syndrome	Halal (23,24)
Neuroectodermal tumor	Sotos syndrome	—	Attributed by several authors to Hook and Reynolds (26), even though no such tumor was reported by them

[a]Originally reported as "mixed parotid tumor." In pathology, a pleomorphic adenoma, the most common salivary gland tumor, is also known as "mixed tumor."
Source: From Cohen (11).

hepatocellular carcinoma, neuroblastoma, acute lymphocytic leukemia, non-Hodgkin lymphoma, vaginal epidermoid carcinoma, small cell carcinoma of the lung, and sacrococcygeal teratoma (1,15,21,25,26,29,31,34,43,46). Tumors found in Sotos syndrome are compared to those associated with Beckwith-Wiedemann syndrome and hemihyperplasia in Table 1–5 of Chapter 1. Hersh et al. (25) found a 2.2% risk for childhood tumors in Sotos syndrome and suggested that this might be an overestimate because of reporting bias.

LABORATORY FINDINGS

A 14% frequency of glucose intolerance has been demonstrated in Sotos syndrome by numerous investigators (7).

DIFFERENTIAL DIAGNOSIS

Several syndromes have been confused with Sotos syndrome. Nevo syndrome (8,36) (Chapter 15) has, in addition to Sotosoid features, generalized edema at birth, severe muscular hypotonia, contractures of the feet, wrist drop, and clinodactyly. The condition has autosomal recessive inheritance. Weaver syndrome (Chapter 7) has a distinctive facial appearance, widened distal long bones, and more accelerated osseous maturation. Bannayan-Riley-Ruvalcaba syndrome (7,9) (Chapter 8) has some Sotosoid features but has distinctive pigmentary spotting of the penis and intestinal polyposis, particularly of the colon. Inheritance is autosomal dominant. Some patients clinically suspected of having Sotos syndrome have been reported with fragile X syndrome (3,48) (Chapter 13). Goldstein et al. (22) observed two patients with overgrowth, congenital hypotonia, nystagmus, strabismus, and mental deficiency; they were thought to bear some resemblance to those with Sotos syndrome.

REFERENCES

1. Abraham JM, Snodgrass GJAI: Sotos' syndrome of cerebral gigantism. Arch Dis Child 44:203–210, 1969.
1a. Agwu JC, Shaw NJ, Kirk J, Chapman S, Ravine D, Cole TRP: Growth in Sotos syndrome. Arch Dis Child 80:339–342, 1999.
2. Allanson JE, Cole TRP: Sotos syndrome: Evolution of facial phenotype. Subjective and objective assessment. Am J Med Genet 65:13–20, 1996.
3. Beemer FA, Veenema H, de Pater JM: Cerebral gigantism (Sotos syndrome) in two patients with fragile (X) syndrome. Am J Med Genet 23:221–226, 1986.
3a. Boman H, Nilson D: Sotos syndrome in two brothers. Clin Genet 18:421–427, 1980.
4. Brown WT, Wisniewski KE, Sudhalter V, Keogh M, Tsiouris J, Miezejeski C, Schaefer GB: Identical twins discordant for Sotos syndrome. Am J Med Genet 79:329–333, 1998.
5. Butler MG, Meany FJ, Kittur S, Hersh JH, Hornstein L: Metacarpophalangeal pattern profile analysis in Sotos syndrome. Am J Med Genet 20:625–629, 1985.
6. Butler MG, Dijkstra PF, Meany FJ: Metacarpophalangeal pattern profile analysis in Sotos syndrome: A follow-up report on 34 subjects. Am J Med Genet 29:143–147, 1988.

7. Cohen MM Jr: A comprehensive and critical assessment of overgrowth and overgrowth syndromes, in H Harris and Hirschhorn K (eds) Advances in Human Genetics. New York, Plenum Press, vol 18, Ch 4, pp 181–303; Addendum, pp 373–376, 1989.
8. Cohen MM Jr: Diagnostic problems in cerebral gigantism. J Med Genet 13:80, 1976.
9. Cohen MM Jr: Overgrowth syndromes: An update. Adv Pediatr 46:441–491, 1999.
10. Cohen MM Jr: Perspectives on overgrowth syndromes. Am J Med Genet 79:234–237, 1998.
11. Cohen MM Jr: Tumors and non-tumors in Sotos syndrome. Am J Med Genet 84:173–175, 1999.
12. Cole T, Allanson J: Letter to the editor: Reply to "Lymphoproliferative Disorders in Sotos Syndrome: Observation in Two Cases". Am J Med Genet 75:226, 1998.
13. Cole TRP, Hughes HE: Sotos syndrome. J Med Genet 27:571–576, 1990.
14. Cole TRP, Hughes HE: Sotos syndrome: A study of the diagnostic criteria and natural history. J Med Genet 31:20–32, 1994.
15. Cole TRP, Hughes HE, Jeffreys MJ, Williams GT, Arnold MM: Small cell lung carcinoma in a patient with Sotos syndrome. Are genes at 3p21 involved in both conditions? J Med Genet 29:338–341, 1992.
16. Corsello G, Giuffrè M: Letter to the editor: Sotos syndrome and lymphoproliferative disorders: Reply to T Cole and J Allanson. Am J Med Genet 75:227, 1998.
17. Corsello G, Giuffrè M, Carcione A, Lo Curto M, Piccione M, Ziino O: Lymphoproliferative disorders in Sotos syndromes: Observation of two cases. Am J Med Genet 64:598–593.
18. Dijkstra PF, Cole TRP, Oorthuys JWE, Venema HW, Oosting J, Nocker RET: Metacarpophalangeal pattern profile analysis in Sotos and Marfan syndrome. Am J Med Genet 51:55–60, 1994.
19. Evans PR: Sotos' syndrome (cerebral gigantism) with peripheral dysostosis. Arch Dis Child 46:199–202, 1971.
19a. Faivre L, Vekemans M, Sanlaville D, Munnich A, Cormier-Daire V: No evidence of unbalanced growth-related gene inheritance in a series of overgrowth syndrome patients. Am J Med Genet 99:166–167, 2001.
20. Faivre L, Viot G, Prieur M, Turleau C, Gosset P, Romana S, Munnich A, Vekemans M, Cormier-Daire V: Apparent Sotos syndrome (cerebral gigantism) in a child with trisomy 20p11.2–p12.,1 mosaicism. Am J Med Genet 91:273–276, 2000.
21. Flaggert JJ III, Heldt LV, Garies FJ: Recurrent giant cell granuloma occurring in the mandible of a patient on high dose estrogen therapy for the treatment of Sotos syndrome. J Oral Maxillofac Surg 45:1074–1076, 1987.
21a. Fryer A, Sweeney E, Donnai D. Sotos syndrome. Two cases with severe scoliosis. 9th Manchester Birth Defects Conference, Manchester, UK, November 7–10, 2000.
21b. Gemelli M, Carlo Stella N, Barberio G, Tortorella G, Mami C, De Luca F: Sindrome di Sotos in due fratelli. Minerva Pediatr 34:983–986, 1982.
22. Goldstein DJ, Ward RE, Moore E, Fremion AS, Wappner RS: Overgrowth, congenital hypotonia, nystagmus, strabismus, and mental retardation: Variant of dominantly inherited Sotos sequence? Am J Med Genet 29:783–792, 1988.
23. Halal F: Male-to-male transmission of cerebral gigantism. Am J Med Genet 12:411–419, 1982.
24. Halal F: Letter to the editor: Cerebral gigantism, intestinal polyposis, and pigmentary spotting of the genitalia. Am J Med Genet 15:161, 1983.
25. Hersh JH, Cole TRP, Bloom AS, Bertolone SJ, Hughes HE: Risk of malignancy in Sotos syndrome. J Pediatr 120:572–574, 1992.
26. Hook EB, Reynolds JW: Cerebral gigantism: Endocrinological and clinical observations of six patients including a congenital giant, concordant monozygotic twins, and a child who achieved adult gigantic size. J Pediatr 70:900–914, 1967.
27. Jaeken J, Vander Schueren-Lodeweyckx M, Eeckels R: Cerebral gigantism syndrome—A report of four cases and review of the literature. Z Kinderheilkd 112:332–346, 1972.
28. Kaneko H, Tsukahara M, Tachibana H, Kurashige H, Kuwano A, Kajii T: Congenital heart defects in Sotos sequence. Am J Med Genet 26:569–576, 1987.
29. Leonard NJ, Cole T, Bhargava R, HonorÈ LH, Watt J: Letter to the editor: Sacrococcygeal teratoma in two cases of Sotos syndrome. Am J Med Genet 95:182–184, 2000.
30. Lin AE, Liu Q, Mannheim GB, Darras BT: Exclusion of growth factor gene mutations as a common cause of Sotos syndrome. Am J Med Genet 98:101–102, 2001.
31. Maldonado V, Gaynon PS, Poznanski AK: Cerebral gigantism associated with Wilms' tumor. Am J Dis Child 138:486–488, 1984.
32. Maroun C, Schmerler S, Hutcheon RG: Child with Sotos phenotype and a 5:15 translocation. Am J Med Genet 50:291–293, 1994.
33. Melo DG, Pina-Neto JM, Acosta AX, Daniel J, de Castro V, Santos AC: Letter to the editor: Neuroimaging and echocardiographic findings in Sotos syndrome. Am J Med Genet 90:432–433, 1999.
33a. Moriyama M, Terashima K, Fukushima Y, Kuroki Y: Urogenital anomalies in patients with Sotos syndrome. Nippon Hinyokika Gakkai Zasshi 75:591–593, 1984.
34. Nance MA, Neglia JP, Talwar D, Berry SA: Neuroblastoma in a patient with Sotos syndrome. J Med Genet 27:130–132, 1990.

35. Naritomi K, Izumikawa Y, Toma R, Chinen Y: A study on natural history of Sotos syndrome (in Japanese). In: *Annual Report of Grant for Maternal Child Health Research from Ministry of Health and Welfare*. pp. 212–213, 1997.
36. Nevo S, Zeltzer M, Benderly A, Levy J: Evidence for autosomal recessive inheritance in cerebral gigantism. J Med Genet 11:158–165, 1974.
37. Noreau DR, Al-Ata J, Jutras L, Teebi AS: Congenital heart defects in Sotos syndrome. Am J Med Genet 79:327–328, 1998.
38. Opitz JM, Weaver DW, Reynolds JF Jr: The syndromes of Sotos and Weaver: Reports and review. Am J Med Genet 79:294–304, 1998.
39. Ruvalcaba RHA, Myhre S, Smith DW: Sotos syndrome with intestinal polyposis and pigmentary spotting of the genitalia. Clin Genet 18:413–416, 1980.
40. Schaefer GB: Letter to the editor: Response to the letter to the editor by Gusmao Melo et al.—"Neuroimaging and Echocardiographic Findings in Sotos Syndrome". Am J Med Genet 90:434, 2000.
41. Schaefer GB, Bodensteiner JB, Bueuler BA: The neuroimaging findings in Sotos syndrome. Am J Med Genet 68:462–465, 1997.
42. Schrander-Stumpel CT, Fryns JP, Hamers GG: Sotos syndrome and de novo balanced autosomal translocation [t(3;6)(p21;p21)]. Clin Genet 37:226–229, 1990.
43. Seyedabadi S, Bard DS, Zuna RE: Epidermoid carcinoma of the vagina in a patient with cerebral gigantism. J Ark Med Soc 78:123–127, 1981.
44. Smith M, Fullwood P, Qi Y, Palmer S, Upadhyaya M, Cole T: No evidence for uniparental disomy as a common cause of Sotos syndrome. J Med Genet 34:10–12, 1997.
45. Sotos JF, Dodge PR, Muirhead D, Crawford JD, Talbot NB: Cerebral gigantism in childhood: A syndrome of excessively rapid growth with acromelic features and a non-progressive neurologic disorder. N Engl J Med 272:109–116, 1964.
46. Sugarman GI, Heuser ET, Reed WB: A case of cerebral gigantism and hepatocarcinoma. Am J Dis Child 131:631–633, 1977.
46a. Townes PL, Sheinen AP: Cerebral gigantism (Sotos syndrome). Evidence for recessive inheritance. Pediatr Res 7:349, 1973.
47. Tsukahara M, Marakami K, Iino H, Tateishi H, Fujita K, Uchida M: Letter to the editor: Congenital heart defects in Sotos syndrome. Am J Med Genet 84:172, 1999.
48. Verloes A, Sacrè J-P, Geubelle F: Sotos syndrome and fragile X chromosomes. Lancet ii:329, 1987.
49. Wajntal A, Koiffman CP: Chromosome aberrations in Sotos syndrome [letter, comment]. Clin Genet 40:472, 1991.
50. Winship IM: Sotos syndrome—autosomal dominant inheritance substantiated. Clin Genet 28:243–246, 1985.
51. Wit JM, Beemer FA, Barth PG, Orthuys JWE, Dijkstra PE, van den Brande JL, Leschot NJ: Cerebral gigantism (Sotos syndrome). Compiled data of 22 cases. Eur J Pediatr 144:131–140, 1985.
52. Zonana J, Sotos JF, Romshe CA, Fischer DA, Elders MJ, Rimoin DL: Dominant inheritance of cerebral gigantism. J Pediatr 91:251–256, 1977.

Weaver Syndrome

In 1974, Weaver et al. (51) reported a syndrome of persistent overgrowth of prenatal onset, accelerated osseous maturation, distinctive craniofacial appearance, developmental delay, widened distal long bones, and camptodactyly (OMIM 277590)[a] (Figs. 7–1 to 7–4).

ETIOLOGIC CONSIDERATIONS

The molecular basis of Weaver syndrome is unknown. Faivre et al. (14a) found no evidence of unbalanced growth-related genes from 78 loci of various chromosomal regions in 9 cases.

Most cases are sporadic. Parent-to-child transmission consistent with autosomal dominant transmission has been recorded on seven occasions (13,20,27a,37,38). Kelly et al. (27a) reported affected half brothers and their father. Affected adults may show few signs of Weaver syndrome except tall stature. Fitch (16,17) published extensive analyses of the syndrome. Ardinger et al. (2) reported seven cases and reviewed the literature. A recent critical review was published by Opitz et al (37) and an updated review is that of Cohen (7). Khosravi et al. (28) tabulated 34 patients and determined the minimal diagnostic criteria for Weaver syndrome. Many cases have been reported (1,2,4,7–9,11–18,20,21–25,28–30,32,35–40,42,44,47,48,51–53). There is a 3:1 male-to-female ratio (2,7,37) and females have been noted to be more mildly affected (2,7,37,47). Features of Weaver syndrome are summarized in Table 7–1 and shown in Figures 7–1 to 7–7.

[a]On-Line Mendelian Inheritance in Man number.

GROWTH AND SKELETAL FINDINGS

Mean birth weight is 4785 g in males and 3883 g in females. Birth length is 56 cm in males and 53 cm in females. Head circumference at birth is 36.6 cm in males and 35.2 cm in females. Final height attainment is 194.2 cm in males and 176.3 cm in females. Skeletal growth is more accelerated than skeletal maturation, resulting in excessive height in adults, in contrast to Sotos syndrome, in which accelerated growth and accelerated maturation occur so that final height attainment is not excessive. Adult weight is 102.2 kg in males and 87.6 kg in females. Adult head circumference is 61 cm in males and 59.5 cm in females (27a,37).

Bone age is remarkably advanced (Fig. 7–1); the growth parameters of head circumference, length, and weight are two to three times the expected rate. Carpal maturation is accelerated over that of phalanges and metacarpals. Other skeletal findings include widened or splayed long bone metaphyses, especially of the femurs, and somewhat mottled epiphyses (Fig. 7–7). The iliac wings may be broad and low (2,7,37). Cervical kyphosis and underdevelopment of the mid-cervical vertebral bodies have been reported, and it has been suggested that cervical spine abnormalities might be a diagnostic clue in a tall parent of a Weaver syndrome child (27a).[b]

[b]Muhonen and Menezes (35) reported cervical spine instability requiring stabilization in a child with Weaver syndrome.

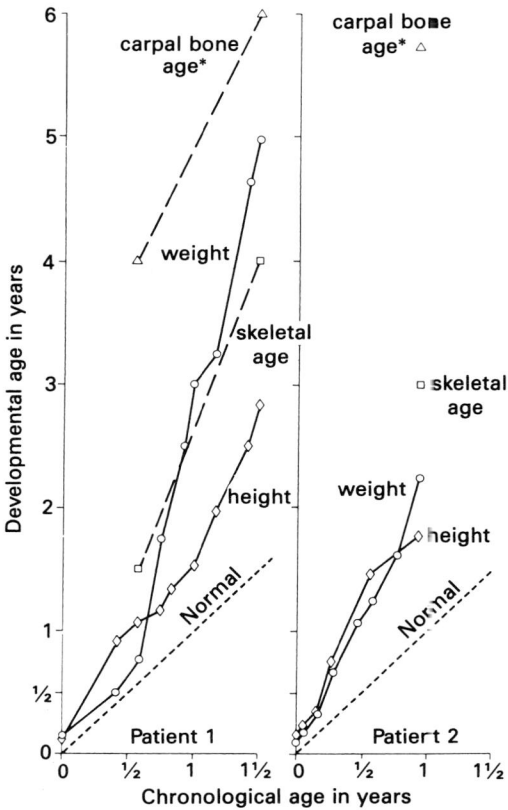

Figure 7–1 Weaver syndrome. Growth rates: Height and weight ages are expressed relative to the 50th centiles for chronological age. Carpal bone age is derived for the wrist centers and skeletal age is an average for the remainder of the skeleton. From Weaver et al. (51).

PERFORMANCE AND CENTRAL NERVOUS SYSTEM

Mild hypertonia or hypotonia is common, and motor development is mildly to moderately retarded. The cry is low-pitched and hoarse. Although the appetite is voracious, hypothalamic dysregulation has not been demonstrated. Difficulty in swallowing or breathing has been noted in several cases. Other findings have included cysts of the septum pellucidum (2 cases); dilation of the ventricles, basal cisterns, sylvian cistern, and interhemispheric fissure, consistent with nonspecific cerebral atrophy (1 case); enlarged vessels and hypervascularization in the areas of the middle and left posterior cerebral arteries (1 case); and pachygyria (1 case) (2,7,18, 37). The wide range of intelligence found with Weaver syndrome and the brain abnormalities reported in some cases suggest that MRI should be considered as part of the work-up.

CRANIOFACIAL FEATURES

Macrocephaly, broad forehead, and flattened occiput are characteristic. Scalp hair is moderately thin. The ears are large and may be mildly dysmorphic or low set (Figs. 7–2 to 7–5). Other features include hypertelorism, long prominent philtrum, relative micrognathia, and redundant nuchal skin folds. Low-frequency findings have been noted such as mild craniofacial asymmetry, upslanting or downslanting palpebral fissures,

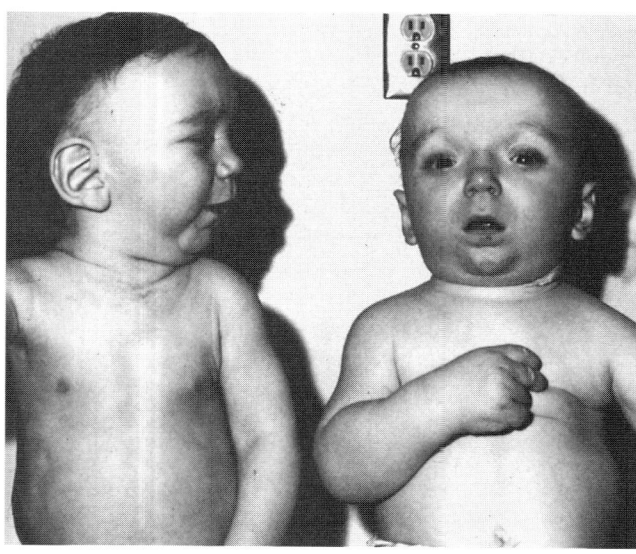

Figure 7–2 Weaver syndrome. **Left**: Patient at 11 months. **Right**: A second patient at 18 months. From Weaver et al. (51).

WEAVER SYNDROME

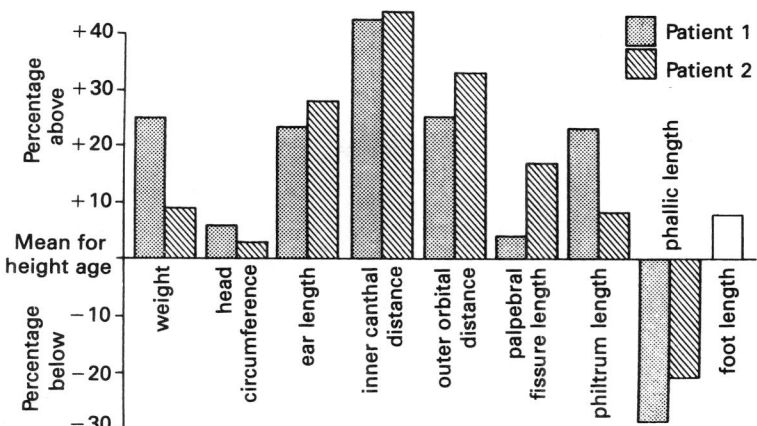

Figure 7–3 Weaver syndrome. Growth parameters in relationship to normal values for height age, demonstrating malproportion for height. The sizes of various parameters are expressed as percentages above or below that expected for height age. Patient 1 was 18 months old with a height age of 34 months, and patient 2 was 11 months old with a height age of 22 months. From Weaver et al. (51).

small palpebral fissures, ptosis, strabismus, and highly arched palate (2,7,37).

LIMBS

Common findings include camptodactyly, prominent finger pads, thin deeply set nails, broad thumbs, clinodactyly of the toes (Fig. 7–6), and limited extension at the elbows and knees. Foot deformities have been noted such as talipes equinovarus, talipes calcaneovalgus, metatarsus adductus, pes adductus, and pes cavus. Deep creases may be observed on the palmar and plantar surfaces (2,7,37).

NEOPLASMS

Mulhonen and Menezes (35) and Huffman et al. (25) reported stage 4S neuroblastoma (Fig. 7–8), which has a favorable prognosis, and spontaneous resolution occurs in more than 90% of the cases. The patient of Muhonen and Menezes (35) was treated with melphalan, vincristine, cyclophosphamide, and dacarbazine and the tumor went into remission. In the patient of Huffman et al. (25), abdominal MRI at 18 months showed a decrease in the size of the neuroblastoma and no evidence of metastases was evident.

Derry et al. (13) reported a malignant ovarian endodermal sinus tumor in a 17-year-old woman. Surgical excision was followed by chemotherapy. She has been well since then and when she was older, she gave birth to a boy with Weaver syndrome (13). Kelly et al. (27a) reported a sacrococcygeal teratoma in a male infant.

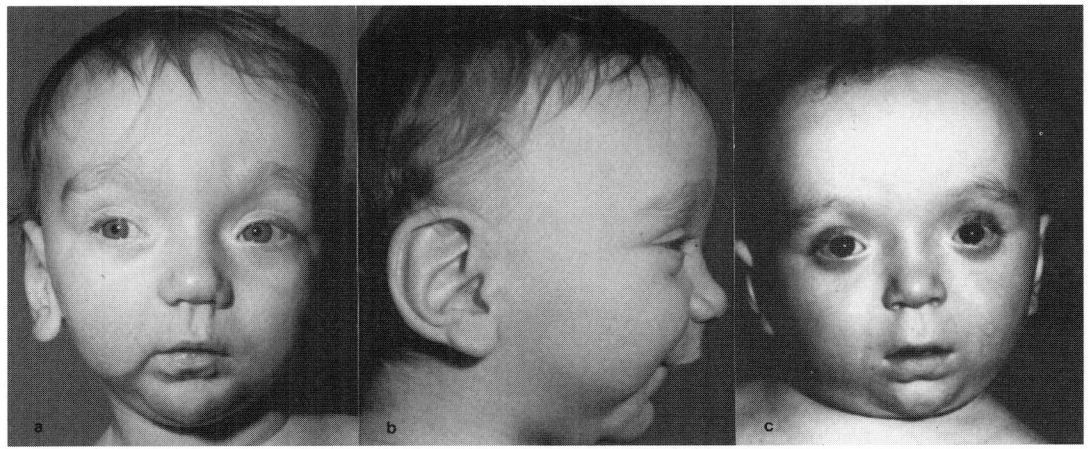

Figure 7–4 Weaver syndrome. **a–c**: Note broad forehead, ocular hypertelorism, large ears, long philtrum, micrognathia. From Weaver et al. (51).

Table 7–1 Features of Weaver Syndrome

Findings	Frequencies
GROWTH	
Prenatal growth excess	16/20
Postnatal growth excess	19/20
Accelerated osseous maturation	19/19
PERFORMANCE	
Hypertonia	10/18
Hypotonia	5/18
Developmental delay	19/19
Hoarse, low-pitched cry	14/17
CRANIOFACIAL	
Broad forehead	18/19
Flat occiput	6/11
Large ears	15/17
Ocular hypertelorism	19/19
Prominent or long philtrum	10/14
Relative micrognathia	17/19
LIMBS	
Camptodactyly	11/16
Prominent fingerpads	6/9
Thin, deeply set nails	9/10
Broad thumbs	4/6
Clinodactyly, toes	4/5
Limited elbow or knee extension	10/13
Widened distal long bones	16/18
Foot deformities[a]	7/10
OTHER	
Excess loose skin	11/12
Umbilical hernia or diastasis recti	12/17
Inguinal hernia	4/14
Inverted nipples	3/4

[a]Talipes equinovarus, talipes calcaneovalgus, metatarsus adductus.
Source: From Ardinger et al. (2).

If we assume 46 reported cases of Weaver syndrome (13,25,27a,37,38), then 4 had tumors (13,25,27a,35), suggesting an approximately 8.7% occurrence; ascertainment bias for reporting such cases may have inflated the risk. Nevertheless, it is clear that neoplasms occur in Weaver syndrome more commonly than expected by chance.

Because two patients with Weaver syndrome have had neuroblastoma, Huffman et al. (25) suggested retroperitoneal ultrasonography every 3 months until age 7—the same protocol recommended for Beckwith-Wiedemann syndrome (6).

CARDIOVASCULAR ANOMALIES

Huffman et al. (25) reported a case of Weaver syndrome with the combination of neoplasia and congenital heart defects (VSD, PDA). The tumors reported by Muhonen and Menezes (35) and Derry et al. (13) were not associated with heart defects. VSD without neoplasia was reported by Weisswichert et al. (53) and by Sarigül et al. (42).

DIFFERENTIAL DIAGNOSIS

Weaver syndrome should be differentiated from Sotos syndrome (Chapter 6), with which it is sometimes confused (37). A few patients cannot

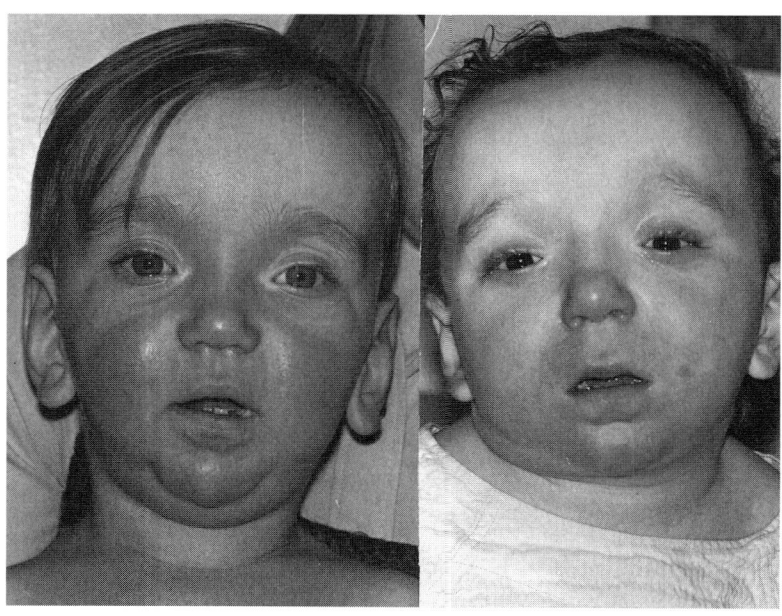

Figure 7–5 Weaver syndrome. Same patients as in Figure 7–4, but older.

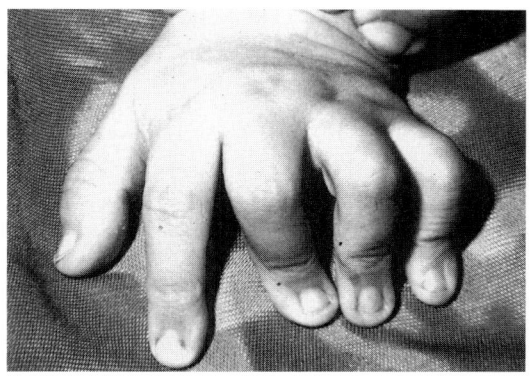

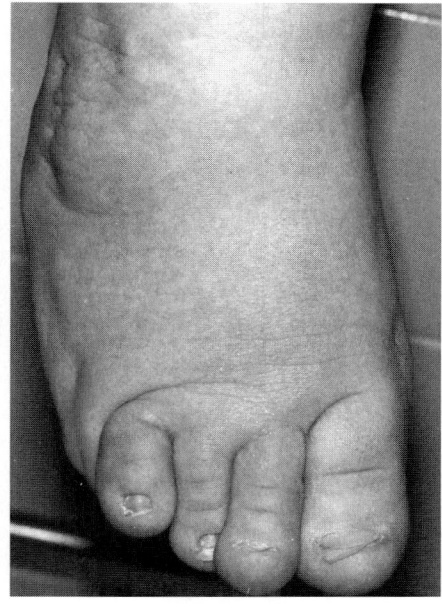

Figure 7–6 Weaver syndrome. **A**: Contractures at proximal interphalangeal joints and deeply set nails. **B**: Clinodactyly with overlapping of fifth toe by fourth toe. Thin, deeply set nails. Repaired talipes equinovarus. From Weaver et al. (51).

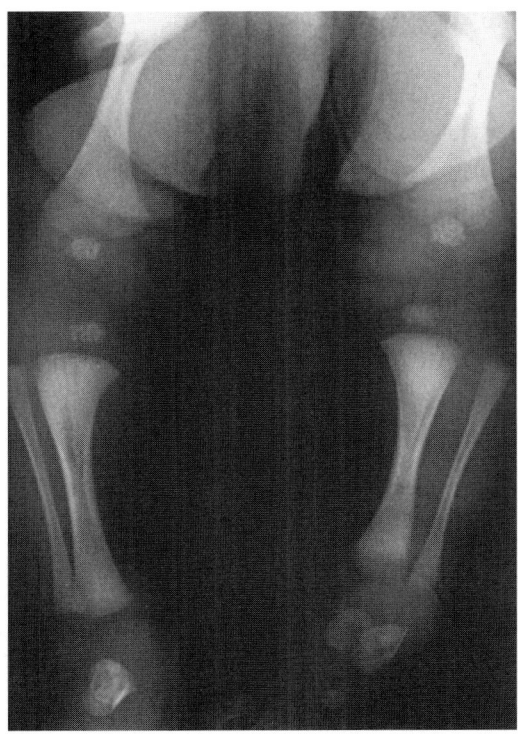

Figure 7–7 Radiograph showing splayed metaphyses and mottled epiphyses. From Huffman et al. (25).

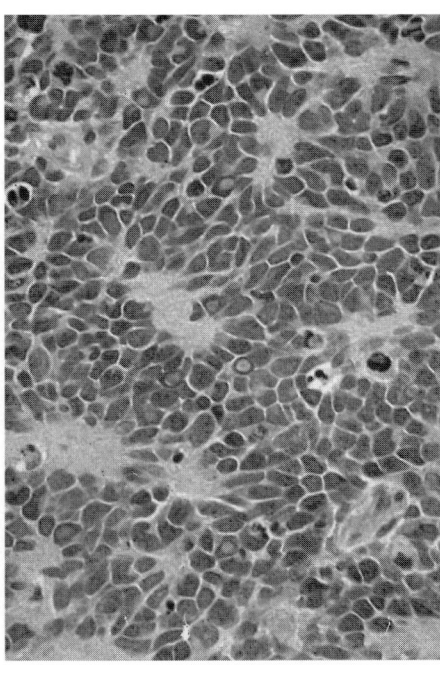

Figure 7–8 Histopathology of neuroblastoma showing rosette formation. From Huffman et al. (25).

be diagnosed confidently as having either Sotos syndrome or Weaver syndrome (37).

There are a number of Weaver-like syndromes and misdiagnosed cases in the literature (3,5, 19,26,27,31,33,34,41,43,45,46,49,50,54). The patient described by Fretzayas et al. (19) had Pallister mosaic tetraploidy i(12p). Case 2 of Majewski et al. (31) is an example of benign familial megalencephaly. A surviving sib first described by Roussounis and Crawford (41) has del(5p) (_1). Asperen et al. (3) reported a mother and son with NF1 and overgrowth with a Weaver-like phenotype. The proband had more than six café-au-lait spots, Lisch nodules, axillary freckling, and numerous neurofibromas. NF1 was confirmed at the molecular level. Perhaps the patient reported by Tsukahara et al. (49) and Kajii and Tsukahara (26a) may represent an example of severe Simpson-Golabi-Behmel syndrome (Chapter 4).

There has been debate about whether certain patients have Weaver syndrome or Marshall-Smith syndrome (see Chapter 19). Shimura et al. (43a) thought their patient had overlapping features; Cohen (7) indicated that Weaver syndrome was more likely. Opitz et al. (37) concluded that the cases of Bosch-Banyeras et al. (5) and Jalaguier et al. (26) probably had Marshall-Smith syndrome.

REFERENCES

1. Amir N, Gross-Kieselstein E, Hirsch H, Lax E, Silverberg-Shale VR: Weaver-Smith syndrome: A case study with long-term follow-up. Am J Dis Child 138:1113–1115, 1984.
2. Ardinger HH, Hanson JW, Harrod MJE, Cohen MM Jr, Tibbles JAR, Welch JP, Young-Wee T, Sommer A, Goldberg R, Shprintzen RJ, Sidoti EJ, Leichtman LG, Hoyme HE: Further delineation of Weaver syndrome. J Pediatr 108:228–235, 1986.
3. Asperen CJ van, Overweg-Plandsoen WCG, Cnossen MH: Familial neurofibromatosis type 1 associated with an overgrowth syndrome resembling Weaver syndrome. J Med Genet 35: 323–327, 1998.
4. Bailey-Wilson JE, Shapira E, Blitzer MG, Braverman N: An unusual case of early overgrowth and congenital anomalies [abstract]. In: American Society of Human Genetics 34th Annual Meeting, Norfolk, Virginia 1983. p. 75A, 1983.
5. Bosch-Banyeras JM, Salcedo S, Lucaya J, Laverde R, Boronat M, Marti-Henneberg C: Accélération du development postnatal, hypertonie, elargissement des phalanges médianes et des metaphyses distales du femur, facies particular: s'agit-il d'un syndrome de Weaver? Arch Fr Pédiatr 35:177–183, 1978.
6. Clericuzio C, D'Angio GL, Duncan M, Green DM, Knudson AG Jr: Recognition and management of childhood cancer syndromes: A systems approach. Am J Med Genet 89:81–90, 1999.
7. Cohen MM Jr: Overgrowth syndromes: An update. Adv Pediatr 46:441–491, 1999.
8. Cohen MM Jr: Overgrowth syndromes. In: *Associated Congenital Anomalies*. M El Shafie and CH Klippel, eds. Williams & Wilkins, Baltimore, pp. 71–104, 1981.
9. Cohen MM Jr: The large-for-gestational age infant in dysmorphic perspective. In: *Clinical Genetics: Problems in Diagnosis and Counseling*. AM Wiley, TP Carter, S Kelly, et al., eds. Academic Press, New York, pp. 153–169, 1982.
10. Cohen MM Jr: A comprehensive and critical assessment of overgrowth and overgrowth syndromes. Adv Hum Genet 18:181–303, 1989.
11. Cole TRP, Dennis NR, Hughes HE: Weaver syndrome. J Med Genet 29:332–337, 1992.
12. Dawood AA, Machado GT, Winship WS: Weaver's syndrome—primordial excessive growth velocity. A case report. S Afr Med J 67:646–648, 1985.
13. Derry CP, Temple IK, Venkat-Raman K: A probable case of familial Weaver syndrome associated with neoplasia. J Med Genet 36:725–728, 1999.
14. Dumíc M, Vukovíc J, Cvitkovíc M, Medica I: Twins and their mildly affected mother with Weaver syndrome. Clin Genet 44:338–340, 1993.
14a. Faivre L, Vekemans M, Sanlaville D, Munnich A, Cormier-Daire V: No evidence of unbalanced growth-related gene inheritance in a series of overgrowth syndrome patients. Am J Med Genet 99:166–167, 2001.
15. Farrell SA, Hughes HE: Brief clinical report: Weaver syndrome with pes cavus. Am J Med Genet 21:737–739, 1985.
16. Fitch N: The syndromes of Marshall and Weaver. J Med Genet 17:174–178, 1980.
17. Fitch N: Update on the Marshall-Smith-Weaver controversy. Am J Med Genet 20:559–562, 1985.
18. Freeman BM, Hoon AH Jr, Breiter SN, Hamosh A: Letter to the editor: Pachygyria in Weaver syndrome. Am J Med Genet 86:395–397, 1999.
19. Fretzayas A, Papanicolaou A, Tzanetakos K, Theodoridis C, Karpathios T: Retarded skeletal maturation in Weaver syndrome. Acta Paediatr Scand 77:930–932, 1988.
20. Freyer A, Smith C, Rosenbloom L, Cole T: Autosomal dominant inheritance of Weaver syndrome. J Med Genet 34:418–419, 1997.
21. Gemme G, Bonioli E, Ruffia G, Lagorio V: The Weaver-Smith syndrome. J Pediatr 97:962–964, 1980.
22. Greenberg F, Wasiewski W, McCabe ERB: Weaver syndrome: The changing phenotype in an adult. Am J Med Genet 33:127–129, 1989.
23. Hall BD: Weaver syndrome: Expanded natural history. Prog Clin Biol Res 200:123–144, 1985.

24. Hoyme HE, West BR, Welsh GW: The Weaver syndrome: Natural history through adulthood. Proc Greenwood Genet Ctr 3:84, 1984.
25. Huffman C, McCandless D, Jasty R, Matloub J, Robinson HB, Weaver DD, Cohen MM Jr: Weaver syndrome with neuroblastoma and cardiovascular anomalies. Am J Med Genet 99:252–255, 2001.
26. Jalaguier J, Montoya F, Germain M, Bonnet H: Advance de la maturation osseuse et syndrome dysmorphique chez deux germains (syndrome de Marshall-Weaver). J Génét Hum 31:385–395, 1983.
26a. Kajii T, Tsukahara M: The Golabi-Rosen syndrome. Letter to the editor. Am J Med Genet 19:819, 1984.
27. Kelly T, Stelling M, Wilson T: Weaver-like syndrome with hyperprogesteronemia and maternal luteoma. Proc Greenwood Genet Ctr 2:128–129, 1983.
27a. Kelly TE, Alford BA, Abel M: Cervical spine anomalies and tumors in Weaver syndrome. Am J Med Genet 95:492–495, 2000.
28. Khosravi M, Weaver DD, Christensen C, McCandless D: Criteria for the Diagnosis of Weaver Syndrome. David W. Smith Workshop on Malformations and Morphogenesis, La Jolla, California, August 2–5, 2000.
29. Kondo I, Mori Y, Kuwajima K: A Japanese male infant with the Weaver syndrome. J Hum Genet 35:257–262, 1990.
30. Kondo I, Mori Y, Kuwajima K: Weaver syndrome in two Japanese children. Am J Med Genet 41:221–224, 1991.
31. Majewski F, Ranke M, Kemperdick H, Schmidt E: The Weaver syndrome: A rare type of primordial overgrowth. Eur J Pediatr 137:277–282, 1981.
32. Meinecke P, Schaefer E, Englbrecht R: The Weaver syndrome in a girl. Eur J Pediatr 141:58–59, 1983.
33. Moreno H, Kirkland R: Another candidate for the overgrowth syndrome [letter]. J Pediatr 85:583, 1974.
34. Moreno HD, Zackai EH, Kaufman HG, Mellman WJ: Case report 18. Syndrome Ident 2:22–25, 1974.
35. Muhonen MG, Menezes AH: Weaver syndrome and instability of the upper cervical spine. J Pediatr 116:596–599, 1990.
36. Nishimura G, Hasegawa T, Nagai T: Propositus with Weaver syndrome and his mildly-affected mother. Implication of nontraditional inheritance. Am J Med Genet 65:249–251, 1996.
37. Opitz JM, Weaver DW, Reynolds JF Jr: The syndromes of Sotos and Weaver: Reports and review. Am J Med Genet 79:294–304, 1998.
38. Proud VK, Braddock SR, Cook L, Weaver DD: Weaver syndrome: Autosomal dominant inheritance of the disorder. Am J Med Genet 79:305–310, 1998.
39. Ramos-Arroyo MA, Weaver DD, Banks ER: Weaver syndrome: A case without early overgrowth and review of the literature. Pediatrics 88:1106–1111, 1991.
40. Rojas-Martínez A, Sánchez-Corona J, García-Cruz MO, Gonzáles-Martínez A, Nazará Z, García-Cruz D: A sporadic case of Weaver syndrome in a female. Dysmorphol Clin Genet 5:23–26, 1991.
41. Roussounis MB, Crawford JJ: Siblings with Weaver syndrome. J Pediatr 102:595–597, 1983.
42. Sarigül A, Yihnaz M, Ates S, Yurdakul Y: A case with Weaver syndrome operated for congenital cardiac defect. Pediatr Cardiol 20:375–376, 1999.
43. Scarano G, Della Monica M, Leonardo F, Neri G: Novel findings in a patient with Weaver or a Weaver-like syndrome. Am J Med Genet 63:378–381, 1996.
43a. Shimura T, Utsumi Y, Fujikawa S, Nakamura H, Baba K: Marshall-Smith syndrome with large bifrontal diameter, broad distal femora, camptodactyly, and without broad middle phalanges. J Pediatr 94:93–95, 1979.
44. Stewart FJ, Cole TRP, Carson DJ, Nevin NC: Diagnosis of Weaver syndrome in a teenage girl. 6th Manchester Birth Defects Conference, Manchester, UK, November 1–4, 1994.
45. Stoll C, Talon P, Mengus L, Roth MP, Dott B: A Weaver-like syndrome with endocrinological abnormalities in a boy and his mother. Clin Genet 28:255–259, 1985.
46. Teebi AS, Sundaresham TS, Hammouri MY, Al-Awadi SA, Al-Saleh QA: A new autosomal recessive disorder resembling Weaver syndrome. Am J Med Genet 33:479–482, 1989.
47. Thompson EM, Hill S, Leonard JV, Pembrey ME: A girl with the Weaver syndrome. J Med Genet 24:232–234, 1987.
48. Trabelsi M, Ben Hariz MD, Monastiri R, Taktak M, Bennaceur B: Le syndrome de Weaver: A propos d'un nouveau cas. Ann Pédiatr (Paris) 37:327–330, 1990.
49. Tsukahara M, Tanaka S, Kajii T: A Weaver-like syndrome in a Japanese boy. Clin Genet 25:73–78, 1984.
50. Turner DR, Downing JW: Anesthetic problems associated with Weaver's syndrome. Br J Anaesth 57:1260–1263, 1985.
51. Weaver DD, Graham CB, Thomas IT, Smith DW: A new overgrowth syndrome with accelerated skeletal maturation, unusual facies, and camptodactyy. J Pediatr 84:547–552, 1974.
52. Weaver DD, Ramos Arroyo MT, Banks E: Delayed onset of the Weaver syndrome. Proc Greenwood Genet Ctr 7:153–154, 1988.
53. Weisswichert PH, Knapp G, Willich E: Accelerated bone maturation syndrome of the Weaver type. Eur J Pediatr 137:329–333, 1981.
54. Williams MS: A semi-unknown case; Is Weaver-like syndrome a separate clinical entity? 19th Annual David W. Smith Workshop on Malformations and Morphogenesis, Whistler, British Columbia, August 6–10, 1998.

Bannayan-Riley-Ruvalcaba Syndrome

Bannayan-Riley-Ruvalcaba syndrome (OMIM 153480)[a] (6) is an autosomal dominant disorder consisting of macrocephaly, vascular malformations, lipomas, hamartomatous polyps of the distal ileum and colon, pigmented macules on the shaft of the penis, and Hashimoto's thyroiditis (6,18).

DELINEATION AND NOMENCLATURE

Ruvalcaba et al. (40) reported two males with macrocephaly, intestinal polyposis, and pigmented spotting of the penis. Bannayan (2) described the combination of macrocephaly with subcutaneous and visceral lipomas and vascular malformations. Riley and Smith (39) observed the association of macrocephaly, pseudopapilledema, and vascular malformations. Cohen (6) and Dvir et al. (13) suggested lumping these three earlier recognized syndromes as a single entity and Cohen (6) suggested combining the names of the first authors of the three original reports to keep learning hurdles to a minimum: "Bannayan-Riley-Ruvalcaba syndrome." Gorlin et al. (18) then demonstrated all three phenotypes in a single family through four generations. PTEN mutations have been found in both Bannayan-Riley-Ruvalcaba syndrome and Cowden syndrome (3,4,30–32) and phenotypic overlap has been described (1,15,16,48). Marsh et al. (32) demonstrated that the PTEN mutational spectrum also involves overlap, suggesting a single genetic entity they called the "PTEN hamartoma-tumor syndrome."

MOLECULAR BIOLOGY OF PTEN

PTEN is a member of the protein tyrosine phosphatase (PTPase) superfamily defined by an invariant signature motif $Cys(X)_5Arg$; within this catalytic domain, cysteine is a catalyst and arginine plays an important role in binding the phosphoryl group of the substrate. PTEN is a tumor suppressor gene that maps to 10q23. It's name is derived from phosphatase (P) and the cytoskeletal protein tensin (TEN). For proper functioning, the phosphatase domain must be intact (7,28).

The PTEN gene consists of nine exons and encodes a protein of 403 amino acids. The signature motif is in the N-terminal domain. The phosphatase active site of PTEN is larger than those observed in other protein phosphatases. The site is important for accommodating the phosphoinositide substrate. PTEN also has a C2 domain that can bind phospholipid membranes. The phosphatase and C2 domains associating across an extensive interface suggest that the C2 domain might serve to position the catalytic domain on the membrane (26) (Fig. 8–1).

PTEN is known to have multiple targets. It can dephosphorylate tyrosine-, serine-, and threonine-phosphorylated peptides. It can also dephosphorylate phosphatidylinositol 3,4,5-trisphosphate [PI(3,4,5)P3], a lipid second messenger

[a]On-Line Mendelian Inheritance in Man number.

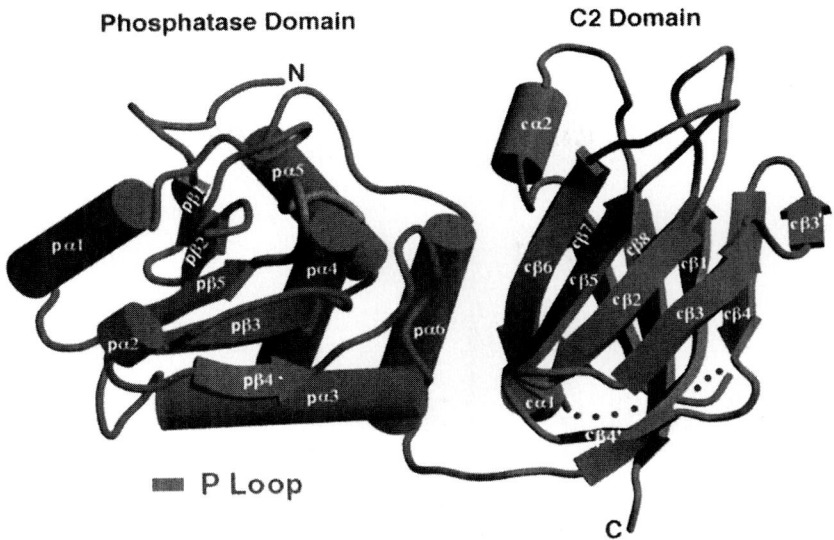

Figure 8–1 PTEN has an N-terminal phosphatase domain and a C-terminal C2 domain. Dotted line indicates region deleted in crystallized protein. From Lee et al. (26).

produced by phosphatidylinositol 3 kinase (PI3K). *PTEN* modulates cell cycle progression and cell survival by regulating PI(3,4,5)P3 and the Akt/protein kinase B (PKB) signaling pathway. *PTEN* dephosphorylates focal adhesion kinase (FAK) and inhibits integrin-mediated cell spreading and cell migration on extracellular matrix proteins such as fibronectin and vitronectin. A general function of *PTEN* appears to be downregulation of FAK and Shc phosphorylation, Ras activity, downstream MAP kinase activation, and associated focal contact formation and cell spreading (Fig. 8–2). Little is known about how PTEN itself is regulated, except that mRNA levels are modulated by TGFβ (19,28,29, 35,44,46).

MUTATIONS

PTEN plays an important role in neoplasia. Deletions and mutations have been found in breast cancer, prostate cancer, glioblastoma, kidney cancer, endometrial carcinoma, malignant melanoma, and thyroid tumors. *PTEN* germline mutations have been identified in Bannayan-Riley-Ruvalcaba syndrome, Cowden syndrome, and phenotypic overlap between the two (1,3,4,30–32,48). Second mutations occur in so-

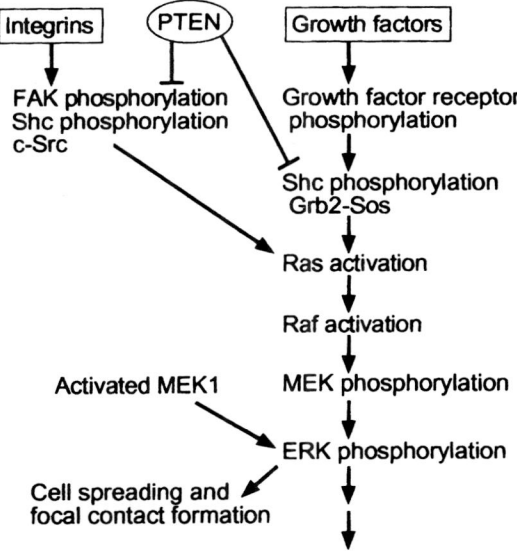

Figure 8–2 Working model of *PTEN* regulatory network. Integrins and growth factors can separately stimulate the Ras/ERK/MAP kinase pathway or function collaboratively. Integrin receptor engagement with FN stimulates FAK, Shc, and c-Src, and they activate pathway. Growth factors can activate pathway through autophosphorylation of growth factor receptors. *PTEN* reduces Shc phosphorylation and its interaction with Grb2, as well as the downstream Ras/ERK common MAP kinase pathway for integrin- and growth factor–mediated signaling, and then affects cell spreading and focal contact formation. Activated MEK1 can partially reverse the latter effects of *PTEN*. From Gu et al. (19).

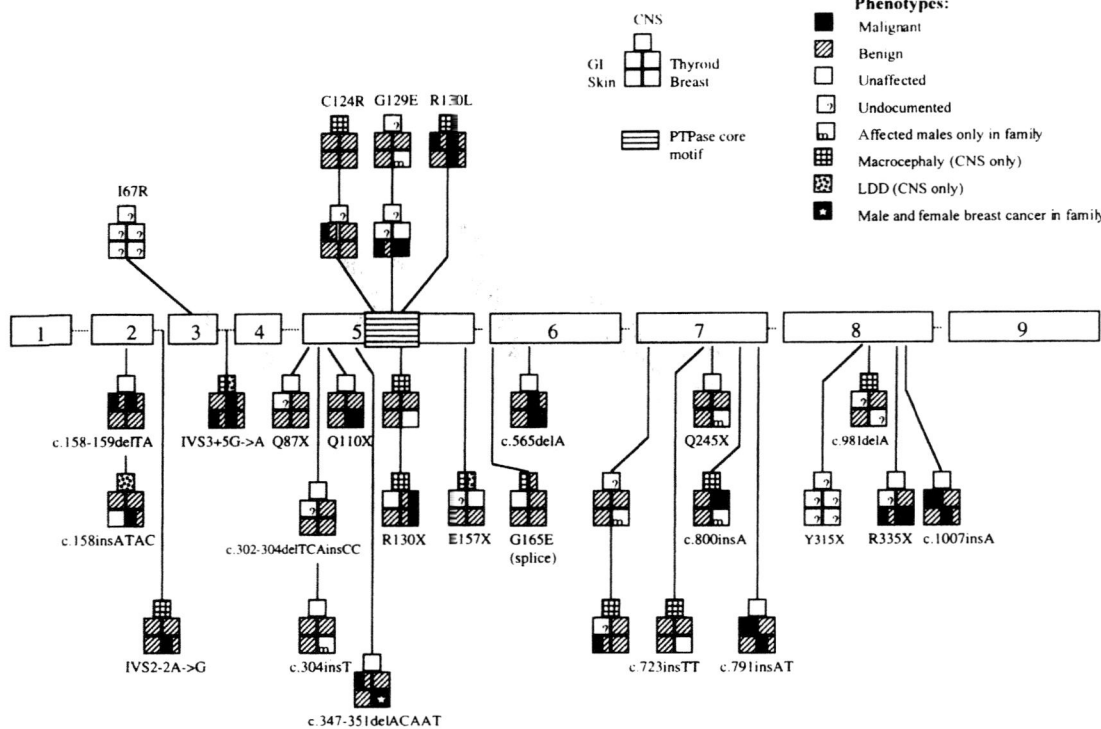

Figure 8–3 PTEN mutations in Bannayan-Riley-Ruvalcaba syndrome and Bannayan-Riley-Ruvalcaba syndrome/Cowden syndrome overlap families. PTPase core motif indicated in exon 5 (horizontal lines). Truncating mutations shown in lower portion of figure. Missense mutations shown in upper portion of figure. Phenotype indicated by shaded box in one of six positions shown in upper right portion of figure. From Marsh et al. (32).

matic cells, inactivating the normal allele by allelic loss or loss of heterozygosity.

PTEN mutations have been identified in 60% of Bannayan-Riley-Ruvalcaba patients ($n = 32$), in 81% of Cowden syndrome patients ($n = 37$), and in 91% of phenotypic overlap patients ($n = 11$)[b] (31,32). Mutations are of the missense, nonsense, deletion, insertion, and splice site types (4,32). Mutations in Bannayan-Riley-Ruvalcaba syndrome and in overlap patients with additional features of Cowden syndrome are shown in Figure 8–3 and summarized in Table 8–1. Mutations are scattered along the length of PTEN except for exons 1, 4, and 9. A hot spot for mutations is the core phosphatase-containing exon 5.

[b]Marsh et al. (32) state that 11 families had phenotypic overlap. However, their Table 1 shows only 9 families with phenotypic overlap.

Marsh et al. (32) found three genotype–phenotype correlations in Bannayan-Riley-Ruvalcaba syndrome patients with or without Cowden syndrome overlap. First, germline mutations were correlated with the presence of lipomas in contrast to Cowden syndrome alone, in which lipomas are rare. Second, germline mutations showed an association with any cancer or with fibroadenoma of the breast. Third, an association was observed between truncating PTEN mutations and cancer or fibroadenoma of the breast.

Identical nonsense mutations have been found with Bannayan-Riley-Ruvalcaba syndrome alone, in Cowden syndrome alone, and in phenotypic overlap between the two: Gln110Stop, Arg130Stop, Arg233Stop, and Arg335Stop (31,32). Clearly, other genetic and/or epigenetic factors must be involved.

Marsh et al. (32) found germline mutations in two Bannayan-Riley-Ruvalcaba syndrome pa-

Table 8–1 PTEN Mutations in Bannayan-Riley-Ruvalcaba Syndrome and in Bannayan-Riley-Ruvalcaba/Cowden Syndrome Overlap

Phenotype[a]	Mutation	Exon
BRRS	Ala34Asp	2
BRRS	Tyr68His	3
BRRS	Cys105Tyr	5
BRRS	324delG[b]	5
BRRS	Arg130Stop[c]	5
BRRS	Ile135Val	5
BRRS	Ser170Arg	5
BRRS	520-544del25[b]	6
BRRS	Arg233Stop	7
BRRS	Pro246Leu	7
BRRS	866insCT[b]	8
BRRS	950-953delTACT[b]	8
BRRS	46,XY,del(10)(q23.3-q24.1)	Gross deletion
BRRS	46,XY,t(10;13)(q23.2;q33)	Balanced translocation
BRRS/CS	Gln110Stop	5
BRRG/CS	Arg130Stop[c]	5
BRRS/CS	441insAdelGG[b]	5
BRRS/CS	987-990delTAAA[b]	8
BRRS/CS	Arg335Stop	8
		Intron
BRRS	209+1G → A	3
BRRS	209+5G → A	3
BRRS	253+2T → C	4
BRRS	634+5G → T	6
BRRS	1027−8G → A	8
BRRS/CS	635−1G → C	6
BRRS/CS	802−4insT	7

[a]BRRS, Bannayan-Riley-Ruvalcaba syndrome; BRRS/CS, features of both Bannayan-Riley-Ruvalcaba syndrome and Cowden syndrome.
[b]These are approximations.
[c]Arg130Stop has been found with Bannayan-Riley-Ruvalcaba syndrome, with Cowden syndrome, and with the combined phenotype.
Source: Data from Marsh et al. (32) and Çelebi et al. (4).

tients *in the absence of additional identifiable PTEN mutations*, suggesting that *PTEN* haploinsufficiency alone may produce *both* developmental defects *and* tumor formation.[e]

Çelebri et al. (4) reported two splice site mutations with partial intron exclusion (one Bannayan-Riley-Ruvalcaba syndrome patient and one Cowden syndrome patient). Splice site mutations with exon skipping have also been found in two patients with Cowden syndrome.

PHENOTYPIC FEATURES

Growth

Birth weight usually exceeds 4000 g and birth length is above the 97th centile. Postnatal growth decelerates, with older children and adults being within the normal range. Head circumference is at least 4.5 SD above the mean (11,12,18,40).

Central Nervous System

Hypotonia, gross motor delay, mild to severe mental deficiency, and cognitive speech delay have been reported in approximately 70% of patients (11,24,33,34,38,42). About 25% exhibit seizures (11,38). Asymmetric motor development has been reported (10,38).[d]

[e]Disruption by alternative mechanisms, such as transcription activation, were not excluded (32).

[d]In Llermitte-Duclos disease, dysplastic gangliocytoma of the cerebellum, which results in cerebellar signs and seizures, is a severe manifestation of some cases of Cowden syndrome, but to date, has not been found with Bannayan-Riley-Ruvalcaba syndrome (14,45).

Muscle

At least 60% of patients have had a myopathic process in the proximal muscles (5,12) that manifests as delayed motor development. Muscle biopsy has shown neutral fat accumulation, predominantly in enlarged type I muscle fibers (9,38). Type II fibers are smaller than normal and contain less fat (9). Muscle-free carnitine levels are reduced (38).

Fryburg et al. (17) described a patient with Bannayan-Riley-Ruvalcaba syndrome who had long-chain 3-hydroxyacyl-CoA dehydrogenase deficiency (LCHAD). Patients deficient in this enzyme are known to exhibit myopathy. Knowledge of *PTEN* mutations for Bannayan-Riley-Ruvalcaba syndrome was not known at the time of Fryburg's study in 1994. In 1999, Otto et al. (37) reported a family with a *PTEN* mutation and found normal enzyme activity. They suggested that LCHAD reported earlier with Bannayan-Riley-Ruvalcaba syndrome might represent either a rare occurrence of two genetic disorders or a gene other than *PTEN* being responsible for the Bannayan-Riley-Ruvalcaba case reported by Fryburg et al. (17).

Craniofacial Features

Macrocephaly is a prominent feature (Fig. 8–4). A few patients have exhibited delayed closure of the anterior fontanelle. Ocular hypertelorism has been noted in some instances. Downslanting palpebral fissures and strabismus or amblyopia are frequently observed. Examination of the eyes under slit lamp has demonstrated prominent Schwalbe lines and clearly visible corneal nerves in approximately 35% of patients. Pseudopapilledema has been found in some cases (11,39,47).

Skin

Pigmented macules are found on the penile shaft in most affected males (Fig. 8–5). This spotting is often subtle and will be missed if not specifically looked for. Cutaneous lipomas with a vascular component are common. They vary in number, size, and location. A few patients have had a smaller number of café-au-lait spots on the trunk and lower extremities (11,18,38).

Gastrointestinal System

Hamartomatous polyps, usually multiple and limited to the distal ileum and colon, may be as-

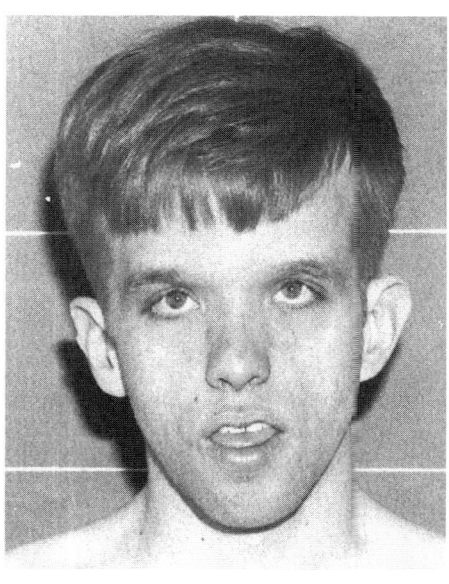
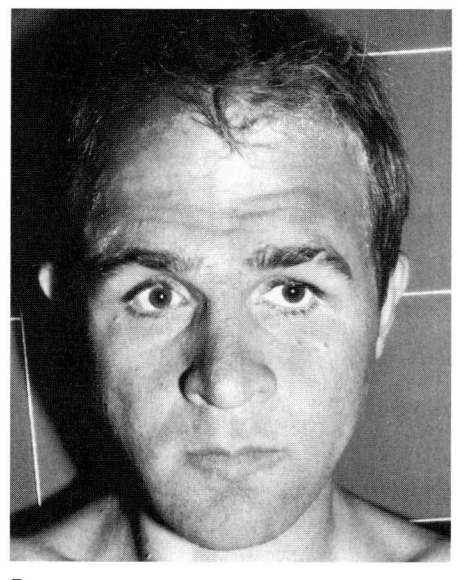

Figure 8–4 Bannayan-Riley-Ruvalcaba syndrome. **A:** Macrocephaly, triangular face, and prominent mandible. **B:** Macrocephaly and prominent mandible. From Ruvalcaba et al. (40).

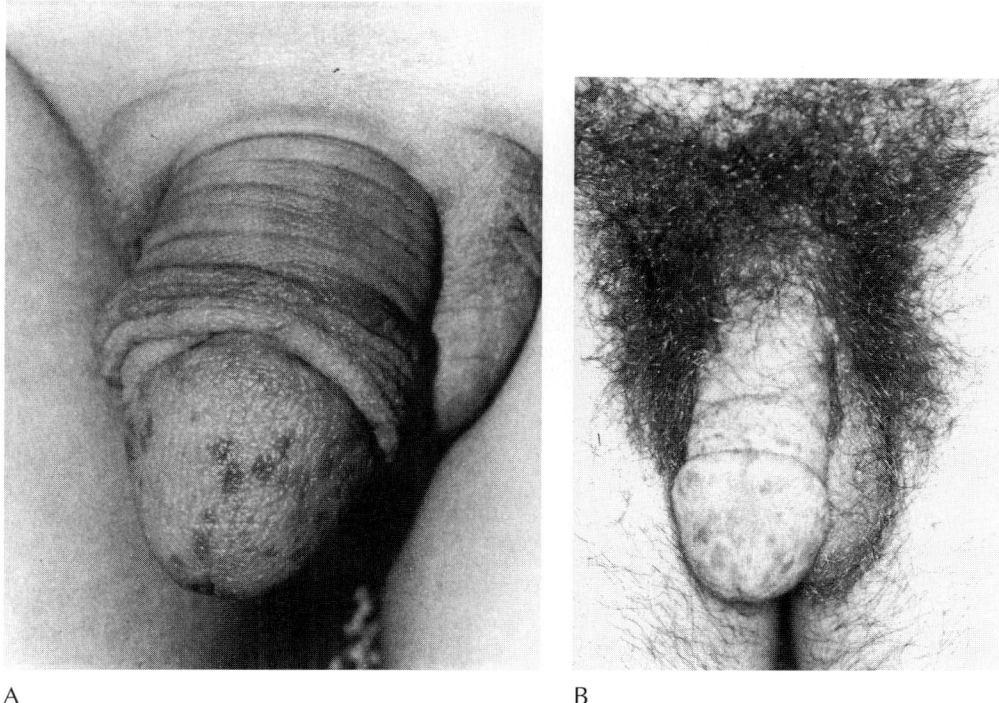

Figure 8–5 Bannayan-Riley-Ruvalcaba syndrome. **A,B:** Pigmented macules on penile shaft. A from DiLiberti et al. (12); B from Ruvalcaba et al. (40).

sociated with intussusception and/or rectal bleeding. They have been found in 45% of all patients. While some became manifested in childhood, others have not become evident until middle age. The spectrum of intestinal pathology includes juvenile polyps, ectopic ganglion cells, and atypical polyps with some features of tubulovillous adenoma. Protein-losing enteropathy has been observed (11,16,18,27,41,43).

Neoplasms

These are usually subcutaneous in location but may be intracranial or osseous in some patients. Lipomas are common (75%) (18,33,47). Aggressive lipomas with serious complications have been noted on occasion (33). Less commonly, capillary, venous, and/or lymphatic malformations are found (18,25,33). Malignant tumors have been noted on occasion, including thyroid tumors and rapid onset of bilateral invasive breast cancer (8). Haggitt and Reid (20) reported a case with ganglioneuromas.

Other Findings

Joint hyperextensibility, pectus excavatum, and scoliosis have been recorded in about 50% of patients (11,23). Adult males have enlarged testes (11,16). Gorlin et al. (18) expanded the syndrome to include Hashimoto's thyroiditis. Rarely, acanthosis-like lesions of the face and accessory nipples have been noted (40).

Laboratory Aids

Electromyography, muscle biopsy, and mutational analysis should be performed on all infants with macrocephaly, normal CT scans, and hypotonia. Patients with Bannayan-Riley-Ruvalcaba syndrome should be monitored for gastrointestinal polyposis and thyroid neoplasms.

DIFFERENTIAL DIAGNOSIS

Macrocephaly is found in Sotos syndrome (Chapter 6), Weaver syndrome (Chapter 7), autosomal dominant macrocephaly, and with nonsyndromal overgrowth (Chapter 18). Lipomas and vascular malformations may be found in Proteus syndrome (Chapter 9) and in hemihyperplasia/multiple lipomatosis syndrome. The patient reported by Okamura et al. (36) appeared to have overlapping manifestations of Bannayan-Riley-Ruvalcaba syndrome, Klippel-Trenaunay syndrome, and Proteus syndrome. The patients reported by Halal (21,22) as having cerebral gigantism have Bannayan-Riley-Ruvalcaba syndrome (see Chapter 6, Table 6–4).

REFERENCES

1. Arch EM, Goodman BK, Van Wesep RA: Deletion of PTEN in a patient with Bannayan-Riley-Ruvalcaba syndrome suggests allelism with Cowden disease. Am J Med Genet 71 489–493, 1997.
2. Bannayan GA: Lipomatosis, angiomatosis and macroencephaly: A previously undescribed congenital syndrome. Arch Pathol 92:1–5, 1971.
3. Çelebi JT, Chen FF, Zhang H, Ping XL, Tsou HC, Peacocke M: Identification of PTEN mutations in five families with Bannayan-Zonana syndrome. Exp Dermatol 8 134–140, 1999.
4. Çelebi JT, Wanner M, Ping XL, Zhang H, Peacocke M: Association of splicing defects in PTEN leading to exon skipping or partial intron retention in Cowden syndrome. Hum Genet 107:234–238, 2000.
5. Christian CL, Fleisher DR, Feldman EJ, Pepkowitz SH, Iafolla AK, DiLiberti JH, Graham JM Jr: Lipid storage myopathy associated with Ruvalcaba-Myhre-Smith syndrome: Treatment with carnitine. Clin Res 39:64A, 1991.
6. Cohen MM Jr: Bannayan-Riley-Ruvalcaba syndrome. Renaming a condition previously thought to represent three separate entities. Am J Med Genet 35:291, 1990.
7. Di Cristofano A, Pesce B, Cordon-Cardo C: Pten is essential for embryonic development and tumour suppression. Nat Genet 19:348–355, 1998.
8. DiLiberti JH: Personal communication, 1986.
9. DiLiberti JH: Correlation of skeletal muscle biopsy with phenotype in the familial macrocephaly syndromes. J Med Genet 29:46–49, 1992.
10. DiLiberti JH, Budden S: Transient motor asymmetry in young children with the Ruvalcaba-Myhre-Smith syndrome. Ninth Annual David W. Smith Workshop and Malformations and Morphogenesis, Oakland, California, August 3–7, 1988.
11. DiLiberti JH, Weleber RG, Budden S: Ruvalcaba-Myhre-Smith syndrome: Case report with probable autosomal-dominant inheritance and additional manifestations. Am J Med Genet 15:491–495, 1983.
12. DiLiberti JH, D'Agostino AN, Ruvalcaba RHA, Schimschock JR: A new lipid storage myopathy observed in individuals with the Ruvalcaba-Myhre-Smith syndrome. Am J Med Genet 18: 163–167, 1984.
13. Dvir M, Beer S, Aladjem M: Heredofamilial syndrome of mesodermal hamartomas, macrocephaly and pseudopapilledema. Pediatrics 81: 287–290, 1988.
14. Eng C, Murday V, Seal S, Mohammed S, Hodgson SV, Chaudray MA, Fentiman IS, Ponder BA, Ecles RA: Cowden syndrome and Lhermitte-Duclos disease in a family: A single genetic syndrome with pleiotropy? J Med Genet 31:458–461, 1994.
15. Fargnoli MC, Orlow SJ, Semel-Concepcion J, Bologna JL: Clinicopathologic findings in the Bannayan-Riley-Ruvalcaba syndrome. Arch Dermatol 132:1214–1218, 1996.
16. Foster MA, Kilkoyne RF: Ruvalcaba-Myhre-Smith syndrome: A new consideration in the differential diagnosis of intestinal polyposis. Gastrointest Radiol 11:349–350, 1986.
17. Fryburg JS, Pelegano JP, Bennett MJ, Bebin EM: Long-chain 3-hydroxyacyl-coenzyme A dehydrogenase deficiency in a patient with the Bannayan-Riley-Ruvalcaba syndrome. Am J Med Genet 52:97–102, 1994.
18. Gorlin RJ, Cohen MM Jr, Condon LM, Burke BA: Bannayan-Riley-Ruvalcaba syndrome. Am J Med Genet 44:307–314, 1992.
19. Gu J, Tamura M, Yamada KM: Tumor suppressor PTEN inhibits integrin- and growth factor–mediated mitogen-activated protein (MAP) kinase signaling pathways. J Cell Biol 143:1375–1383, 1998.
20. Haggitt RC, Reid BJ: Hereditary gastrointestinal polyposis syndromes. Am J Surg Pathol 10: 871–887, 1986.
21. Halal F: Male-to-male transmission of cerebral gigantism. Am J Med Genet 12:411–419, 1982.
22. Halal F: Letter to the editor: Cerebral gigantism, intestinal polyposis, and pigmentary spotting of the genitalia. Am J Med Genet 15:161, 1983.
23. Hayashi Y, Ohi R, Tomita Y, Chiba T, Matsumoto Y, Chiba T: Bannayan-Zonana syndrome associated with lipomas, hemangiomas, and lymphangiomas. J Pediatr Surg 27:722–723, 1992.
24. Higginbottom MC, Schultz P: The Bannayan syndrome: An autosomal dominant disorder consisting of macrocephaly, lipomas, heman-

giomas, and risk for intracranial tumors. Pediatrics 69:632–634, 1982.
25. Klein JA, Barr RJ: Bannayan-Zonana syndrome associated with lymphangiomyomatosis lesions. Pediatr Dermatol 7:48–53, 1990.
26. Lee J-O, Yang H, Georgescu M-M, Di Cristofano A, Maehama T, Shi Y, Dixon JE, Pandolfi P, Pavletich NP: Crystal structure of the *PTEN* tumor suppressor: Implications for its phosphoinositide phosphatase activity and membrane association. Cell 99:323–334, 1999.
27. Lowichik A, White FV, Timmons CF, Weinberg AG, Gunasekaran TS, Nathan K, Coffin CM: Bannayan-Riley-Ruvalcaba syndrome: Spectrum of intestinal pathology including juvenile polyps. Pediatr Dev Pathol 3:155–161, 2000.
28. Maehama T, Dixon JE: *PTEN*: A tumour suppressor that functions as a phospholipid phosphatase. Trends Genet 9:125–128, 1999.
29. Maehama T, Dixon JE: The tumor suppressor, *PTEN/MMAC1*, dephosphorylates the lipid second messenger, phosphatidylinositol 3,4,5-trisphosphate. J Biol Chem 13375–13378, 1998.
30. Marsh DJ, Dahia PLM, Zheng Z, Liaw D, Parsons R, Gorlin RJ, Eng C: Germline mutations in *PTEN* are present in Bannayan-Zonana syndrome. Nat Genet 16:333–334, 1997.
31. Marsh DJ, Coulon V, Lunetta KL, Rocca-Serra P, Dahia PLM, Zheng Z, Liaw D, Caron S, Cuboue B, Lin AY, Richardson AL, Bonnetblanc J-M, Bressieux J-M, Cabarrot-Moreau A, Chompret A, Damange L, Eeles RA, Yahanda AM, Fearon ER, Fricker J-P, Gorlin RJ, Hodgson SV, Huson S, Lacombe D, LePrat F, Odent S, Toulouse C, Olopade OI, Sobol H, Tishler S, Woods CG, Robinson BG, Weber HC, Parsons R, Peacocke M, Longy M, Eng C: Mutation spectrum and genotype–phenotype analyses in Cowden disease and Bannayan-Zonana syndrome, two hamartoma syndromes with germline *PTEN* mutation. Hum Mol Genet 7:507–517, 1998.
32. Marsh DJ, Kum JB, Lunetta KL, Bennett MJ, Gorlin RJ, Ahmed SF, Bodurtha J, Crowe C, Curtis MA, Dasouki M, Dunn T, Feit H, Geraghty MT, Graham JM Jr, Hodgson SV, Hunter A, Korf BR, Manchester D, Miesfeldt S, Murday VA, Nathanson KL, Parisi M, Pober B, Romano C, Tolmie JL, Trembath R, Winter RM, Zackai EH, Zori RT, Weng L-P, Dahia PLM, Eng C: *PTEN* mutation spectrum and genotype–phenotype correlations in Bannayan-Riley-Ruvalcaba syndrome suggest a single entity with Cowden syndrome. Hum Mol Genet 8:1461–1472, 1999.
33. Miles JH, Zonana J, MacFarlane J, Aleck KA, Bawle E: Macrocephaly with hemangiomas: Bannayan-Zonana syndrome. Am J Med Genet 19:225–234, 1984.
34. Moretti-Ferreira D, Koiffmann CP, Souza DH, Diament AJ, Wajntal A: Macrocephaly, multiple lipomas and hemangiomata (Bannayan-Zonana syndrome): Genetic heterogeneity or autosomal dominant locus with at least two different allelic forms? Am J Med Genet 34:548–551, 1989.
35. Myers MP, Stolarov JP, Eng C, Li J, Wang SI, Wigler MH, Parsons R, Tonks NK: *P-TEN*, the tumor suppressor from human chromosome 10q23, is a dual-specificity phosphatase. Proc Natl Acad Sci USA 94:9052–9057, 1997.
36. Okumura K, Sasaka Y, Ohyama M, Nishi T: Bannayan syndrome–generalized lipomatosis associated with megalencephaly and macrodactyly. Acta Pathol Jpn 36:269–277, 1986.
37. Otto LR, Boriack RL, Marsh DJ, Kum JB, Eng C, Burlina AB, Bennett MJ: Long chain L hydroxyacyl-CoA dehydrogenase (LCHAD) deficiency does not appear to be the primary cause of lipid myopathy in patients with Bannayan-Riley-Ruvalcaba syndrome (BRRS). Am J Med Genet 83:3–5, 1999.
38. Powell BR, Budden SS, Buist NRM: Dominantly inherited megalencephaly, muscle weakness, and myoliposis: A carnitine-deficient myopathy within the spectrum of the Ruvalcaba-Myhre-Smith syndrome. J Pediatr 123:70–75, 1993.
39. Riley HD, Smith WR: Macrocephaly, pseudopapilledema and multiple hemangiomata. Pediatrics 26:293–300, 1960.
40. Ruvalcaba RHA, Myhre S, Smith DW: Sotos syndrome with intestinal polyposis and pigmentary changes of the genitalia. Clin Genet 18:413–416, 1980.
41. Sachatello CR, Hahn IS, Carrington CP: Juvenile gastrointestinal polyposis in a female infant: Report of a case and review of the literature of a recently recognized syndrome. Surgery 75:107–114, 1974.
42. Saul RA, Stevenson RE: Are Bannayan syndrome and Ruvalcaba-Myhre-Smith syndrome discrete entities? Proc Greenwood Genet Ctr 5:3–7, 1986.
43. Saul RA, Stevenson RE, Bley R: Mental retardation in the Bannayan syndrome. Pediatrics 69:642–644, 1982.
44. Sun H, Lesche R, Li D-M, Liliental J, Zhang H, Gao J, Gavrilova N, Mueller B, Liu X, Wu H: *PTEN* modulates cell cycle progression and cell survival by regulating phosphatidylinositol 3,4,5,-trisphosphate and Akt/protein kinase B signaling pathway. Proc Natl Acad Sci USA 96:6199–6204, 1999.
45. Sutphen R, Diamond TM, Minton SE, Peacocke M, Tsou HC, Root AW: Severe Lhermitte-Duclos disease with unique germline mutation of *PTEN*. Am J Med Genet 82:290–293, 1999.

46. Tamura M, Gu J, Danen HJ, Takino T, Miyamoto S, Yamada KM: *PTEN* interactions with focal adhesion kinase and suppression of the extracellular matrix-dependent phosphatidylinositol 3-kinase/Akt cell survival pathway. J Biol Chem 274:20693–20703, 1999.
47. Zonana J, Rimoin DL, Davis DC: Macrocephaly with multiple lipomas and hemangiomas. J Pediatr 89:600–603, 1976.
48. Zori RT, Marsh DJ, Graham GE, Marliss EB, Eng C: Germline *PTEN* mutation in a family with Cowden syndrome and Bannayan-Riley-Ruvalcaba syndrome. Am J Med Genet 80:399–402, 1998.

Proteus Syndrome

Proteus syndrome (OMIM 176920)[a] is a complex and variable disorder consisting of overgrowth of the hands and/or feet, asymmetry of the limbs, connective tissue nevi, epidermal nevi, vascular and lymphatic malformations, and cranial hyperostoses. The syndrome was first delineated by Cohen and Hayden (33) who reported a newly recognized disorder in two similar patients. Cohen and Hayden (33) distinguished the condition from neurofibromatosis and Klippel-Trenaunay syndrome. Four years later, Wiedemann et al. (115) reported four patients and named the condition after the Greek God Proteus, who could change his shape to avoid capture. About 100 cases have been recorded and perhaps 100 more unreported patients are being followed in medical clinics (8a,11,27,33,109a). Many publications bearing the name "Proteus syndrome" in the title *do not*, in fact, describe patients with Proteus syndrome because they do not meet the diagnostic criteria (10,109a) (see Publications and the Diagnosis of Proteus syndrome, below). Such references, with few exceptions, are not cited in this chapter.

PHENOTYPE

The phenotype is extremely variable; possible findings are listed in Table 9–1. Uncommon and unusual abnormalities have been reported, which are listed together with pertinent references in Table 9–2. Lipomas and vascular malformations of the capillary and venous types occur frequently in Proteus syndrome. Infrequent neoplasms have also been recorded and these are compiled with appropriate references in Tables 9–3 and 9–4.

UNDERSTANDING PROTEUS SYNDROME AND NEUROFIBROMATOSIS, UNMASKING THE ELEPHANT MAN, AND STEMMING ELEPHANT FEVER

There has been long-standing confusion between Proteus syndrome and neurofibromatosis (NF1). Connective tissue nevi found in Proteus syndrome are distinct from lesions found in neurofibromatosis (28) (Table 9–5, Figs. 9–1 and 9–2). Cohen (24,31,32) provided evidence that Joseph Carey Merrick, pejoratively known as the "Elephant Man," had Proteus syndrome and not, as previously thought, neurofibromatosis.

Joseph Merrick was born in 1862 in Leicester, the obstetric history apparently having been normal. At birth he had no obvious congenital abnormalities. The family history was negative for neurofibromatosis. Both parents and two subsequent siblings had no evidence of the disorder. Overgrowth began to develop at about 18 months of age and progressed to adulthood. When he was 22 years of age, his case was fully described by Sir Frederick Treves (89,109), who referred to him as "John" rather than by his real

[a]On-Line Mendelian Inheritance in Man number.

Table 9–1 Possible Findings in Proteus Syndrome

SKIN

Connective tissue nevi (see Table 9–5)
Epidermal nevi

DISPROPORTIONATE OVERGROWTH

Limbs
   Arms/legs/digits
Skull
   Hyperostoses
Vertebrae
   Megaspondylodysplasia (low frequency)
Viscera
   Spleen/thymus (low frequency)

DISREGULATED ADIPOSE TISSUE

Lipomas
Regional absence of fat

VASCULAR MALFORMATIONS

Capillary malformations
Venous malformations

LUNGS

Cystic lung alterations (12%–13%)
Progressive diffuse cystic pulmonary disease (low frequency)

CENTRAL NERVOUS SYSTEM

Mental deficiency (20%)
Seizures (13%)
Brain malformations

OTHER ABNORMALITIES (LOW FREQUENCY)

Neoplasms (see Table 9–3)
Facial phenotype with seizures and severe mental deficiency (see text and Table 9–9)
Epibulbar dermoids (see Table 9–2)
Craniosynostosis (see Table 9–2)
Renal anomalies (see Table 9–2)

Source: Adapted from Cohen (27) and Biesecker et al. 10).

name, Joseph. When Treves met Merrick, he was earning a living by exhibiting himself as an "Elephant Man." Merrick told Treves of an accident his mother had experienced during her pregnancy when she was knocked down by an elephant at a circus—the alleged cause of Merrick's condition.

In the case of Joseph Merrick, there is no evidence of café-au-lait spots in adulthood, which surely would have been recognized and described by clinicians of the stature of those who examined him, such as the dermatologist Radcliffe Crocker (35). In contrast, multiple café-au-lait spots are present in over 99% of patients with neurofibromatosis (NF1) (96). No evidence of neurofibromas has come forth either. What is clear is that Merrick was normal at birth and went on to develop more severe manifestations than those usually encountered with neurofibromatosis.

Merrick had the following features of Proteus syndrome: macrocephaly; hyperostoses of the skull (Fig. 9–3); asymmetric long-bone overgrowth; macrodactyly; thickened skin and subcutaneous tissue, particularly of the hands and feet, including moccasin-type plantar hyperplasia (connective tissue nevi) (Fig. 9–4); and other unspecified subcutaneous masses (Table 9–6). Mental deficiency is a variable feature, so Merrick's normal mentation is fully compatible with Proteus syndrome.

Besides neurofibromatosis, other skeletal diagnoses have been entertained including Maffucci syndrome, Paget's disease of bone, pyarthrosis, and fibrous dysplasia. In 1965 Bean (7) suspected that Merrick might have had Maffucci syndrome. On his next visit to London, he studied Merrick's skeleton at the Medical Museum of the London Hospital and arranged for radiographs to be taken, which he brought back to the United States for review by some of his colleagues. The diagnosis of Maffucci syndrome was not confirmed. One radiologist named Gillis found some of the lesions consistent with but not diagnostic of Maffucci syndrome; other areas were suggestive of Paget's disease, and still other areas were diagnostic of neurofibromatosis (8). Felson, another radiologist, indicated that Merrick's radiographs could best be interpreted by three concurrent diagnoses: neurofibromatosis, polyostotic fibrous dysplasia, and destruction of the left hip by pyarthrosis, possibly tuberculous in nature (8).

Felson indicated that Merrick's macrodactyly was undoubtedly related to plexiform neurofibromas involving the periosteum. He noted that Merrick's scoliosis did not have the acute angle usually observed with neurofibromatosis and was most likely related to destruction of the left hip joint from a documented episode of severe trauma in childhood (8). Felson observed that the radiographic appearance of the right femur taken in isolation would have been attributed to Paget's disease by most radiologists. However, because the patient was a young adult and because the other changes in the skeleton were unlike those of Paget's disease, Felson (8) was reluctant to add a fourth diagnosis to the three he

Table 9–2 Uncommon and Unusual Findings in Proteus Syndrome

CENTRAL NERVOUS SYSTEM
Macrocephaly
  Cohen and Hayden (33)
  Wiedemann et al. (115)
  Malamitsi-Puchner et al. (75)
Hemimegalencephaly
  Cohen and Hayden (33)
  Rizzo et al. (98)
  Newman et al. (85)
Hydrocephalus
  Cohen and Hayden (33)
  Cohen (32)
  Malamitsi-Puchner et al. (75)
  Malamitsi-Puchner et al. (76)
  Mayatepek et al. (78)
Cortical atrophy
  Mayatepek et al. (78)
Polymicrogyria
  Cohen (32)
  Newman et al. (85)
  Gilbert-Barness et al. (43)
Absent corpus callosum
  Mayatepek et al. (78)
Arachnoid cyst of posterior fossa
  Cohen (27)

EYE[a]
Strabismus
  Biesecker et al. (11)
  Clark et al. (19)
  Fay and Schow (40)
  Kontras (66)
  Malamitsi-Puchner et al. (76)
  Pawlaczyk and Sioda (90)
  Samlaska et al. (100)
  Wiedemann et al. (115)
  Newman et al. (85)
Nystagmus
  Burke et al. (16)
  Fay and Schow (40)
  Malamitsi-Puchner et al. (76)
  Viljoen et al. (111)
High myopia
  Cohen and Hayden (33)
  Burgio and Wiedemann (15)
  Newman et al. (85)
Retinal pigmentary abnormalities
  Burke et al. (16)
  Gilbert-Barness et al. (43)
Retinal detachment
  Cohen and Hayden (33)
  Mayatepek et al. (78)
  Lessner and Margo (73)
Cataract
  Cohen and Hayden (33)
  Mayatepek et al. (78)
Posterior segment hamartomas
  Burke et al. (16)
  Viljoen et al. (111)
  Kontras (66)
Epibulbar tumor
  Cohen and Hayden (33)
  Cohen (27)
  Smeets et al. (106)
  Costa et al. (34)
  Burke et al. (16)
  Bouzas et al. (14)
  Gilbert-Barness et al. (43)
Eyelid hamartomas
  Lessner and Margo (73)
Eyelid ptosis
  Fay and Schow (40)
Retinal coloboma
  Cohen (32)
  Mayatepek et al. (78)
Glaucoma
  Mayatepek et al. (78)
  Rizzo et al. (98)
Pale optic disk
  Cohen and Hayden (33)
Anisocoria
  Cohen and Hayden (33)
Heterochromia irides
  Cohen and Hayden (33)
  Burke et al. (16)

CARDIOVASCULAR SYSTEM
Cardiomyopathy and myocardial mass
  Shaw et al. (104)
Complex congenital heart defects
  Mayatepek et al. (78)

SPLEEN
Enlarged spleen
  Biesecker et al. (10)
  Biesecker et al. (11)
  Ceelen et al. (17)

THYMUS
Enlarged thymus
  Biesecker et al. (10)
  Biesecker et al. (11)

KIDNEY
Nephrogenic diabetes insipidus
  Hotamisligil and Ertogan (63)
Unilateral nephromegaly
  Clark et al. (19)
  Hornstein et al. (61)
Duplicated renal collecting system
  Clark et al. (19)
Hydronephrosis
  Cohen (27)

GENITAL SYSTEM
Clitoromegaly
  Pawlaczyk and Sioda (90)
Macropenis
  Viljoen et al. (112)
Macro-orchidism
  Viljoen et al. (112)
Cryptorchidism
  Viljoen et al. (112)
Ambiguous genitalia
  Frydman et al. (42)

(continued)

Table 9–2 Uncommon and Unusual Findings in Proteus Syndrome (cont.)

SKIN AND MUCOSA

Absent breast development
  Viljoen et al. (112)
Premature breast development
  Viljoen et al. (111)
  Viljoen et al. (112)
  Newman et al. (85)
Rectal polyposis
  Lamireau et al. (71)
  Biesecker (9)

DENTITION

Enamel hypoplasia, unusual distribution
  Mason and Roberts (77)
Hypoplastic teeth
  Smeets et al. (106)
Dental anomalies
  Smeets et al. (106)
  Shaw et al. (104)
  Viljoen et al. (112)
Malocclusion
  Cohen and Hayden (33)
  Clark et al. (19)
  Fay and Schow (40)
  Viljoen et al. (111)
  Viljoen et al. (112)

SKELETAL SYSTEM

Cervical spine fusion
  Nishimura and Kozlowski (86)
Angular kyphosis with spinal stenosis
  Skovby et al. (105)
Clinodactyly
  Cohen (32)
Cubitus valgus
  Clark et al. (19)
Radial head subluxation
  Nishimura and Kozlowski (86)
Pectus excavatum
  Kontras (66)
Hip dysplasia
  Clark et al. (19)
  Malamitsi-Puchner et al. (75)
  Viljoen et al. (111)
Coxa valga
  Malamitsi-Puchner et al. (75)
Coxa vara
  Costa et al. (34)
Coxa plana
  Nishimura and Kozlowski (86)
Genu recurvatum
  Cohen and Hayden (33)

Absent patella
  Clark et al. (19)
Tibial bowing
  Costa et al. (34)
Fibular bowing
  Hornstein et al. (61)
Heel valgus
  Clark et al. (19)
  Cohen (32)
  Cohen and Hayden (33)
  Hornstein et al. (61)
Gap between first and second toes
  Skovby et al. (105)
  Clark et al. (19)
Craniosynostosis
  Cohen (27)
  Biesecker et al. (11)
  Hornstein et al. (61)
  Mayatepek et al. (78)
Hyperostosis, external auditory canal
  Cohen (27)
  Biesecker et al. (10)
  Smeets et al. (106)
  Pawlaczyk and Sioda (90)
  Gilbert-Barness et al. (43)
Nasal hyperostoses
  Cohen and Hayden (33)
  Cohen (32)
Alveolar hyperostoses
  Smeets et al. (106)
Highly arched palate
  Wiedemann et al. (115)
  Fay and Schow (40)
  Kontras (66)
  Viljoen et al. (111)
  Viljoen et al. (112)
  Malamitsi-Puchner et al. (76)
Mandibular prognathism
  Cohen and Hayden (33)
  Fay and Schow (40)
  Clark et al. (19)

OTHER

Muscular atrophy
  Fay and Schow (40)
  Costa et al. (34)
  Pawlaczyk and Sioda (90)
  Clark et al. (19)
Mixed mesenchymal bronchial hamartoma
  Costa et al. (34)
Vocal cord nodule
  Samlaska et al. (100)

a"Enlarged eye" has been described a number of times (33,40,76,78,111) and, depending on the particular case, could refer to ocular proptosis, buphthalmos, or skeleto-orbital distortion from hyperostoses or craniosynostosis.

already had. He emphasized that Merrick's hyperostotic skull lesions and perhaps some of his long-bone changes could not be attributed to neurofibromatosis per se, but could result from polyostotic fibrous dysplasia, noting that the café-au-lait spots, pseudoarthroses, and sexual precocity occurred in both conditions. He also cited the few known examples in the medical literature of documented neurofibromatosis and fibrous dysplasia in the same patient (24). Neurofibromatosis is common, and given the large number of reported cases in the literature and

Table 9–3 Uncommon Neoplasms in Proteus Syndrome

Tumor [no. of cases] and References (ref. no.)	Age at Tumor Diagnosis (yrs)	Sex
Meningioma [3]		
Aylsworth et al. (3)	Teenage	Male
Maassen and Voigtländer (74)	33	Female
Bale et al. (5)	22	Male
Multiple meningiomas [3]		
Bouzas et al. (14)	27	Female
Horie et al. (60)	46	Female
Gilbert-Barness et al. (43)	22	Female
Optic nerve tumor [1]		
Aylsworth et al. (3)	Teenage	Male
Pinealoma [1]		
Pearson and Hoyme (91) (case 2)	16	Male
Monomorphic adenoma (parotid gland) [2]		
Cohen and Hayden (33) (case 1)	9	Female
Kontras (66)[a]	5.5	Male
Intraductal papillomas and epithelial hyperplasia (breast) [1]		
Cohen (32) (case 4)	17	Female
Unilateral breast hyperplasia [1]		
Cohen (25)	25	Female
Goiter (thyroid) [1]		
Viljoen et al. (111) (case 6)[b]	20	Female
Cyst or cystadenoma (ovary) [7]		
Maassen and Voigtländer (74) (cysts)	30	Female
Bouzas et al. (14) (bilateral cysts)	16	Female
Kousseff (67) (cyst)	3.5	Female
Skovby et al. (105) (case 1) (serous cystadenoma)	11	Female
Minnesota Dermatological Society Meeting (81) (mucinous cystadenoma)	18	Female
Gordon et al. (45) (case 2) (bilateral serous cystadenomas)	6	Female
Boccone et al. (12) (bilateral serous cystadenomas)	5	Female
Leiomyoma		
Maassen and Voigtländer (74) (multiple tumors) (uterus) [1]	30	Female
Horie et al. (60) (single tumor) (bladder) [1]	37	Female
Giant cyst (kidney) [1]		
Nishimura and Kozlowski (86) (case 1)	17	Male
Bale et al. (5) (same patient as above)		
Sacrococcygeal teratoma [1]		
Zachariou et al. (116)	5	Male
Mesothelioma [2]		
Gordon et al. (45) (case 1) (probable diagnosis) (peritoneal surfaces)	5.5	Male
Malamitsi-Puchner et al. (75) (tunica vaginalis of testis)	4	Male
Demetriades et al. (37) (same patient as Malamitsi-Puchner et al.) (75)		
Papillary adenocarcinoma (testis) [1]		
Hornstein et al. (61) (case 2)	4	Male
Papillary adenoma (appendix testis) [1]		
Hornstein et al. (61) (case 1)	14	Male

(continued)

Table 9–3 Uncommon Neoplasms in Proteus Syndrome (cont.)

Tumor [no. of cases] and References (ref. no.)	Age at Tumor Diagnosis (yrs)	Sex
Cystadenoma (bilateral) (epididymis) [1]		Male
Nishimura and Kozlowski (86) (case 1)	12	
Bale et al. (5) (same patient as	22	
Nishimura and Kozlowski (86)		
Endometrial carcinoma [1]		
Cohen (25)	25	Female

[a]Observed after publication.
[b]Thyroid goiter reported by Viljoen et al. (111, case 6) is probably secondary to iodine deficiency.

Source: Updated from Cohen (27) and Gordon et al. (45). The case described by Haramoto et al. (55) (multiple meningiomas?) and Horie et al. (60) (leiomyoma) are discussed in the section titled "Clinical Aspects of Somatic Mosaicism."

Table 9–4 Multiple Tumors in the Same Patient

Tumor	Reference
Meningioma and optic nerve tumor	Aylsworth et al. (3)
Multiple meningiomas	Gilbert-Barness et al. (43)
Multiple meningiomas and leiomyoma (bladder)	Horie et al. (60)
Multiple meningiomas and bilateral ovarian cysts	Bouzas et al. (14)
Monomorphic adenoma (parotid) and intraductal papillomas (breast)	Cohen and Hayden (33)
	Cohen (32)
Meningioma, multiple leiomyomas (uterus), and ovarian cysts	Maassen and Voigtländer (74)
	Nishimura and Kozlowski (86)
Meningioma, bilateral cystadenomas (epididymis), and giant cyst (kidney)	Bale et al. (5) (same patient as Nishimura and Kozlowski (86)
Bilateral ovarian serous cystadenomas	Gordon et al. (45)
Bilateral ovarian serous cystadenomas	Boccone et al. (12)
Endometrial carcinoma and unilateral breast hyperplasia	Cohen (25)

Table 9–5 Comparison of Connective Tissue Nevus in Proteus Syndrome and Neurofibroma in Neurofibromatosis

Characteristics	Proteus Syndrome (Connective Tissue Nevus)	Neurofibromatosis (Neurofibroma)
Surface pattern	Cerebriform[a]	Smooth or creased, or wrinkled
Consistency	Firm	Soft, movable
Histology	Highly collagenized fibrous connective tissue	Delicate connective tissue
Location	Skin	Skin and internal organs
Frequency	Some cases[b]	Rare on foot
Clinical diagnosis	Pathognomonic when present	Almost always suggestive of plexiform neurofibroma

Source: From Cohen (28).

[a]In the incipient stage, the lesion may not necessarily appear very cerebriform, but this surface pattern does evolve with time.
[b]When present, the lesion is pathognomonic for Proteus syndrome in the same way that axillary freckling indicates neurofibromatosis, if it happens to be present.

the natural reporting bias that favors more unusual cases, the simultaneous occurrence of neurofibromatosis and fibrous dysplasia in the same patient would be expected to occur several times by chance alone.

Felson's interpretation of a destructive hip joint lesion resulting from a childhood episode of hip disease following severe trauma (8) does fit with the known facts of Merrick's childhood. Other skeletal findings such as macrodactyly and asymmetric overgrowth of long bones are just as characteristic of Proteus syndrome as they are of neurofibromatosis. In fact, they occur more commonly with Proteus syndrome and tend to

PROTEUS SYNDROME

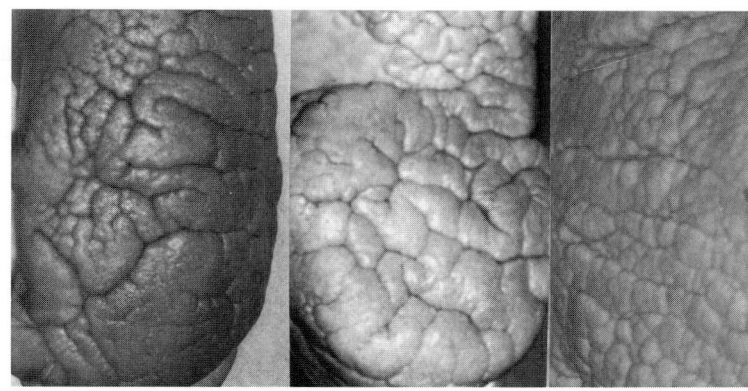

Figure 9–1 Cerebriform surface of connective tissue nevi in Proteus syndrome. Left: Plantar surface of one patient. Center: Plantar surface of another patient. Right: Abdominal surface of a third patient. From Cohen (28).

be more severe (24). Thus, in overall perspective, the skeletal findings for Joseph Merrick support the diagnosis of Proteus syndrome and coincidentally occurring hip disease secondary to childhood trauma.

Families of children with Proteus syndrome who become aware that Joseph Merrick had Proteus syndrome can be told that he represents the most extreme example known and that no other patients to date have had Merrick's degree of disfigurement.

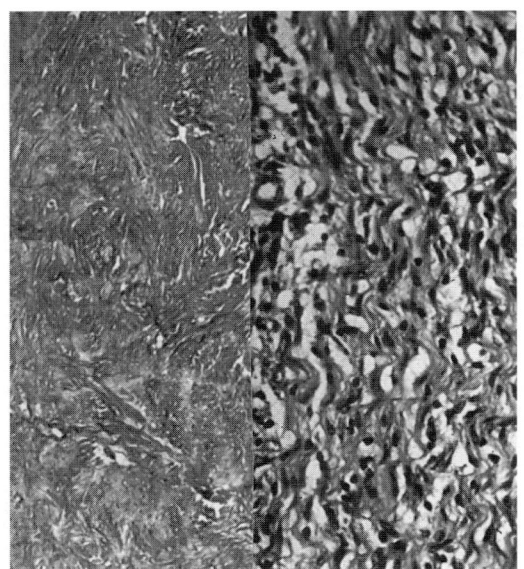

Figure 9–2 Comparative connective tissue patterns. Left: Highly collagenized connective tisse nevus of Proteus syndrome. Right: Delicate connective tissue of neurofibroma. Note cellular component. From Cohen (28).

The story of Joseph Merrick, pejoratively known as the "Elephant Man," has generated great interest not only among doctors (41,92) but also among authors (64,82), playwrights, journalists (95,113), musicians (65), and lay persons. Merrick has been the subject of two books (64,82). It has been the subject of a well-known movie, "The Elephant Man," and a play by the same title. Physicians have also written about the "Elephant Woman" (41) and the "Elephant Man of Cambridge" (92). Doctors and journalists alike have spoken of "Elephant Man's disease" (95), and singer Michael Jackson offered $1 million to the London Hospital for Joseph Merrick's skeleton (65). Truly, such wide interest is a sociological phenomenon that can only be called "elephant fever" (EF). The terms "Elephant Man" and "Elephant Man's Disease" are pejorative and should not be used. Cohen (32) made a plea for stemming elephant fever by taking the EF out of NF!

ETIOLOGIC CONSIDERATIONS

Somatic Mosaicism

Somatic mosaicism lethal in the nonmosaic state, an etiologic hypothesis for Proteus syndrome, was postulated by Happle (49,51). Mosaicism may arise either from a genetic half chromatid mutation or from early somatic mutation. Characteristics of such a disorder include sporadic occurrence, 1:1 sex ratio, mosaic distribution of lesions, and variable extent of involvement, but never diffuse involvement of the entire body or an entire organ system (49). Two known

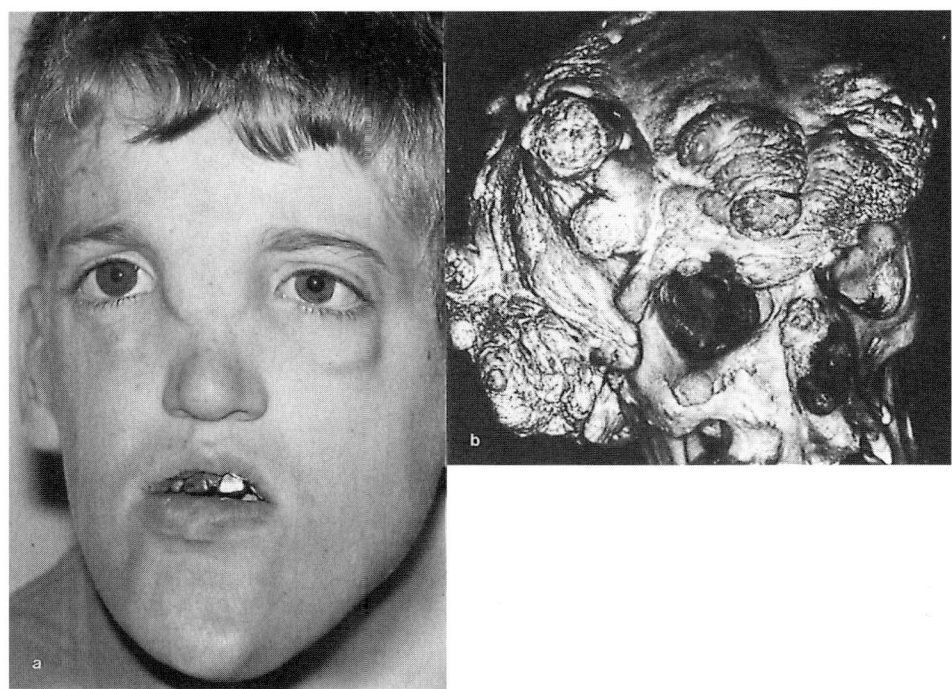

Figure 9–3 Hyperostoses of the skull. **a:** Age 12 years. Hyperostoses of nasal bridge, left infraorbital region, and mandible. **b:** Age 29 years. Skull of Joseph Merrick showing advanced hyperostoses. From Cohen (32).

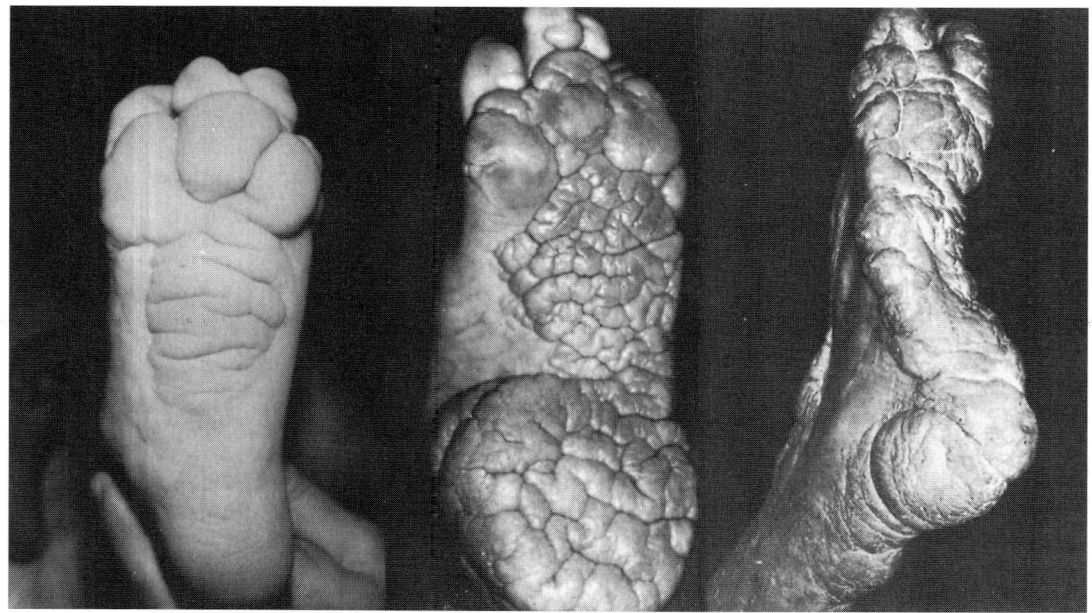

Figure 9–4 Evolution of plantar connective tissue nevus. Left: Age 5 and 1/2 years. Center: A second patient at age 12 years. Right: Age 29 years. Plaster cast of Joseph Merrick's foot. From Cohen (32).

Table 9–6 Comparison of Findings in Proteus Syndrome and Neurofibromatosis

Findings	Proteus Syndrome	Neurofibromatosis, type 1 (NF1)
Café-au-lait spots	−[a]	+
Axillary freckling	−	+
Epidermal nevi	+	−
Connective tissue nevi	+	−
Lisch nodules	−	+
Vascular malformations	+[b]	−[b]
Lipomas	+	−[c]
Skull hyperostoses	+	−
Macrocephaly	+	+
Craniofacial asymmetry	+	+
Limb overgrowth	+[d]	+
NF1 mutations	−	+

[a]An occasional patient with Proteus syndrome has been reported with a single café-au-lait spot.

[b]Vascular malformations are much more common in Proteus syndrome than in NF1.

[c]Lipomas are common in Proteus syndrome, but occur rarely in NF1. Rarely, liposarcoma has been noted with NF1, but has not been reported to date in Proteus syndrome.

[d]Limb overgrowth is much more common and more pronounced in Proteus syndrome than in NF1.

instances of monozygotic twins discordant for Proteus syndrome (59,103) lend support to the hypothesis of somatic mosaicism. DNA fingerprinting has shown single-band differences in one of these pairs of monozygotic twins discordant for Proteus syndrome. Differences have also been found in the normal and affected areas of another Proteus patient (103).

Two purported instances of transmission from parent to child (44,69) are not convincing. In both cases, neither the parent nor the child had Proteus syndrome. A de novo mosaic chromosome abnormality was found in another patient, suggesting that possibly the gene involved might reside in the 1q11 → 25 region (101), but it is extremely doubtful that the patient had Proteus syndrome.

Happle (51,52) discussed the possibility of "paradominant inheritance," should a rare example of familial Proteus syndrome be recorded in the future. According to this hypothesis (52), heterozygosity for a paradominant mutation would confer phenotypic normality and the allele may be transmitted unperceived for generations. The gene carrier would exhibit Proteus syndrome when a somatic mutation occurred during embryogenesis, giving rise to a cell line that would be either hemizygous, from allelic loss, or homozygous, from a point mutation. On rare occasions, more than one relative might be affected. Because the trait is neither simply mendelian nor entirely nonmendelian but sometimes tends to imitate dominant transmission, Happle (52) proposed the term "paradominance."

Molecular Speculation

At this writing, molecular definition of Proteus syndrome is still unknown, but because of rapid progress in molecular biology in general and recent clarification of some of the overgrowth syndromes in particular (Beckwith-Wiedemann syndrome, Simpson-Golabi-Behmel syndrome, Bannayan-Riley-Ruvalcaba syndrome, and neurofibromatosis), a molecular breakthrough for Proteus syndrome can be anticipated in the near future. The following speculations may or may not have some bearing on the anticipated molecular breakthrough.

Although the gene and gene product remain unknown to date, a mutation-altering tissue growth factor or receptor response may be involved. Rudolph et al. (99) speculated that disproportionate growth of tissues in Proteus syndrome might be related to local imbalance of insulin-like growth factor binding proteins (IGF-BPs), which have been hypothesized by Clemmons et al. (20) to modulate the growth-promoting effects of insulin-like growth factors (IGFs) at the cellular level. Relaxation of imprinting could also be considered in syndromes characterized by local overgrowth (99).

It is possible to consider a tumor suppressor gene as a possible cause for Proteus syndrome. One allele might mutate in a somatic cell, resulting in the somatic mosaicism of Proteus syndrome, producing overgrowth and vascular malformations. A second hit on the other allele might be responsible for lipomas and various uncommonly occurring neoplasms.

One possible gene that may be considered is the high (electrophoretic) mobility group protein gene *HMGIC* in the multiple aberration region (MAR) at 12q15. Eight different benign solid tumors have been associated with this gene (2,38,102), including lipomas, which are common in Proteus syndrome, and salivary gland tumors, leiomyomas, and lung hamartoma, which have been recorded in a few instances of Proteus syndrome. Other genes in MAR might possibly be involved and a variety of malignant tumor types have been associated with 12q13–q15 (38,102).

The suggestion of *PTEN* mutations as a cause of Proteus syndrome has not borne fruit (6a,117)

NATURAL HISTORY

Although birthweight may be increased in Proteus syndrome with some newborns weighing 4000 g or more, normal birthweight and even small-for-gestational-age infants have been observed. At birth, patients with Proteus syndrome are usually normal or show mild to moderate alterations, hyperplasias, or hamartoses. Vascular malformations may be present. Patients with highly significant hyperplastic overgrowth of the limbs at birth are very unlikely to have Proteus syndrome. Most often they have Klippel-Trenaunay syndrome or hemihyperplasia/multiple lipoma syndrome. The most remarkable postnatal growth in Proteus syndrome occurs during the first few years of life. However, a few patients may even be short during childhood. The syndrome is characterized by disproportionate overgrowth of bone and soft tissue. Somatic growth during adolescence and final height attainment are apparently normal. Bone and soft tissue overgrowth tend to plateau after adolescence (10,11,19,27,45), although there are some exceptions and an occasional neoplasm has been noted from age 20 to 30 or older (Table 9–3).

CAUSES OF PREMATURE DEATH

At least 17 cases of premature death have been identified (9,19,25,32,34,37a,45,60,66,78,85,98, 105,105a). Of the cases summarized in Table 9–7, males have been affected more commonly than females (3.25:1). Nine cases occurred in children under 10 years of age. Four cases were found in teenagers. The remaining patients died at ages 24, 25, 29, and 52 years, respectively (20a). Although ascertainment bias is possible, the number of premature deaths is significant because only 200 cases of Proteus syndrome have been published. Biesecker (9,9a,10 11,105a) and Cohen (20a,25,32,33,105), who have had extensive experience with a large number of patients, have been aware of premature deaths for some time. However, it is only in recent years that Cohen and Biesecker have become aware of the magnitude of the problem.

Pulmonary embolism was the cause of death in five cases and might have been the cause in two other cases. Other respiratory deaths have occurred in three cases: respiratory emphysematous pulmonary disease associated with numerous cysts of the lungs, ventilatory failure secondary to massive rib overgrowth, and laryngospasm. Central nervous system deaths have also occurred: during an epileptic seizure and from a large cerebellar abscess (20a).

Vascular abnormalities are predisposing factors for pulmonary embolism. Patients with Proteus syndrome can have capillary, venous, and lymphatic malformations in addition to varicose veins (10,11,32,33). Surgical convalescence is another important factor. Premature death following surgery occurred in 4 of 17 cases (Table 9–7); spinal surgery was involved in 2 of the cases. Patients with severe Proteus syndrome who are relatively immobile or nonambulatory are also at increased risk. Postmortem examinations were not available in four instances of unexplained death (20a).

In Klippel-Trenaunay syndrome, pulmonary embolism may be encountered in about 10% of children ($n = 47$) (100a), and the risk is particularly increased postoperatively. However, vascular malformations tend to be more extensive in Klippel-Trenaunay syndrome than in Proteus syndrome. Furthermore, Klippel-Trenaunay sydrome is much more common than Proteus syndrome (768 operated cases for Klippel-Trenaunay syndrome vs. about 200 reported cases of Proteus syndrome[b]) (24a). Thus, the premature deaths recorded in Table 9–7 appear to be significant.

Patients with Proteus syndrome and/or their parents should make their health care providers aware of the risk of deep venous thrombosis and pulmonary embolism. Biesecker and his colleagues (9a,105a) observed that symptoms warranting investigation include calf pain, calf or leg swelling, shortness of breath, and chest pain. Patients undergoing surgical procedures should be evaluated by a hematologist to determine coag-

---

[b]There are also thousands of unoperated Klippel-Trenaunay syndrome patients either in the literature or found in clinics, whereas there are 250 Proteus syndrome patients either in the literature or found in clinics (24a).

Table 9–7 Causes of Premature Death in Proteus Syndrome

Cause or Circumstance of Death	Age at Death (years)	Sex	Significant History
Pulmonary embolism	25	Male	Varicose veins of lower limbs at 16 years; portal vein thrombosis at 19 years; right iliac vein occlusion at 24 years; unrelenting headache, recurrent pulmonary emboli, and acute episode of breathlessness
Pulmonary embolism	9	Male	Leg pain 2 weeks prior to final illness and shortness of breath on day of arrest
Pulmonary embolism	18	Female	Treatment for sinusitis and refractory otitis media when unexpectedly arrested; autopsy showed extensive embolus at bifurcation of main pulmonary artery and thrombi in veins of left popliteal fossa
Pulmonary embolism	2	Male	Surgical convalescence; widespread lymphaticovenous malformations
Pulmonary embolism	8	Female	Surgical convalescence for spinal surgery for T2 to T4 stenosis with profuse bleeding from friable bones
Postoperative death[a]	11	Male	Died postoperatively after spinal fusion (? pulmonary embolism)
"Suffocation"	29	Male	Cause of death attributed to asphyxia, although no autopsy record found; death occurred in 1890 (? pulmonary embolism)
Respiratory emphysematous pulmonary disease	18	Male	Numerous cysts of the lungs found at autopsy
Pneumonia	4 years, 10 months	Male	Ventilatory failure secondary to massive overgrowth of ribs
Pneumonia and congestive heart failure	16.5 months	Male	Synostosis of sagittal and lambdoid sutures; hydrocephalus; questionable agenesis of corpus callosum; vascular malformations of chest and abdomen; varicosities of right popliteal area; cardiac catheterization showed dilated superior vena cava, small right ventricle, small pulmonary arteries, dilated left ventricle, stenotic aortic valve, dilated ascending aorta with slight coarctation of descending portion
Laryngospasm	14	Male	Mental deficiency; uncooperative while being given liquid medication during surgical convalescence; aspiration
Unexplained death	3	Male	Died during sleep: no autopsy; history of obstructive breathing
Died during epileptic seizure	1	Male	Hemimegalencephaly, hypodensity of periventricular white matter, hypotonia, severe mental retardation, epileptic seizures, varicose veins, vascular malformation
Cerebellar abscess secondary to otitis media	5 years, 6 months	Male	Profound developmental retardation, hemimegalencephaly, ventricular dilation, capillary and venous malformations, lipomas of thorax and abdomen. Autopsy showed large cerebellar abscess, polymicrogyria, heterotopic gray matter nodules
Died suddenly while sleeping	5 years, 7 months	Male	Breath-holding spells; episode of apnea following surgical extubation for orthopedic procedure; apneic episodes developed subsequently with possible seizures; autopsy showed mesothelioma infiltrating diaphragm, omentum, pelvic area, scrotum, and mesenteric lymph nodes; PDA; cyst-like spaces around left lateral ventricle
Sepsis with cerebral abscesses	52	Female	Multiple meningiomas; vascular malformations and bony overgrowth overlapped intracranial region
Unexplained death[b]	24	Female	

[a] Patient reported by Kontras (66) whose death was described by a personal communication from Kontras to Costa et al. (34) after Kontras's report.
[b] Case 4 reported by Cohen (32). Death occurred after publication of report.

Source: Data based on Slavotinek et al. (105a); Eberhard (37a); Skovby et al. (105) (Patient 1); Kontras (66); Costa et al. (34); Cohen (32); Newman et al. (85) (Case 1); Clark et al. (19) (Patient 2); Mayatepek et al. (79); Rizzo et al. (98); Gordon et al. (45) (Patient 1); Horie et al. (60); Cohen (25) (Patient 1); Table from Cohen (20a).

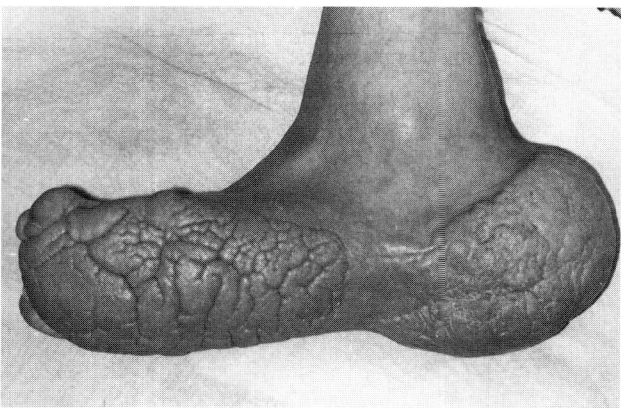

Figure 9–5 Connective tissue nevus. Plantar hyperplasia resulting in moccasin lesion. From Cohen (32).

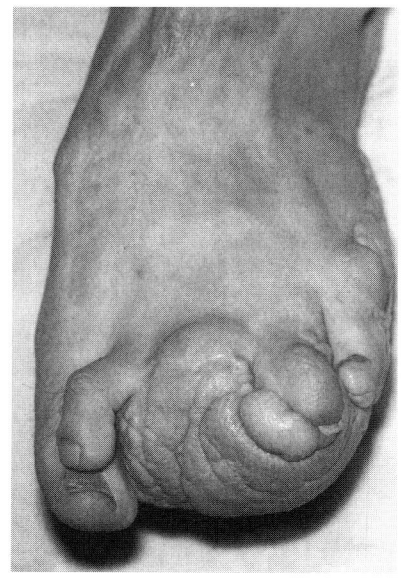

Figure 9–6 Connective tissue nevus. Plantar overgrowth resulting in malposed toes. From Cohen (32).

ulopathic potential and whether antithrombotic prophylaxis is indicated.

CLINICAL FEATURES

Connective Tissue Nevi

Connective tissue nevi are common and are facultative, not obligatory—i.e., they may or may not be present. They have been recorded most frequently on the plantar surface of the feet (Figs. 9–5 and 9–6), but can also be found on the hands (Fig. 9–7), abdomen (Fig. 9–8), and nose (27). When present, a connective tissue nevus (Fig. 9–1) is almost pathognomonic for Proteus syndrome.

Histologically, connective tissue nevi are characterized by highly collagenized connective tissue. They are easily distinguished from neurofibromas (Figs. 9–2 and 9–9) (28,32). A few isolated examples of connective tissue nevi have been recorded but the patients have subse-

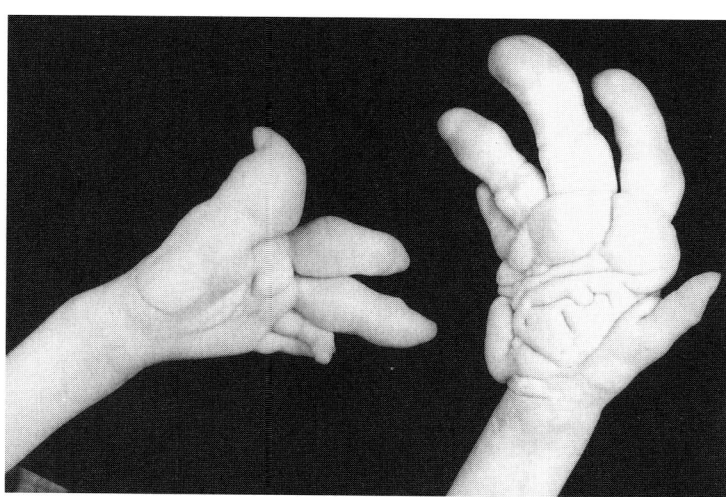

Figure 9–7 Connective tissue nevi, open palms of both hands. Courtesy of N. O'Doherty, Dublin, Ireland.

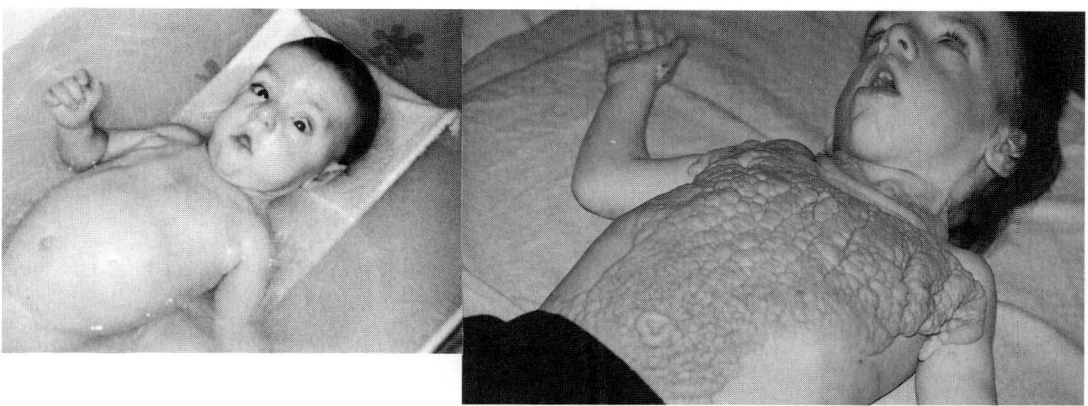

Figure 9–8 Left: Normal chest and abdomen of infant who later manifested Proteus syndrome. Right: Same child age at age 4 and 1/2 years with extensive connective tissue nevus of chest and abdomen.

quently been shown to have had Proteus syndrome (110, see his Fig. 2, middle). If there are isolated examples, particularly involving the feet, they must be extremely rare. Botella-Estrada et al. (13) reported such a case but showed no photographs. Furthermore, these authors used the term "collagenoma" and suggested that it may appear as an acquired lesion, as a hereditary trait, or as part of tuberous sclerosis. The lack of histopathologic confirmation and the heterogeneity described cast doubt on whether these authors were discussing the same lesion as that found in Proteus syndrome.

Epidermal Nevi and Other Skin Lesions

Epidermal nevi are etiologically and pathogenetically heterogeneous (48). In Proteus syndrome, nevi are evident in early life and may be found on the neck (Fig. 9–10), trunk (Figs. 9–11 and 9–12), or extremities. Lesions may be linear, whorled, or verrucous and, in some cases, may exhibit abrupt midline margins (10,11,19, 33,34,111,112). Infrequently, a single café-au-lait spot may be observed. Areas of patchy dermal hypoplasia and of hypopigmentation have also been noted (32,33,47,54,100,111,112,115). Coexistence of lesions can be found in some cases.

Vascular Malformations

Vascular malformations may be of the capillary, venous, or lymphatic type, or may occur as combined channel anomalies, e.g., capillary and venous channels or capillary, venous, and lym-

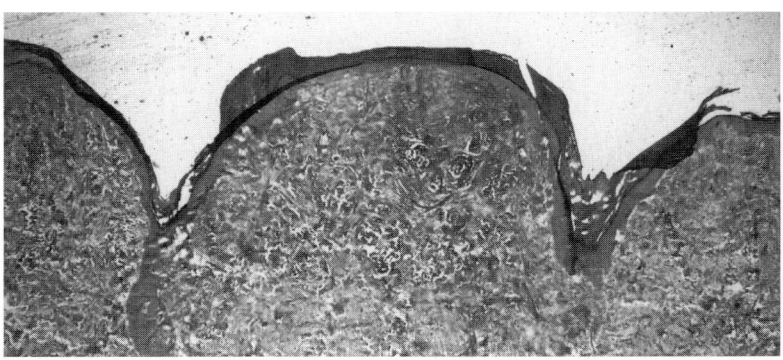

Figure 9–9 Biopsy of plantar connective tissue nevus. Densely collagenized fibrous connective tissue covered by a layer of hyperkeratinized stratified squamous epithelium. Note gyriform patterning of the surface. Keratin folding and V-shaped keratin defect are artifacts. Hematoxylin and eosin, ×40. From Cohen (32).

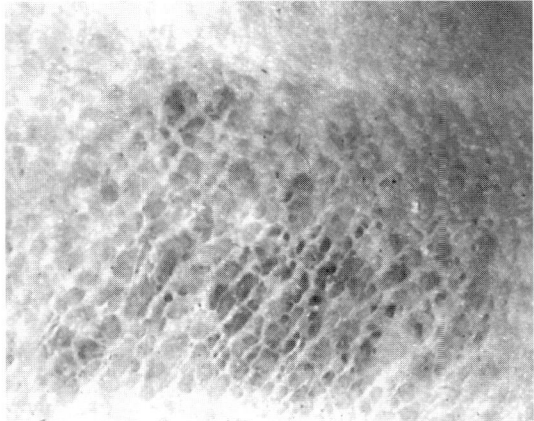

Figure 9–10 Epidermal nevus of neck. From Cohen and Hayden (33).

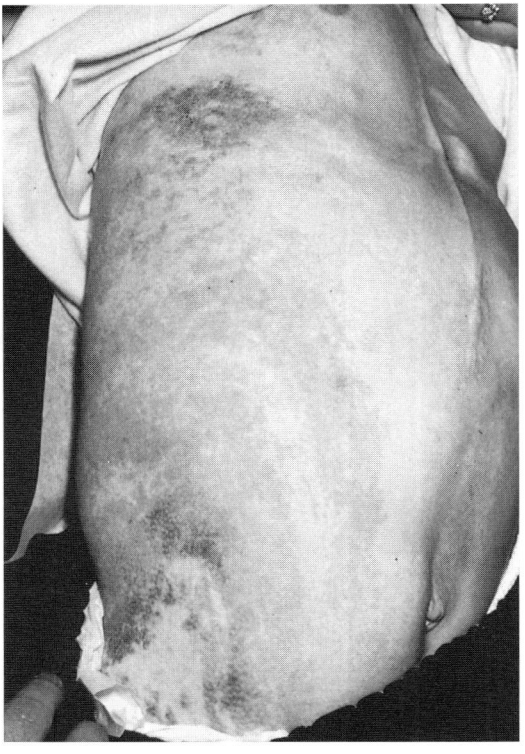

Figure 9–11 Extensive epidermal nevus of trunk. From Biesecker et al. (10).

phatic channels (Fig. 9–13). They are developmental anomalies lined by flat endothelium exhibiting a normal, slow rate of turnover. They grow proportionately with the patient; they never regress, but they can expand. So-called combined tumors such as "angiolipomas" probably do not occur; they probably represent lipomas with a vascular stroma. So-called "lymphohemangioma" is a misnomer for combined lymphatic–capillary malformation. Varicose veins have been reported in the hypogastric and inguinal region and on the legs (Fig. 9–14) (10,11,26,32,33,40,66,83,84,115).

Lipomas and Dysregulation of Adipose Tissue

Lipomas in Proteus syndrome (Fig. 9–15) are composed principally of mature adipocytes. Decreased and increased fat can be found in the

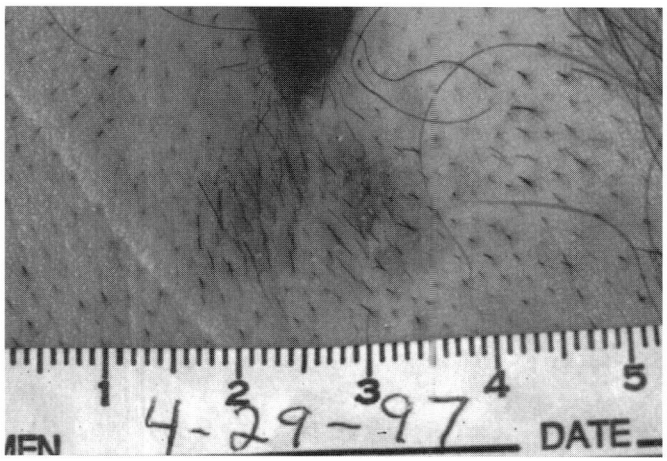

Figure 9–12 Small periumbilical epidermal nevi.

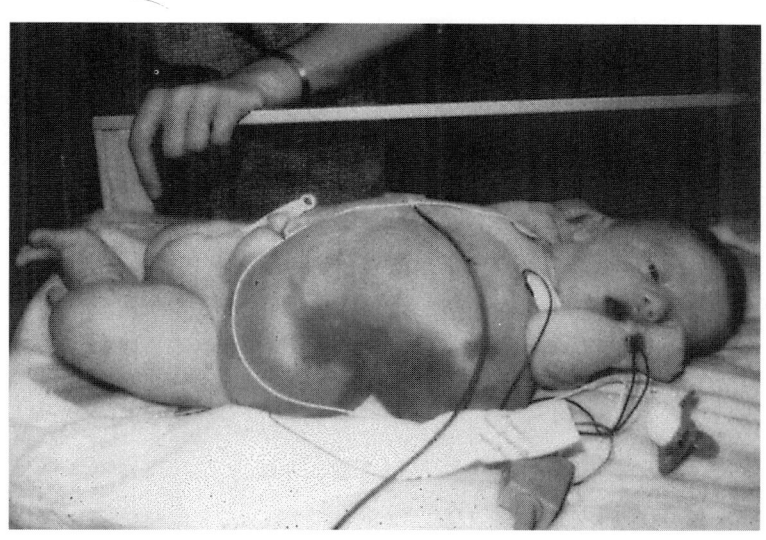

Figure 9–13 Large capillary malformation.

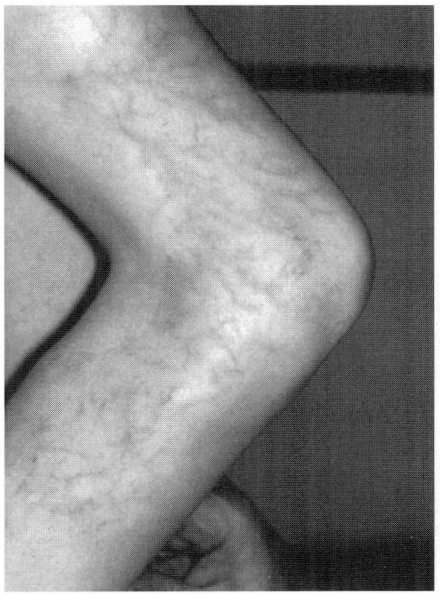

Figure 9–14 Varicose veins of the leg in a 12-year-old boy with Proteus syndrome.

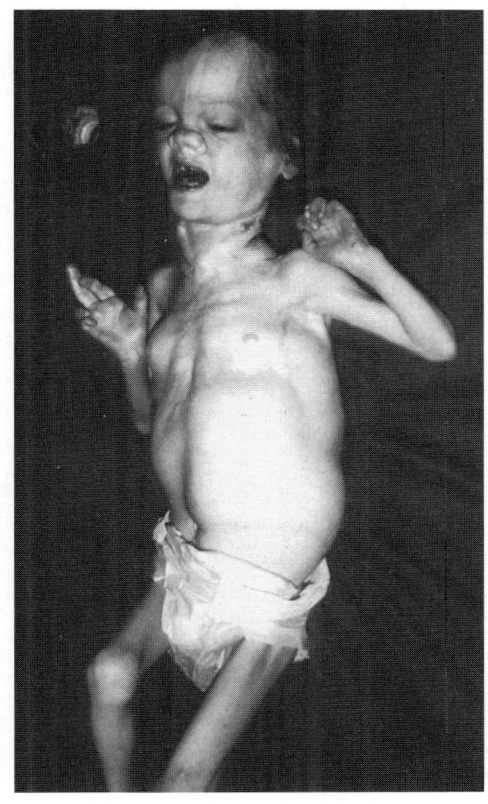

Figure 9–15 Proteus syndrome patient at 5 and 1/2 years of age with large lipomas of the left abdomen and right breast. From Cohen (32).

OVERGROWTH SYNDROMES

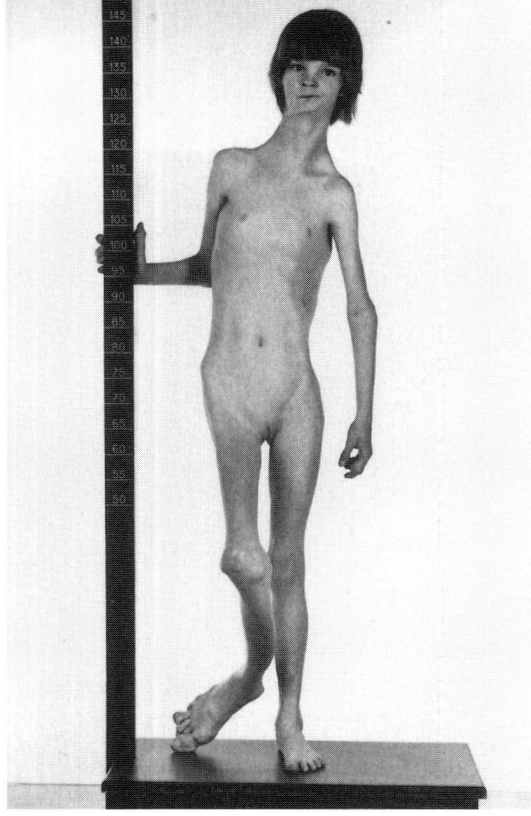

Figure 9–16 Dysregulation of adipose tissue in patient with Proteus syndrome. Note long, thin neck, thin arms, and asymmetric lower limbs. From Skovby et al. (105).

same patient at different sites in the body, indicating dysregulation of adipose tissue (Fig. 9–16) (19,27,47,50,63,105). Lipomas may be confined or infiltrative. Although histopathologic examination always shows benign adipose tissue cells, the location of lesions is of great importance. Superficial lesions tend to be confined and may be self-limited in growth, although this is not always the case. On the other hand, intra-abdominal and intrathoracic lipomas have increased potential for invasive behavior, despite benign histologic appearance (34). Infiltration of the spinal canal has been reported (62,105).

Unusual Tumors

Cohen (27) and Gordon et al. (45) showed that several unusual types of tumors are occasionally associated with Proteus syndrome (Figs. 9–17 to 9–19): ovarian cystadenoma (most commonly unilateral; two cases bilateral; Fig. 9–17), various types of testicular tumors, central nervous system tumors (particularly meningiomas), and monomorphic adenoma of the parotid gland (Fig. 9–19). Other overgrowth syndromes are also known to be associated with infrequently occurring tumors, e.g., embryonal rhabdomyosarcoma in Beckwith-Wiedemann syndrome. Bilateral cystadenomas of the ovary are rare in children and adolescents and therefore of

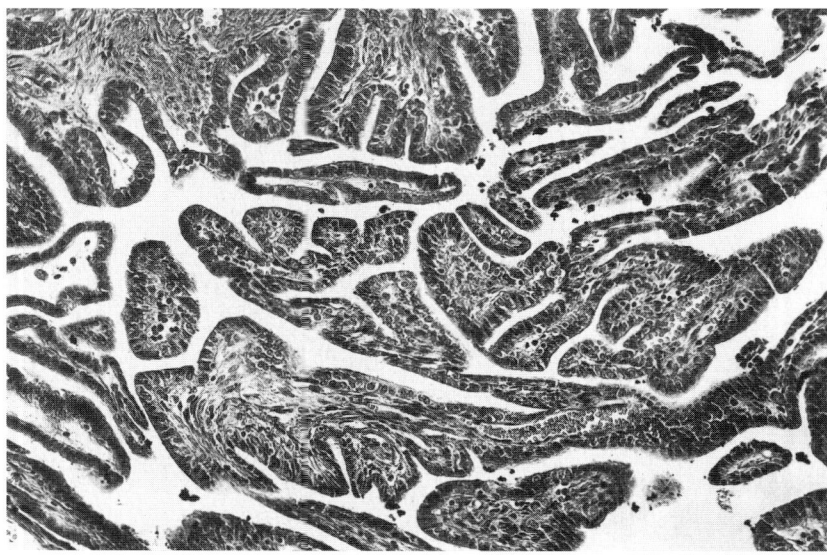

Figure 9–17 Serous cystadenoma of ovary from 6 and 1/2-year-old girl with Proteus syndrome.

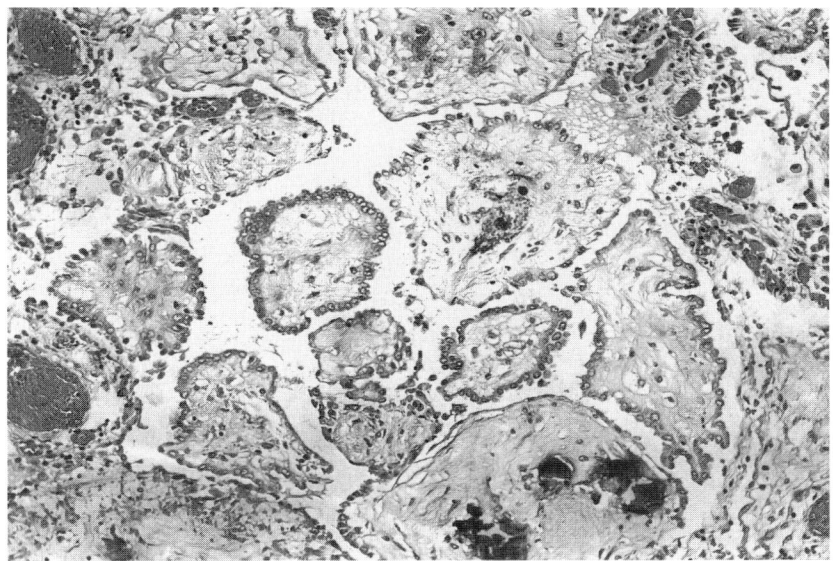

Figure 9–18 Papillary neoplasm most likely of mesothelial origin at autopsy in 5 and 1/2 year-old boy with Proteus syndrome. Tumor involved inferior surface of diaphragm infiltrating into the musculature. Tumor was also found in the omentum, in the pelvic area, within the scrotum, and within some of the mesenteric lymph nodes.

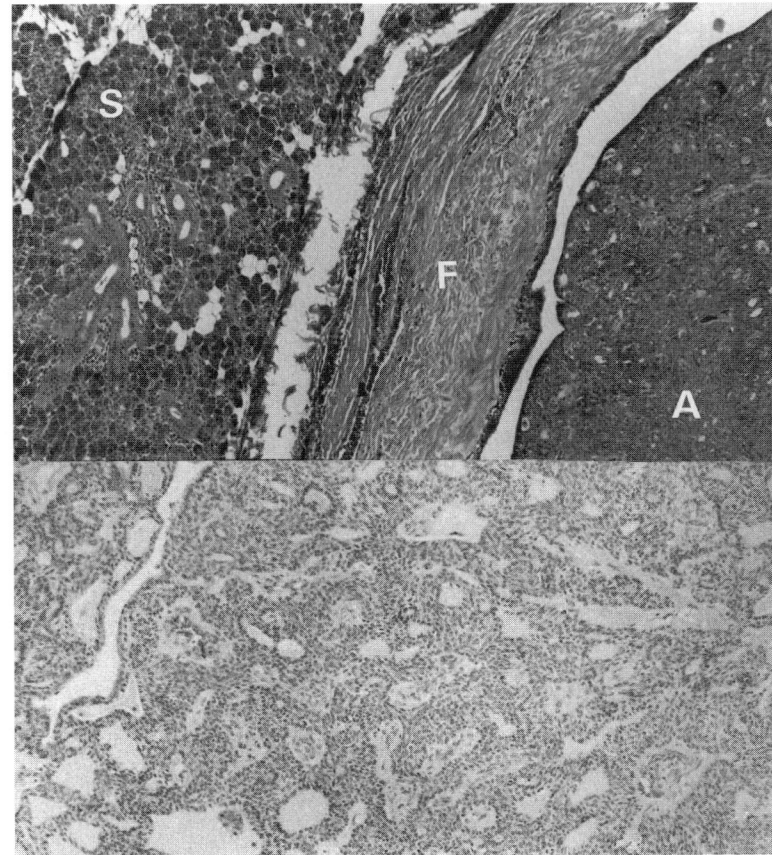

Figure 9–19 Monomorphic adenoma of parotid gland in 9–year-old girl with Proteus syndrome. **Top:** Low-power field showing normal parotid gland tissue (S) and monomorphic adenoma (A) separated by fibrous connective tissue (F). Hematoxylin and eosin, ×160. **Bottom:** High-power field showing histopathologic features of monomorphic adenoma. Note regular adenomatous patterning. Hematoxylin and eosin, ×250. From Cohen (32).

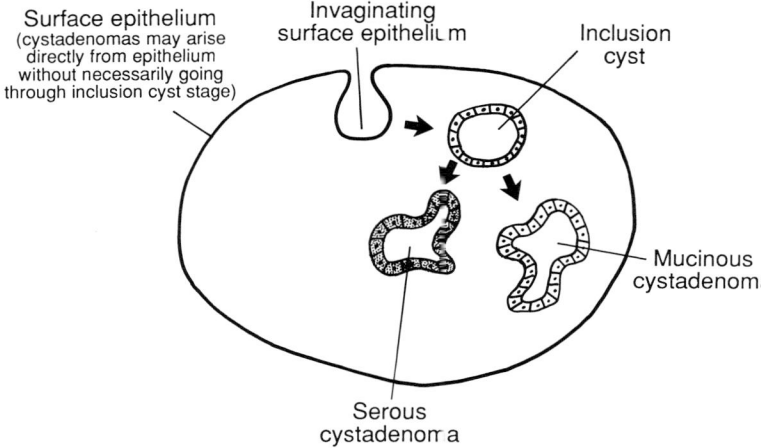

Figure 9–20 Relationship between ovarian surface epithelium, inclusion cysts, and cystadenomas. From Gordon et al. (45).

diagnostic value in Proteus syndrome. In adults, bilateral ovarian involvement is found in a significant percentage of cystadenocarcinomas (45). Monomorphic adenoma of the parotid gland is very uncommon, occurring most frequently in elderly men. The presence of this tumor in two adolescent girls with Proteus syndrome (27,33,45) is highly significant. Unusual tumors are listed in Table 9–3. Multiple tumors are found in some cases and are listed in Table 9–4. Multiple meningiomas have been recorded in three instances (14,43,60).

Perhaps ovarian cysts and cystadenomas (several cases, Table 9–3) have a common histogenic origin. They may arise from the surface epithelium of the ovary by invagination followed by formation of inclusion cysts. The cysts may remain as cysts or undergo further transformation to become cystadenomas, either serous or mucinous (56,57) (Fig. 9–20). It is also conceivable that

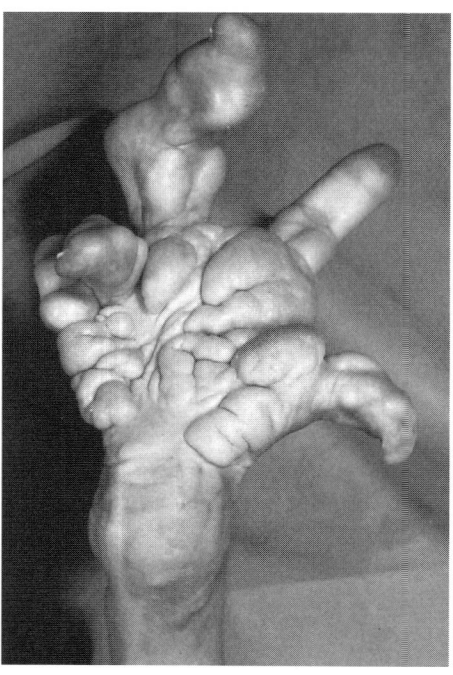

Figure 9–21 Severe digital overgrowth. Note soft tissue overgrowth on palm. From Biesecker et al. (11).

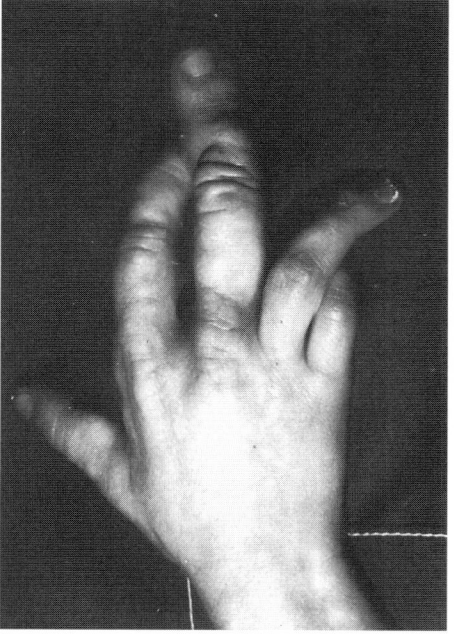

Figure 9–22 Macrodactyly in 5 and 1/2 year-old boy. From Cohen (32).

PROTEUS SYNDROME

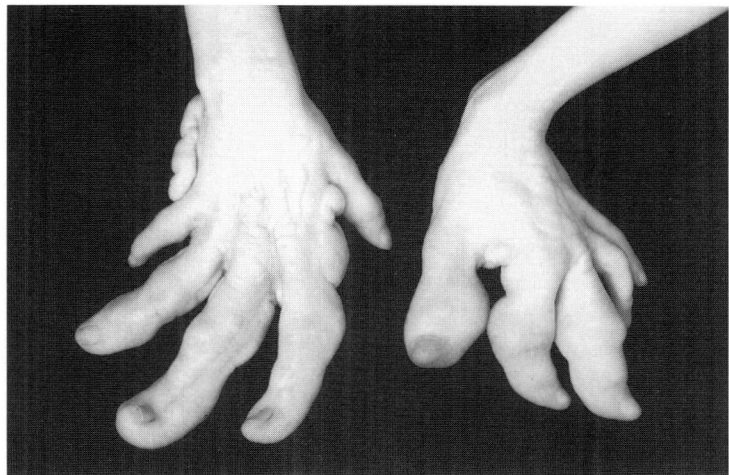

Figure 9–23 Overgrowth of fingers on both hands. Palmer surface shown in Figure 9–7. Courtesy of N. O'Doherty, Dublin, Ireland.

some cystadenomas may develop directly from the ovarian surface epithelium without going through an earlier cystic stage.

Skeletal Abnormalities

Disproportionate overgrowth, commonly asymmetric in nature, can involve the arms, legs, hands, feet, and digits (Figs. 9–21 to 9–24) (10,11,32). Scoliosis and kyphoscoliosis are common (19,32,40,61,78,86,111,115). Genua valga has also been observed (19,34,61,86) and heel valgus has been noted in a number of instances (19,32,33,61). Megaspondylodysplasia is also common; cervical (Fig. 9–25), thoracic, or lumbar vertebrae may be affected (4,10,85,115). When the cervical vertebrae are involved, the neck can appear elongated (40,66,105); the ap-

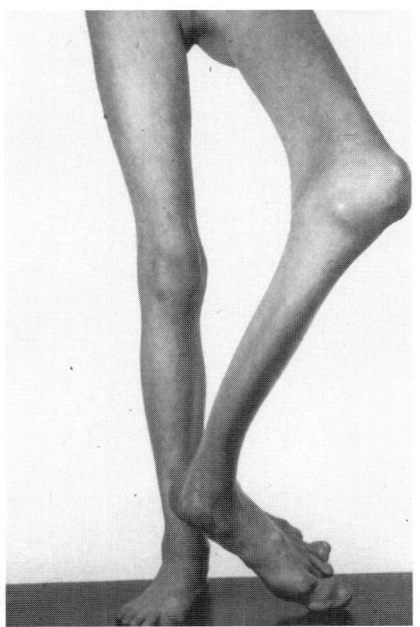

Figure 9–24 Asymmetry of lower limbs with overgrowth of left foot, which has a connective tissue nevus on its plantar surface that cannot be seen in this view.

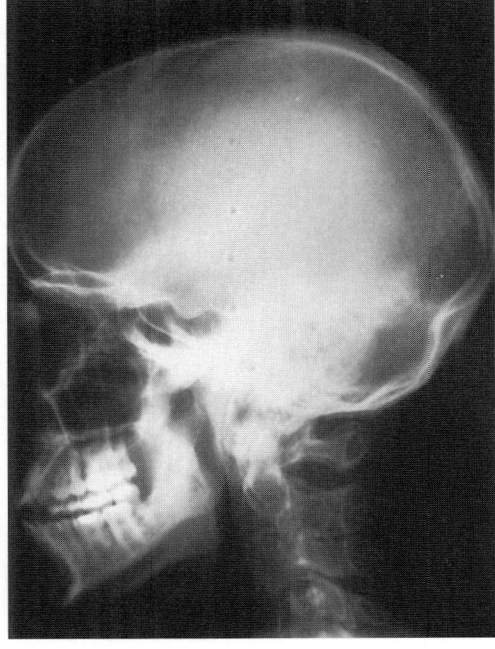

Figure 9–25 Megaspondylodysplasia of cervical vertebrae. From Biesecker et al. (10).

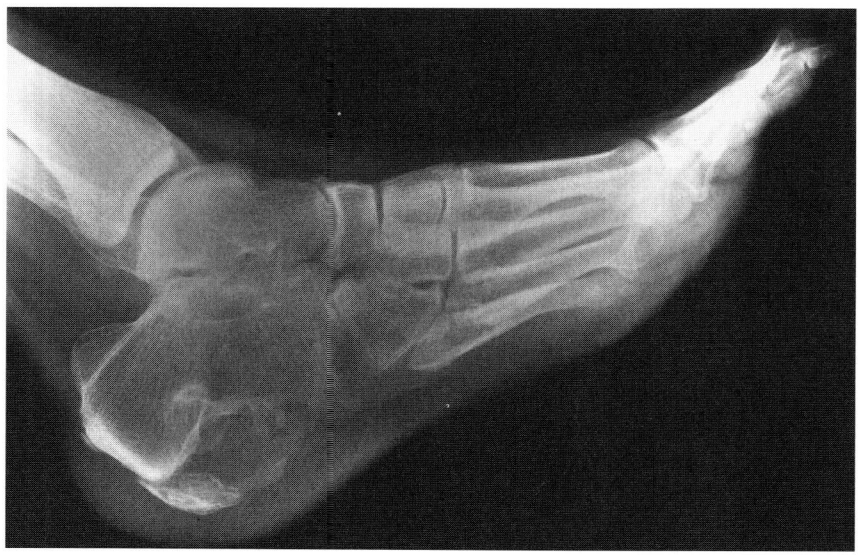

Figure 9–26 Alterations in talus and navicular bones. Note also overgrowth of metatarsals and phalanges. From Biesecker et al. (11).

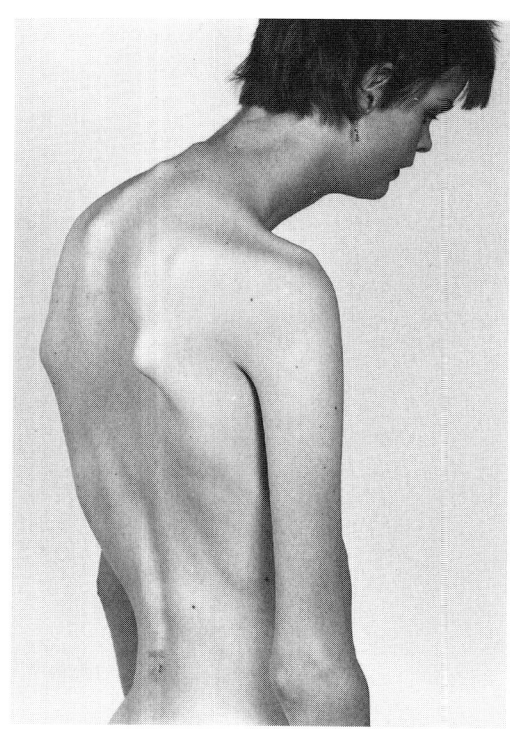

Figure 9–27 Proteus syndrome patient with angular thoracic kyphosis. Age 11 years. From Skovby et al. (105).

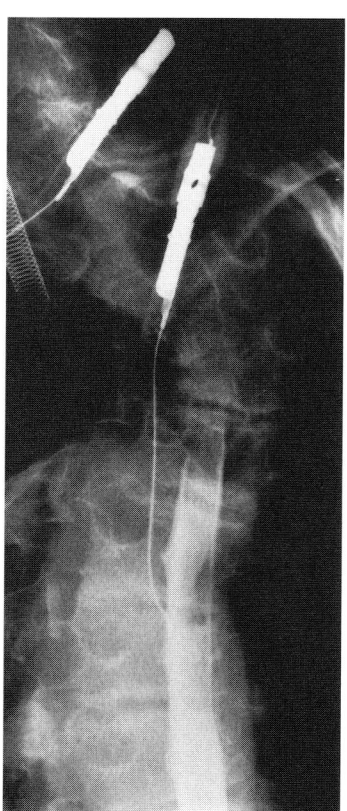

Figure 9–28 Myelogram of patient shown in Figure 9–27. Note lack of contrast material at angle of kyphosis. MRI demonstrated cord compression from T2 to T4. From Skovby et al. (105).

Table 9–8 Types of Abnormal Craniofacial Growth

Type[a]	Relative Frequency	Effect	Comment
Hyperostoses	Common	Major effect	Progressive enlargement, asymmetry, and disfigurement of skull
Cranial hemihyperplasia	Uncommon	Major effect	Calvarial remodeling secondary to hemimegalencephaly
Craniosynostosis	Rare	Major effect	Usually coronal synostosis; sagittal, metopic, and/or lambdoid involvement also recorded
Unilateral condylar hyperplasia	Probably common	Usually minor effect; rarely major effect	Overgrowth of condylar cartilage

[a]Four types of abnormal growth can act singly or in various combinations. Facial phenotype accompanying mental deficiency and, in some cases, seizures and/or brain malformations may override severe craniofacial distortion produced by these four modes of abnormal bone growth (see Table 9–9).

Source: Adapted from Cohen (27) and Kreiborg et al. (68).

pearance of the neck can be exaggerated by dysregulation of adipose tissue with decreased neck fat (Fig. 9–16). Overgrowth may affect other bones such as the metatarsals (Fig. 9–26) (11) and the ribs (19,85). Bony protuberances of the hands and feet (11,32) (hyperostoses, vide infra) have been observed (19,33,111,112,115) and, on occasion, the long bones of the legs and arms may be involved.

Uncommon findings have included cervical spine fusions (86), angular kyphosis with spinal stenosis (Figs. 9–27 and 9–28) (105), clinodactyly (32), cubitus valgus (19), radial head subluxation (86), elbow ankylosis (115), pectus excavatum (66), hip dysplasia (19,75,111), coxa valga (75), coxa vara (34), coxa plana (86), genu recurvatum (33), absent patella (19), tibial bowing (34), fibular bowing (61), and a gap between the first and second toes (105).

Cohen (27) and Kreiborg et al. (68) studied abnormal growth of the craniofacial skeleton. The variability can be explained by four unusual modes of growth that occur with different frequences and act either singly or in combination: (a) hyperostoses, (b) unilateral condylar hyperplasia, (c) abnormal cranial remodeling secondary to hemimegalencephaly, and (d) craniosynostosis (Table 9–8; Figs. 9–29 to 9–35).

Hyperostoses are bony overgrowths that are not true tumors. Cohen (27,32) used the term hyperostoses in preference to exostoses and osteomas; the latter two terms should be avoided because both have somewhat different patterns of osseous organization. Hyperostoses may occur in calvarial, facial, nasal, alveolar, and mandibular bone. They may be small or they may grow to be large in size, producing striking asymmetry. They are most common in the calvaria and least common in nasal and alveolar bone.

Hyperostosis of the external auditory canal is uncommon in Proteus syndrome (32,33) (Table 9–2). It may occur in surfers, in some instances or as an isolated abnormality of unknown cause. Nevertheless, when present with a few other manifestations of Proteus syndrome, its diagnostic value can have great signficance in mildly affected patients (27,106).

Highly arched palate (40,66,76,111,112) and mandibular prognathism (19,33,40) have been noted in some cases.

Facial Phenotype with Mental Deficiency

Cohen (27) described a facial phenotype in Proteus syndrome patients with mental deficiency and, in some cases, seizures and/or brain malformations. Manifestations include dolichocephaly, long face, minor downslanting of the palpebral fissures and/or minor ptosis, low nasal bridge, wide or anteverted nares, and an open mouth at rest (Figs. 9–36 and 9–37). These facial manifestations may even override the severe craniofacial distortion produced by bony overgrowth in some cases. Patients with this facial phenotype who have severe mental deficiency, sometimes with seizures and/or brain malformations, are illustrated in several publications: Cohen (32; see his case 2, Fig. 5, right), Cohen

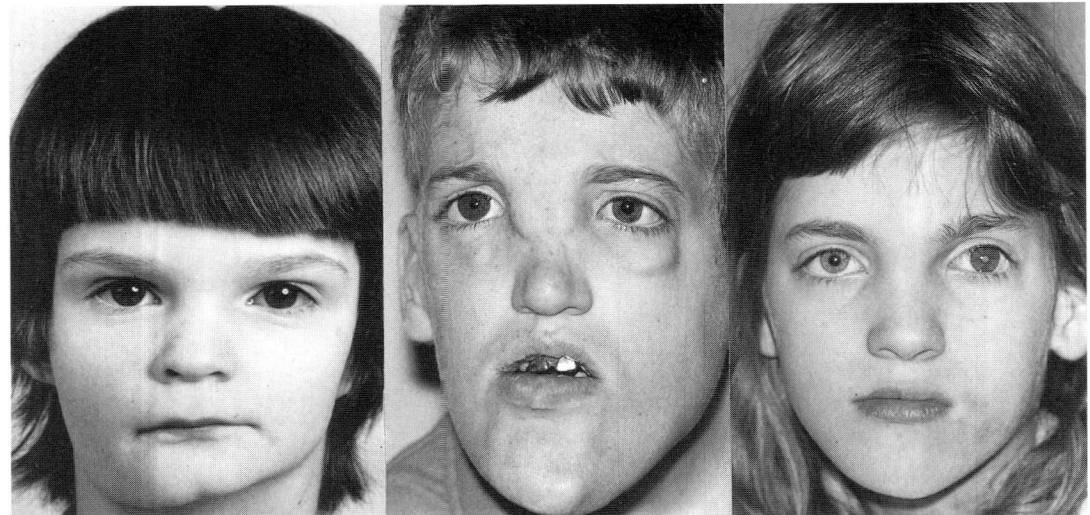

Figure 9–29 Left: Asymmetric mandible. From Kreiborg et al. (68). Center: Macrocephaly, hyperostoses of nasal bridge, left infraorbital region, and mandible that is asymmetric and prognathic. From Cohen (32). Right: Asymmetric eye size, anisocoria, heterochromia irides, cataract in right eye, and mild asymmetry of lower face. From Cohen (32).

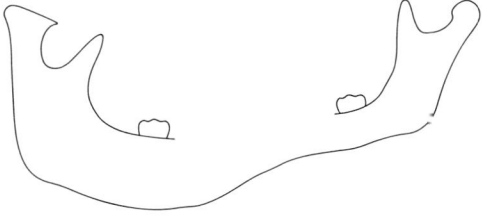

Figure 9–30 Tracing of asymmetric mandible from panorex radiograph of patient shown in Figure 9–29 (left). Note unilateral enlargement of condyle and ramus. From Kreiborg et al. (68).

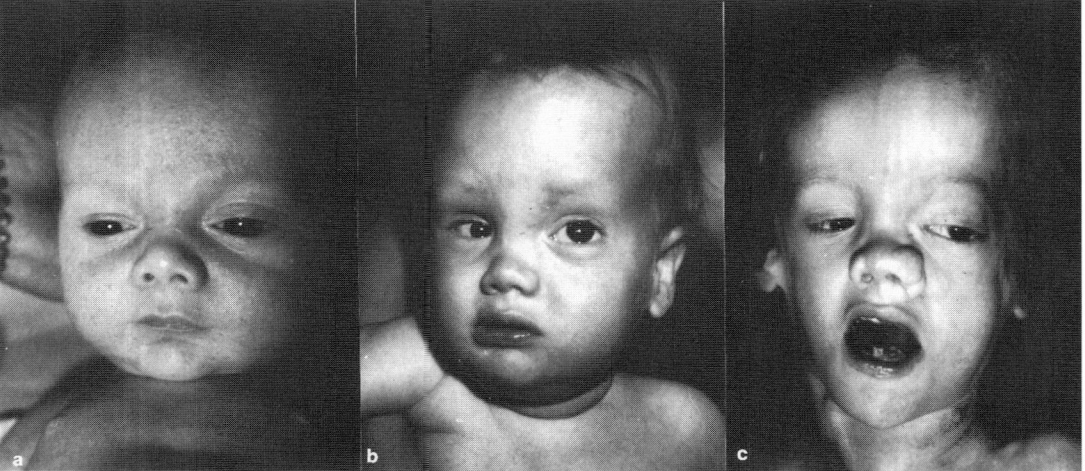

Figure 9–31 Evolution of facial dysmorphism in patient with Proteus syndrome. **a:** age 1 month; **b:** age 5 months; **c:** Age 5 and 1/2 years. Note connective tissue nevus on left side of nose. From Cohen (32).

PROTEUS SYNDROME

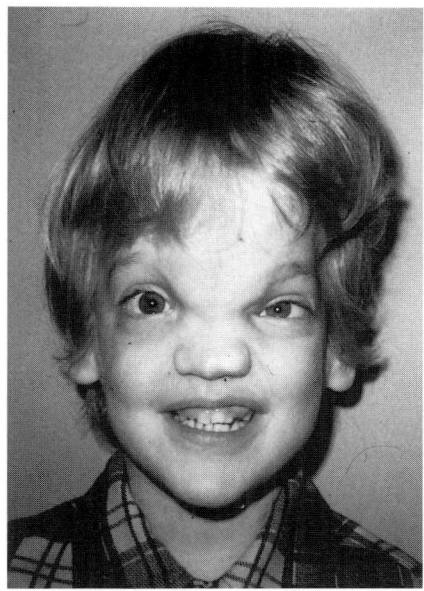

Figure 9–32 Prominent forehead with bilateral hyperostoses of nasal bridge. From Cohen (27).

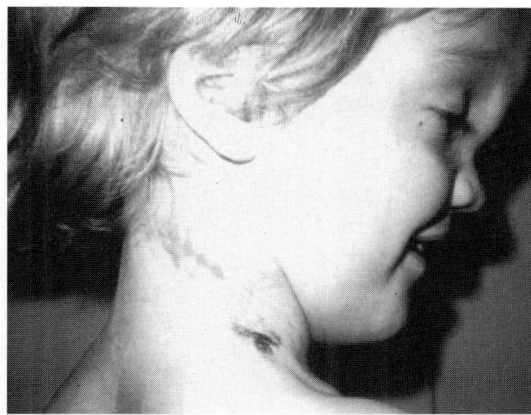

Figure 9–33 Same patient as shown in Figure 9–32. Epidermal nevus of neck. From Cohen (27).

(27; see his case 1, Fig. 1), Mayatepek et al., (78), and Rizzo et al. (98).

Spleen and Thymus

Although limb overgrowth is most common in Proteus syndrome, perhaps any organ may be involved. An uncommon manifestation, found in four patients, is pronounced splenomegaly (Fig. 9–38); one instance was associated with a history of reduced platelet counts. Another uncommon manifestation is enlargement of the thymus (10,11,17).

Central Nervous System

Intelligence may be normal, although some degree of mental deficiency has been evident in about 20% of cases and seizures have been documented in approximately 13%. However, a number of patients have had brain malformations (27). Cohen and Hayden (33) reported a patient with macrocephaly, hydrocephalus, and an estimated IQ of 30–40. Cohen (32) reported hemimegalencephaly, ventricular dilatation, severe mental deficiency, and seizures. Autopsy showed polymicrogyria and heterotopic gray matter nodules in the subcortical and periventricular white matter (Fig. 9–39). Bizarre neurons were found deep in the cortex and white matter. Cohen (27) reported a third patient with severe mental deficiency and seizures accompanied by hydrocephalus and an arachnoid cyst of the posterior fossa. Malamitsi-Puchner et al. (76) described macrocephaly, enlarged ventricles, and asymmetry of the frontal horns in associa-

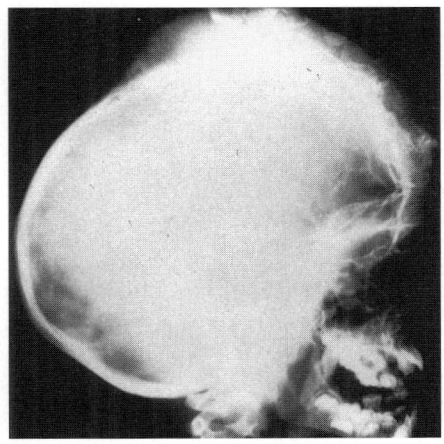

Figure 9–34 Same patient as shown in Figures 9–32 and 9–33. Marked hyperostosis of skull. Patient also had craniosynostosis, hyperostosis of the external auditory canal, epibulbar dermoid, and epidermal nevus of axilla. Arms, legs, hands, and feet were normal. From Cohen (27).

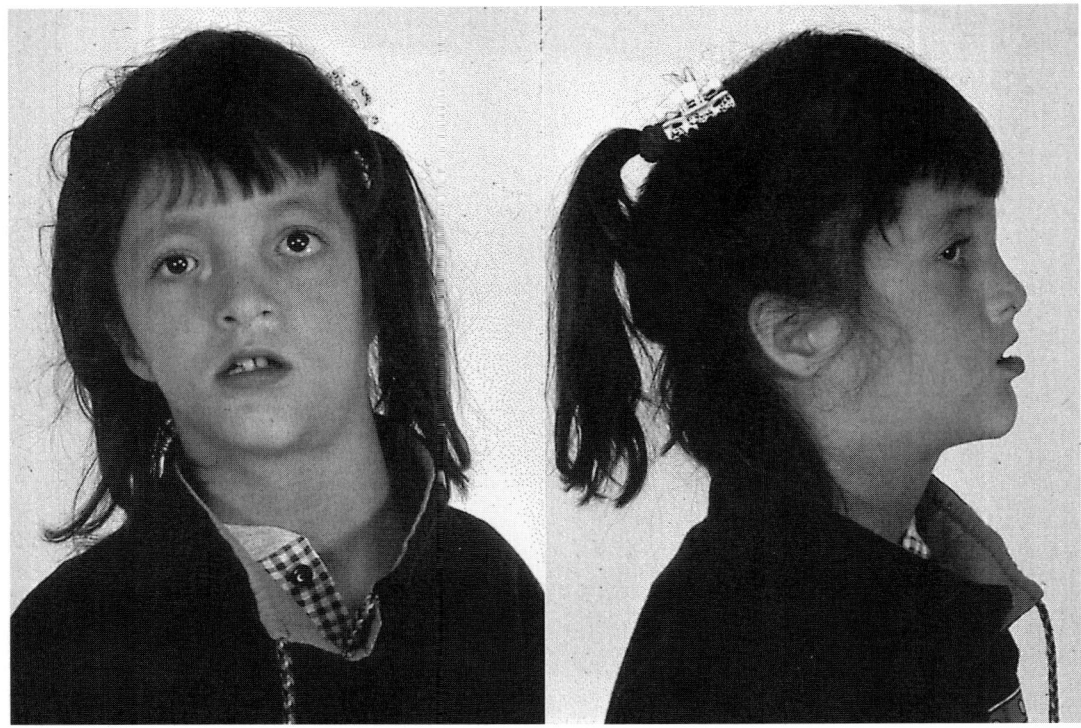

Figure 9–35 Proteus syndrome patient with synostosis of coronal suture.

tion with seizures. Mayatepek et al. (78) noted on computed tomography (CT) dilated ventricles, cortical atrophy, and possible absence of the corpus callosum. Rizzo et al. (98) reported severe mental deficiency, seizures, hemimegalencephaly, and a head circumference above the 97th centile. The CT showed hypodensity of the periventricular white matter.

Ocular Abnormalities

Many ocular manifestations in Proteus syndrome have been reported (14,16,36a,73); these are reviewed in Table 9–2 together with appropriate references. De Becker et al. (36a) suggested that several findings result from severe maldevelopment and malfunction of the neuroretina, including strabismus, nystagmus, high myopia, retinal pigmentary abnormalities, retinal detachment, cataracts, and posterior segment hamartomas. The most commonly recorded ocular findings have been strabismus and epibulbar tumors. Enlarged eye is not recorded in Table 9–2. Although it has been described several times, the term could refer to ocular proptosis, buphthalmos, or skeleto-orbital distortion from hyperostoses or craniosynostosis.

Bouzas et al. (14) indicated that ocular findings were insufficiently described in many reports of Proteus syndrome and suggested that the true frequency of various abnormalities is unknown. Cohen (25) reviewed all published papers of presumed Proteus syndrome and concluded that a number of them did not describe Proteus syndrome. Because of anecdotal and nonsystematic study of the eyes in Proteus syndrome and because of the ascertainment bias inherent in literature reports, the number of cases of each manifestation does not appear in Table 9–2. Of the references cited in the table, spurious reports of Proteus syndrome in the literature have also been avoided.

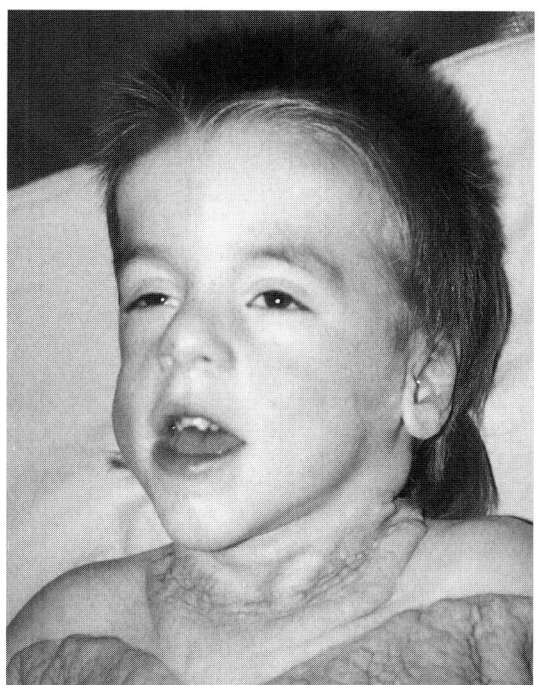

Figure 9–36 Facial phenotype in Proteus syndrome patient with mental deficiency and a history of seizures. Note dolichocephaly, long face, mild downslanting of palpebral fissures, ptosis, low nasal bridge, anteverted nares, and open mouth. From Cohen (27).

Pulmonary Abnormalities

Hotmisligil (62) estimated that about 16% of patients had pulmonary abnormalities ($n = 55$). Cystic anomalies (Fig. 9–40) were reported in two patients by Wiedeman et al. (115); one patient had progressive dyspnea at rest and frequent superinfection. About 12%–13% of patients have had such cystic lung changes. Serious and potentially lethal lung involvement has been emphasized by Newman et al. (85).

Other abnormalities such as tumors and skeletal defects may contribute to pulmonary problems. Pneumonia has been reported in patients with neoplastic impingement on the chest. Scoliosis and megaspondylodysplasia are common, and, if severe, may contribute to restrictive pulmonary disease (10,27). Clark et al. (19, patient 2) reported a patient who died of pneumonia complicated by ventilatory failure secondary to massive rib overgrowth.

Renal Abnormalities

A variety of renal abnormalities have been recorded, including nephrogenic diabetes insipidus, kidney cysts, vascular malformations of the bladder and kidney, ureterectasis, heminephromegaly, duplicated renal collecting system, and hydronephrosis (27,62,63).

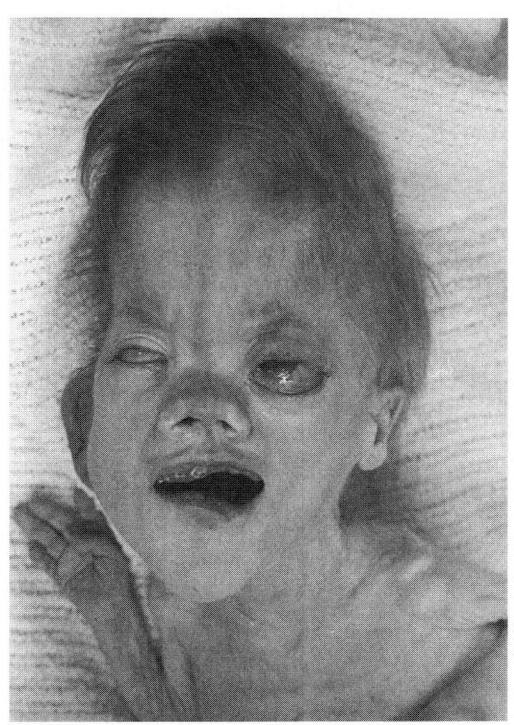

Figure 9–37 Facial phenotype in Proteus syndrome patient at 16 months. Patient had developmental delay, seizures, mild hydrocephalus, craniosynostosis involving the sagittal and lambdoid sutures, hemihyperplasia of the face, marked left proptosis with posterior subcapsular cataract, and retinal detachment. Patient also had vascular malformations, lipomas, and complex congenital heart defects. Note dolichocephaly, long face, mild downslanting of right palpebral fissure with ptosis, low nasal bridge, wide nose, anteverted nares, and open mouth. Facial phenotype overrides severe craniofacial distortion. From Mayatepek et al. (78).

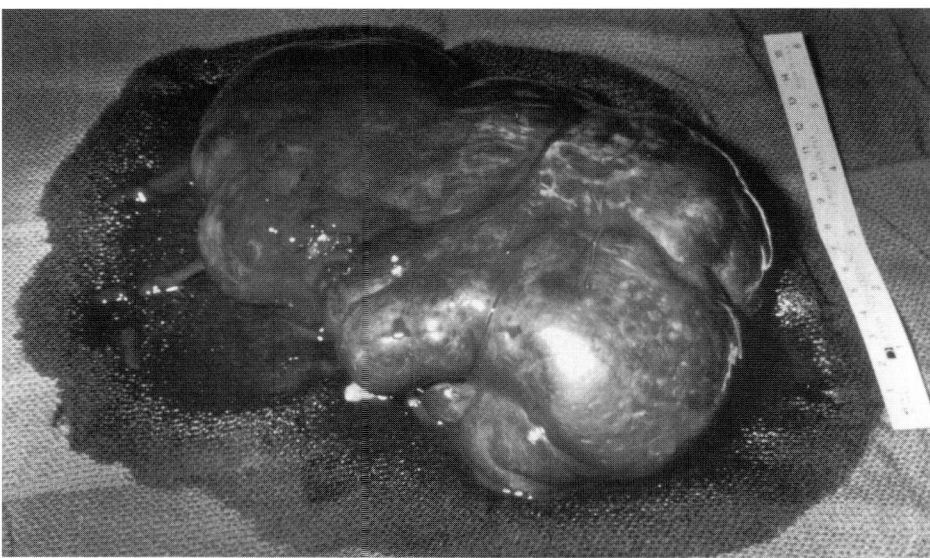

Figure 9–38 Huge spleen removed at surgery from a patient with Proteus syndrome who had thrombocytopenia. From Biesecker et al. (10).

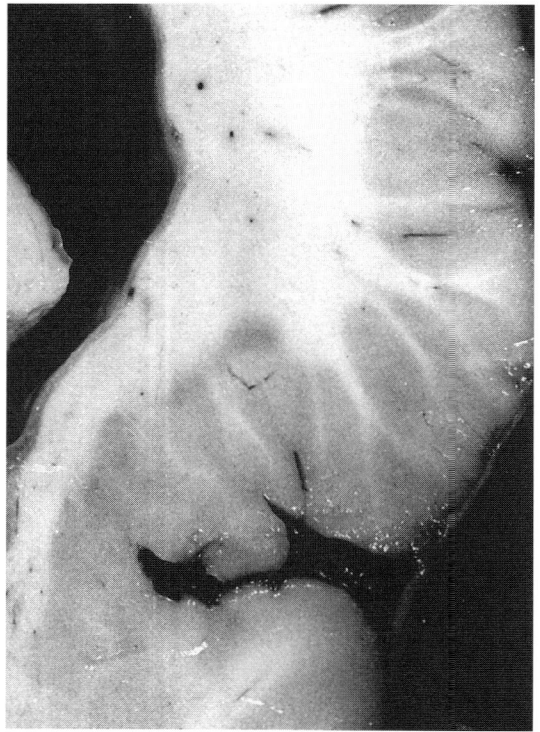

Figure 9–39 Section through right posterior parietal lobe of Proteus syndrome patient who died at 5 and 1/2 years with a cerebellar abscess secondary to otitis media. Note complicated, abortive gyral formations characteristic of polymicrogyria. From Cohen (32).

Other Abnormalities

Rectal polyposis has been found in two patients (Fig. 9–41) (9,71). Muscular atrophy (19,34,40, 90), mixed mesenchymal bronchial hamartoma (34), and a vocal cord nodule (100) have been noted.

CLINICAL ASPECTS OF SOMATIC MOSAICISM

Mosaic distribution of lesions and variable extent of involvement implies that criteria for the diagnosis of Proteus syndrome should be loose rather than overly rigid (27,106). Wiedemann and Burgio (114) suggested that encephalocraniocutaneous lipomatosis (ECCL) might represent a more localized form of Proteus syndrome. Comparison of individual cases of ECCL (1,79, 97) shows a continuum, not two distinct entities that share some common manifestations. For example, in ECCL, cutaneous, craniofacial, and meningeal lipomas (usually unilateral) occur, but cutaneous lipomas below the head and neck and visceral involvement have been found in some cases. One patient had a moderately sized capillary malformation of the right antecubital fossa extending to the upper arm (87a). Other patients

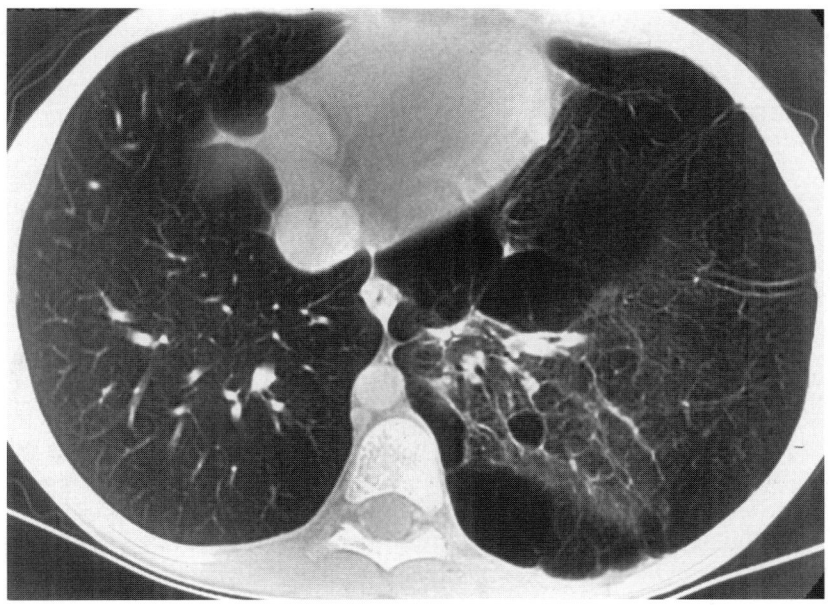

Figure 9–40 Axial computed tomography image of Proteus syndrome patient showing cystic malformations of lung. From Biesecker et al. (11).

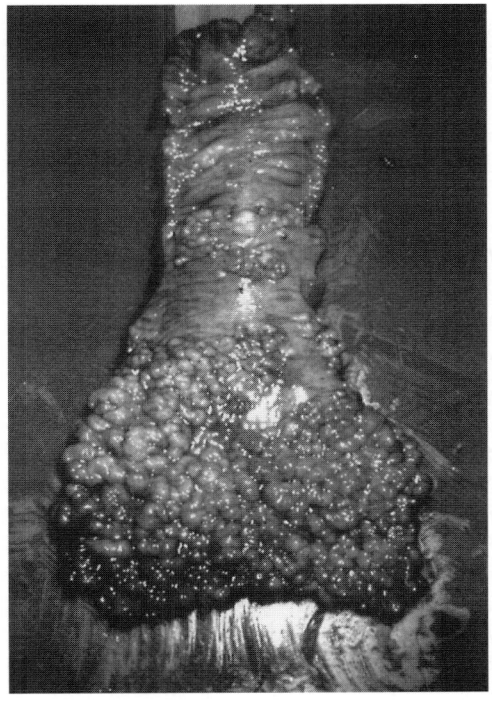

Figure 9–41 Rectal polyposis. Courtesy of L.G. Biesecker, Bethesda, Maryland.

have had mental deficiency, seizures, malformations of the central nervous system, epibulbar dermoids, connective tissue nevi, and focal alopecia. In some instances, hyperostoses of the calvaria have been noted. All of these defects, except possibly focal alopecia, have been seen in Proteus syndrome. Happle (53) believes that Proteus syndrome and ECCL are separate entities. The association of ECCL with an *NF1* mutation, reported by Legius et al. (72), is likely coincidental.

Five other examples or possible examples of regional Proteus syndrome are reviewed here. Although patients with limited regional involvement may be particularly difficult to diagnose, the patients discussed below have a sufficient number of clinical features to suggest the diagnosis of Proteus syndrome (see Diagnostic Criteria, below).

Cohen (27) reported a patient whose features were confined mostly to the head and neck. Manifestations included epidermal nevi on the neck and in the axilla, an epibulbar dermoid, hyperostoses of the calvaria, nasal bridge, and auditory canal, and craniosynostosis. The arms, legs, hands, and feet were normal.

Smeets et al. (106) observed a patient with hyperostoses of the parieto-occipital area frontal bone, nasal bridge, alveolar ridges, and auditory canal. A scleral tumor was present. The arms, legs, hands, and feet were normal.

Cohen (27) described a patient with a large connective tissue nevus of the chest and abdomen, brain abnormalities, mental deficiency, and the facial phenotype that accompanies the latter two abnormalities. Clinodactyly of the fingers and crowding of the toes were noted. The arms, legs, hands, and feet were otherwise normal.

Haramoto et al. (55) reported a patient with craniofacial involvement. Findings included epidermal nevus-like skin ("sebaceous nevus-like skin"), orbital and cranial hyperostosis, subcutaneous and orbital lipomatosis, and bony thickening of the meninges. Although not examined histologically, osseous meningeal thickening was thought to represent an unusual type of meningioma or other type of overgrowth. The arms, legs, hands, and feet were normal except for a capillary malformation on the sole of the right foot. It should be noted that other patients with Proteus syndrome have had documented meningiomas (3,5,14,43,60,74) (Table 9–3).

Horie et al. (60) observed a patient with hemihyperplasia on the right side of the face. Other findings included lipomatosis on the right side of the face, scalp, lip, oral mucosa, and tongue. Intracranial manifestations consisted of thickening of the cranial bones, a lipoma on the left side of the cerebellar peduncle, a venous malformation, and multiple meningiomas. A leiomyoma of the bladder was extirpated at 37 years of age. The arms, legs, hands, and feet were normal. Of the five other patients with Proteus syndrome known to have meningioma (3,5,14,43,74), multiple meningiomas were found in two cases (14,43) (Table 9–3). Furthermore, one case had multiple leiomyomas of the uterus in addition to meningioma (74) (Table 9–4).

Nishimura and Nishimura (87) reported a patient with juxtasutural cranial hyperostoses together with a cardiac tumor that on MRI suggested a lipomatous lesion. Juxtasutural hyperostoses have also been observed on the Proteus syndrome patients discussed by Smeets et al. (106) and by Cohen (27, case 2). Shaw et al. (104) noted a Proteus syndrome patient with a cardiac tumor accompanied by diffuse septal hypertrophy.

PUBLICATIONS AND THE DIAGNOSIS OF PROTEUS SYNDROME

Many publications bearing the name "Proteus syndrome" in the title do not, in fact, describe patients with Proteus syndrome. Several problems are apparent. First, misdiagnosis of Klippel-Trenaunay syndrome and hemihyperplasia/lipomatosis syndrome as Proteus syndrome is common (see Differential Diagnosis, below). Second, some reported patients have hemihyperplasia with associated abnormalities that do not fit into any known diagnostic category and probably represent provisionally unique pattern syndromes. Third, *patients with Proteus syndrome at birth are usually normal or show mild to moderate alterations, hyperplasias, or hamartoses. Progressive asymmetric overgrowth evolves postnatally. Patients with highly significant hyperplastic overgrowth of limbs at birth are very unlikely to have Proteus syndrome.* Fourth, many published reports have either too little documentation or too few photographs or both to establish a diagnosis of Proteus syndrome with certainty. Fifth, some publications, particularly in the surgical literature, discuss clinical problems in a series of Proteus and Klippel-Trenaunay syndrome patients without distinguishing the two in analysis. Finally, some papers that tabulate the frequencies of various abnormalities found in Proteus syndrome cite papers that do not describe Proteus syndrome despite the appelation in the title of the article.

Two other types of problems are described here. First, a reverse diagnostic situation is found with so-called "Thanos syndrome," a condition that does not exist; in fact, such patients have Proteus syndrome (30). Second, a number of patients with overgrowth and associated abnormalities not reported as having Proteus syndrome nevertheless have other disorders that are so intriguing that the manifestations of each are summarized for differential diagnostic purposes.

Thanos Syndrome Does Not Exist

Some patients with striking hyperostoses of the skull and facial bones and other manifestations of Proteus syndrome have been diagnosed as having "Thanos syndrome." The term has been applied so often that a history of how and why the name was introduced should, hopefully, put the matter to rest (30).

"Thanos syndrome" has been referred to in several publications. In 1977, in a table of craniosynostosis syndromes, Cohen listed this condition as "Pederson syndrome," naming it after Dr. G. Pederson, who sent him a consultation by correspondence in 1975 (23). He used the same term in another craniosynostosis table 2 years later (21). In 1977, Thanos et al. (108) published a short report of the same patient. Cohen (22) later used the term "Thanos syndrome" on a provisional basis because a synoptic description of the patient was then available (108) and no other similar patients were known at that time. With the delineation of Proteus syndrome and the formulation of a hypothesis of somatic mosaicism, the significance of the patient's craniosynostosis and hyperostoses became clear. The patient had, in addition, epidermal nevi, epibulbar dermoids, and hyperostosis of the external auditory canal. Craniosynostosis is now known to be a low-frequency abnormality in Proteus syndrome (27). At least four patients with craniosynostosis are known to be associated with Proteus syndrome (Table 9–2). In a later paper, Cohen (27, case 2) published a clinical case history of the original ("Thanos syndrome"/"Pederson syndrome") patient and demonstrated diagnostic criteria for Proteus syndrome. A similar patient with Proteus syndrome was reported by Christianson and Van Allen (18).

Some Intriguing Non–Proteus Syndrome Patients

Several reported patients have had hemihyperplasia and other abnormalities that are not examples of Proteus syndrome but represent either other known diagnoses or newly recognized syndromes. (a) hemihyperplasia, hemimegalencephaly, polydactyly, and syndactyly (94);[c] (b) macrodactyly, megalencephaly, generalized lipomatosis, polypoid lesions of the small intestine, and frond-like projections of Peyers patches (88); (c) cranial hemihyperplasia with nevoid streaks (36,80); and (d) epidermal nevi with localized cranial defects (58).

Raman et al. (93) reported a patient with cystic bony lesions of the frontal and infraorbital regions, firm swelling of the tongue showing chondromyxoid metaplasia, epidermal cyst, tonsillar enlargement, unilateral enlargement of the mandible, and, surprisingly, hyperostosis of the left external auditory canal.

Zhou et al. (117) reported a male patient with marked hemihyperplasia at birth, epidermal nevi in whorls and plaques on the right side of his body, arteriovenous malformations, lipomas, and macrocephaly. He was found to have a *PTEN* mutation (Arg335Stop) (see Chapter 8, Table 8-1).

DIAGNOSTIC CRITERIA, DIFFERENTIAL DIAGNOSIS, AND PATIENT EVALUATION

Although much has been learned about Proteus syndrome in recent years (8a,10,11,27), knowledge is evolving rapidly. Thus, the recommendations in this section about diagnostic criteria should be considered tentative because future clinical and molecular studies may necessitate modification.

Diagnostic Criteria

Clinical diagnostic criteria are summarized in menu form in Table 9–9 (10). General criteria are mandatory, regardless of specific manifestations in a given patient. Specific criteria, based on category signs A, B, or C, must be met (10). Although many manifestations have been recorded in Proteus syndrome (Tables 9–1 to 9–4), only those thought to be of diagnostic value are listed. The single category sign in A appears to be sufficient for diagnosis. Either two category signs from B or three from C also appear

---

[c]The patient has features suggestive of macrocephaly–cutis marmorata syndrome (81a) (see Chapter 15).

Table 9–9 Diagnostic Criteria for Proteus Syndrome

FOR DIAGNOSIS			
	General criteria (mandatory)	+	Specific criteria (category signs)
	Mosaic distribution of lesions Progressive course Sporadic occurrence		Either 1 from A or 2 from B or 3 from C

Category Signs	Manifestations	Relative Frequency (C = Common, U = Uncommon)
A.	1. Connective tissue nevus	C
B.	1. Epidermal nevus	C
	2. Disproportionate overgrowth	
	(one or more)	
	Limbs	
	Arms/legs	C
	Hands/feet/digits	C
	Skull	
	Hyperostoses	C
	External auditory meatus	
	Hyperostosis	U
	Vertebrae	
	Megaspondylodysplasia	C
	Viscera	
	Spleen/thymus	U
	3. Specific tumors before end of second decade	
	(either one)	
	Bilateral ovarian cystadenomas	U
	Parotid monomorphic adenoma	U
C.	1. Dysregulated adipose tissue	
	(either one)	
	Lipomas	C
	Regional absence of fat	C
	2. Vascular malformations	
	(one or more)	
	Capillary ma formation	C
	Venous malformation	C
	Lymphatic malformation	C
	3. Facial phenotype	U
	Dolichocephaly	
	Long face	
	Minor downslanting of palpebral fissures	
	and/or minor ptosis	
	Low nasal bridge	
	Wide or anteverted nares	
	Open mouth at rest	

Source: From Biesecker et al. (10).

to be sufficient for diagnosis. At the present time, the use of combined partial criteria from B and C is not recommended. For example, it is uncertain that one category sign from B combined with two category signs from C would be sufficient to establish diagnosis.

Differential Diagnosis

Various syndromes considered in the differential diagnosis (10) are listed in Table 9–10, but not in order of importance. Rather, they are grouped for convenience as vascular syndromes, syndromes with pigmentation, and lipomatoses. The two disorders most commonly confused with Proteus syndrome are Klippel-Trenaunay syndrome and hemihyperplasia/lipomatosis syndrome. Misdiagnosis of these two conditions as Proteus syndrome is common primarily because of confusion about the variability of Proteus syndrome (10). Of 16 patients referred to an NIH Proteus Evaluation Study, the diagnosis could

Table 9–10 Differential Diagnosis

Klippel-Trenaunay syndrome
Parkes Weber syndrome
Maffucci syndrome
Neurofibromatosis, type 1
Epidermal nevus syndromes[a] (formerly epidermal nevus syndrome or Solomon syndrome)
Bannayan-Riley-Ruvalcaba syndrome
Hemihyperplasia/lipomatosis syndrome
Familial lipomatosis
Symmetrical lipomatosis
Encephalocraniocutaneous lipomatosis (see Clinical Aspects of Somatic Mosaicism, below)

[a]Known to be etiologically and pathogenetically heterogeneous rather than being a single entity (48).

Source: From Biesecker et al. (10).

only be confirmed in 10 cases; the other 6 had Klippel-Trenaunay syndrome or hemihyperplasia/multiple lipomatosis syndrome (11).

Hemihyperplasia with multiple lipomas is a distinct subset of hemihyperplasia. Cutaneous capillary malformation may occur in some instances. Mild to moderate signs are present at birth. Progressive overgrowth does not occur; rather, it tends to be commensurate with growth of the child (11).

Besides hemihyperplasia/lipomatosis syndrome, several other conditions also have lipomatosis. These include autosomal dominant multiple lipomatosis (107), monomelic macrodystrophic lipomatosis (6), symmetrical lipomatosis (39), congenital aggressive thoracic lipomatosis (70)[d], pelvic lipomatosis (39), and lipoblastomatosis (39). Lipomas may occur in Gardner syndrome in association with osteomas of the frontal bone, maxilla, or mandible.

Other disorders with vascular malformations and soft tissue and skeletal overgrowth include Klippel-Trenaunay, Parkes Weber, and Maffucci syndromes. Klippel-Trenaunay syndrome is a "slow-flow" vascular malformation involving lower or upper limbs and/or trunk. The vascular malformations are always combined: capillary, lymphatic, and venous. An MRI with gadolinium can be used to differentiate venous from lymphatic anomalies. Overgrowth is also present at birth and is commonly severe, in contrast to Proteus syndrome, in which overgrowth is usually

[d]Cases 1 and 3. Their Case 2 is an example of hemihyperplasia/lipomatosis syndrome.

mild or absent at birth. Parkes Weber syndrome is a "fast-flow" vascular malformation involving the upper/lower limbs and is characterized by a diffuse, often confluent, capillary blush, warmth, and underlying arteriovenous shunts. In Maffucci syndrome, the vascular anomalies are commonly venous and occur together with enchondromas. These tumors have not been found in Proteus syndrome (24a,29,83,84) (see Chapters 10 and 11).

Other well-defined epidermal nevus syndromes include sebaceous nevus syndrome and CHILD syndrome, which are clearly differentiated from Proteus syndrome. These and other less well-defined epidermal nevus syndromes are discussed by Happle (48).

Type 1 neurofibromatosis and Bannayan-Riley-Ruvalcaba syndrome are distinct from Proteus syndrome and are understood at the molecular level, with mutations occurring in the *NF1* and *PTEN* genes, respectively (26). Neurofibromas have not been reported in Proteus syndrome, although a single café-au-lait spot may be encountered on occasion. Meningioma, either single or multiple, can be found in Proteus syndrome (3,5,14,43,60,74) or as an isolated tumor or in neurofibromatosis, type 2 (42a, 118). Bannayan-Riley-Ruvalcaba syndrome is characterized by macrocephaly, lipomas, capillary malformations, polyposis of the colon and rectum, pigmented macules of the penis, and Hashimoto thyroiditis (46) (see Chapters 8 and 12).

Guidelines for Patient Evaluation

Guidelines for evaluation of patients are listed in Table 9–11 (10). High-resolution chest CT

Table 9–11 Guidelines for Patient Evaluation

Serial clinical photography
Initial skeletal survey with targeted follow-up radiographs
MRI of all clinically affected areas; chest and abdomen in absence of symptoms
Dermatology consultation; biopsy when indicated
Orthopedic consultation; operation when indicated
Ongoing genetic/pediatric management
Other consultations as indicated
Referral to family support group[a]

[a]Contact Ms. Kimberly Hoag, Proteus Syndrome Foundation, 6235 Whetstone Drive, Colorado Springs, CO 80918. E-mail: abscit@aol.com; www.kumc.edu/gec/support/proteus.htm.

Source: From Biesecker et al. (10).

may be useful to evaluate pulmonary cystic malformations. This is particularly true for patients who develop persistent atelectasis or pneumonia or symptoms of pulmonary insufficiency. Newman et al. (85) estimated that 12%–13% of patients have cystic lung abnormalities which, in some cases, may lead to cystic emphysematous pulmonary disease. Even in the absence of symptoms, an abdominal MRI is important to rule out intra-abdominal lipomas, which, if present, can be aggressive. Cranial MRI may be useful to characterize CNS anomalies associated with seizures or developmental delay. Chromosome analysis may possibly show a translocation or deletion that might suggest a candidate gene Finally, other consultations may include, as indicated, pediatric neurology, ophthalmology, or hematology. The coordination of care by an experienced geneticist and genetics counselor is useful because the rarity of Proteus syndrome precludes familiarity of its manifestations by many specialists. Peters and Biesecker (91a) found symptoms of depression in about 23% of parents of children with Proteus syndrome, suggesting referral for appropriate treatment when indicated.

REFERENCES

1. Al-Mefty O, Fox JL, Sakati N, Bashir R, Probst F: The multiple manifestations of the encephalocranocutaneous lipomatosis syndrome. Child Nerv Syst 3:132–134, 1987.
2. Asher HR, Schoenberg Fejzo M, Tkachenko A, Zhou X, Fletcher JA, Weremowicz S, Morton CC, Chada K: Disruption of the architectural factor HMGI-C. DNA-binding at hook motifs fused in lipomas to distinct transcriptional regulatory domains. Cell 82:57–65, 1995.
3. Aylsworth AS, Powers SK, Kahler SG: The Proteus syndrome with parental consanguinity. Proc Greenwood Genet Ctr 7:216, 1988.
4. Azouz EM, Costa T, Fitch N: Radiologic findings in the Proteus syndrome. Pediatr Radiol 17:481–485, 1987.
5. Bale PM, Watson G, Collins F: Pathology of osseous and genitourinary lesions of Proteus syndrome. Pediatr Pathol 13:797–809, 1993.
6. Bansal VP, Harmit S: Monomelic macrodystrophia lipomatosa. Int J Orthopaed 13:77–79, 1989.
6a. Barker K, Martinez A, Wang R, Bevan S, Murday V, Shipley J, Houlston R, Harper J: PTEN mutations are uncommon in Proteus syndrome. J Med Genet 38:480–481, 2001.
7. Bean WB: Book review. Arch Intern Med 115:502, 1965.
8. Bean WB, Felson B, Dolan KD: A nonletter from the editor and a case for all seasons. Semin Roentgenol 17:153–162, 1982.
8a. Biesecker LG: The multifaceted challenges of Proteus syndrome. JAMA 285:2240–2243, 2001.
9. Biesecker LG: Personal communication, 1997.
9a. Biesecker LG: Pulmonary embolism. Proteus Syndrome Foundation Newsletter 7(7):7, 2000.
10. Biesecker LG, Happle R, Mulliken JB, Weksberg R, Graham JM Jr, Viljoen DL, Cohen MM Jr: Proteus syndrome: Diagnostic criteria, differential diagnosis, and patient evaluation. Am J Med Genet 84:389–395, 1999.
11. Biesecker LG, Peters KF, Darling TN, Choyke P, Hill S, Schimke N, Cunningham M, Meltzer P, Cohen MM Jr: Clinical differentiation between Proteus syndrome and hemihyperplasia: Description of a distinct form of hemihyperplasia. Am J Med Genet 79:311–318, 1998.
12. Boccone L, Marica M, Faa G, Licciardi S, Barletta A, Cecchetto G, Ninfo V, D'Amore AC: Un caso di sindrome di Proteus con cistoadenoma ovarico. Genetics Meeting, Spoleto, Italy, 1997.
13. Botella-Estrada RB, Alegre V, Sanmartin O, Ros C, Adolfo A: Isolated plantar cerebriform collagenoma. Arch Dermatol 127:1589–1590, 1991.
14. Bouzas EA, Krasnewich D, Koutroumanidis M, Papadimitriou A, Marini JC, Kaiser-Kupfer MI: Ophthalmologic examination in the diagnosis of Proteus syndrome. Ophthalmology 100:334–338, 1993.
15. Burgio GR, Wiedemann H-R: Further new details on the Proteus syndrome. Eur J Pediatr 143:71–73, 1994.
16. Burke JP, Bowell R, O'Doherty N: Proteus syndrome: Ocular complications. J Pediatr Ophthalmol Strabismus 25:99–102, 1988.
17. Ceelen W, De Waeke J, Kunnen M, de Hemptinne B: Non-operative management of a splenic laceration in a patient with Proteus syndrome. J Accid Emerg Med 14:111–113, 1997.
18. Christianson AL, Van Allen MI: Brief clinical report: Sutural exostoses, rib hyperostoses, craniosynostosis, mental retardation with focal fat deposition: Proteus syndrome? Am J Med Genet 66:150–153, 1996.
19. Clark RD, Donnai D, Rogers J, Cooper J, Baraitser M: Proteus syndrome: An expanded phenotype. Am J Med Genet 27:99–117, 1987.
20. Clemmons DR, Camacho-Hubner C, Jones JI, McCusker RH, Busby WH: Insulin-like growth factor binding proteins: Mechanisms of action at the cellular level. In: *Modern Concepts of Insulin-like Growth Factors*. EM Spencer, ed. Elsevier, New York, pp. 475–486, 1991.
20a. Cohen MM Jr: Causes of premature death in Proteus syndrome. Am J Med Genet 101:1–3, 2001.

21. Cohen MM Jr: Craniosynostosis and syndromes with craniosynostosis: Incidence, genetics, penetrance, variability, and new syndrome updating. Birth Defects 15(5B):13–63, 1979.
22. Cohen MM Jr: *Craniosynostosis: Diagnosis, Evaluation, and Management.* Raven Press, New York, pp. 561–563, 1986.
23. Cohen MM Jr: Genetic perspectives on craniosynostosis and syndromes with craniosynostosis. J Neurosurg 47:886–898, 1977.
24. Cohen MM Jr: Invited historical comment: Further diagnostic thoughts about the Elephant Man. Am J Med Genet 29:777–782, 1988.
24a. Cohen MM Jr: Klippel-Trenaunay syndrome. Am J Med Genet 93:171–175, 2000.
25. Cohen MM Jr: Personal observations, 1998.
26. Cohen MM Jr: Perspectives on overgrowth syndromes. Am J Med Genet 79:234–237, 1998.
27. Cohen MM Jr: Proteus syndrome: Clinical evidence for somatic mosaicism and selective review. Am J Med Genet 47:645–652, 1993.
28. Cohen MM Jr: Putting a foot in one's mouth or putting a foot down: Nonspecificity v. specificity of the connective tissue nevus in Proteus syndrome. Proc Greenwood Genet Ctr 14:11–13, 1995.
29. Cohen MM Jr: Some neoplasms and some hamartomatous syndromes: Genetic considerations. Int J Oral Maxillofac Surg 27:363–369, 1998.
30. Cohen MM Jr: Thanos syndrome does not exist. Am J Med Genet 86:101, 1999.
31. Cohen MM Jr: The Elephant Man did not have neurofibromatosis. Proc Greenwood Genet Ctr 6:187–192, 1986.
32. Cohen MM Jr: Understanding Proteus syndrome, unmasking the Elephant Man, and stemming elephant fever. Neurofibromatosis 1:260–280, 1988.
33. Cohen MM Jr, Hayden PW: A newly recognized hamartomatous syndrome. Birth Defects 15(5B): 291–296, 1979.
34. Costa T, Fitch N, Azouz EM: The Proteus syndrome: Report of two cases of pelvic lipomatosis. Pediatrics 76:984–989, 1985.
35. Crocker HR: *Diseases of the Skin: A Review of 15,000 Cases of Skin Disorders.* Lewis, London, 1905.
36. Dean JCS, Cole GF, Appleton Burn JRE, Roberts SA, Donnai D: Cranial hemihypertrophy and neurodevelopmental prognosis. J Med Genet 27:160–164, 1990.
36a. De Becker I, Gajda DJ, Gilbert-Barness E, Cohen MM Jr: Ocular manifestations of Proteus syndrome. Am J Med Genet 92:350–352, 2000.
37. Demetriades D, Hager J, Nikolaides N, Malamitsi-Puchner A, Bartsocas CS: Proteus syndrome: Musculoskeletal manifestations and management: A report of two cases. J Pediatr Orthop 12:106–113, 1992.
37a. Eberhard DA: Two-year-old boy with Proteus syndrome and fetal pulmonary thromboembolism. Pediatr Pathol 14:771–779, 1994.
38. Elkahloun AG, Bittner M, Hoskins K, Gemmill R, Meltzer PS: Molecular cytogenetic characterization and physical mapping of 12q13–15 amplification in human cancers. Genes Chromosom Cancer 17:205–214, 1996.
39. Enzinger FM, Weiss SW: *Soft Tissue Tumors.* C.V. Mosby, St. Louis, 1995.
40. Fay JT, Schow SR: A possible cause of Maffucci's syndrome: Report of a case. J Oral Surg 26:739–744, 1968.
41. Floyd A, Percy-Lancaster R: The elephant woman. Neurofibromatosis associated with pseudarthrosis of the humerus. J Bone Joint Surg (Br) 69: 121–123, 1987.
42. Frydman M, Kauschansky A, Varsano I: Brief clinical report: Ambiguous genitalia in the Proteus syndrome. Am J Med Genet 36:511–512, 1990.
42a. Giangaspero F, Guiducci A, Lenz FA, Mastronardi L, Burger PC: Meningioma with meningioangiomatosis: A condition mimicking invasive meningiomas in children and young adults. Report of two cases and review of the literature. Am J Surg Pathol 27:872–875, 1999.
43. Gilbert-Barness E, Cohen MM Jr, Opitz JM: Multiple meningiomas, craniofacial hyperostosis and retinal abnormalities in Proteus syndrome. Am J Med Genet 93:234–240, 2000.
44. Goodship J, Redfearn A, Milligan D, Gardner-Medwin D, Burn J: Transmission of Proteus syndrome from father to son? J Med Genet 28:781–785, 1991.
45. Gordon PL, Wilroy RS, Lasater OE, Cohen MM Jr: Neoplasms in Proteus syndrome. Am J Med Genet 57:74–78, 1995.
46. Gorlin RJ, Cohen MM Jr, Condon LM, Burke BA: Bannayan-Riley-Ruvalcaba syndrome. Am J Med Genet 44:307–314, 1992.
47. Happle R: Elattoproteus syndrome: Delineation of an inverse form of Proteus syndrome. Am J Med Genet 84:25–28, 1999.
48. Happle R: How many epidermal nevus syndromes exist? A clinicogenetic classification. J Am Acad Dermatol 25:550–556, 1991.
49. Happle R: Lethal genes surviving by mosaicism: A possible explanation for sporadic birth defects involving the skin. J Am Acad Dermatol 16:899–906, 1987.
50. Happle R: Letter to the editor: Lipomatosis and partial lipohypoplasia in Proteus syndrome: A clinical clue for twin spotting? Am J Med Genet 56:332–333, 1995.
51. Happle R: Mosaicism in human skin: Understanding the patterns and mechanisms. Arch Dermatol 129:1460–1470, 1993.
52. Happle R: Paradominant inheritance: A possible explanation for Becker's pigmented hairy nevus. Eur J Dermatol 2:39–40, 1992.

53. Happle R: Personal communication, 1998.
54. Happle R, Steijlen PM, Theile V, Karitzky D, Tinschert S, Albrecht-Nebe H, Küster W: Patchy dermal hypoplasia as a characteristic feature of Proteus syndrome. Arch Dermatol 133:77–80, 1997.
55. Haramoto U, Kobayashi S, Ohmori K: Hemifacial hyperplasia with meningeal involvement: A variant of Proteus syndrome? Am J Med Genet 59:164–167, 1995.
56. Hertig AT, Gore H: Female genitalia. In: *Pathology*, Vol. 2. WAD Anderson, ed. Mosby, St. Louis, pp. 1488–1577, 1971.
57. Hertig AT, Gore HM: Ovarian cystoma as of germinal epithelial origin: A histogenic classification. Rocky Mt Med J 55:47–50, 1958.
58. Ho N, Roig C, Diadori P: Epidermal nevi and localized cranial defects. Am J Med Genet 83:187–190, 1999.
59. Holmes LB: Personal communication, 1997.
60. Horie Y, Fujita H, Mano S, Kuwajima M, Ogawa K: Regional Proteus syndrome: Report of an autopsy case. Pathol Int 45:530–535, 1995.
61. Hornstein L, Bove KE, Towbin RB: Linear nevi, hemihypertrophy, connective tissue hamartomas and unusual neoplasms in children. J Pediatr 110:404–408, 1987.
62. Hotamisligil GS: Proteus syndrome and hamartoses with overgrowth. Dysmorphol Clin Genet 4:87–102, 1990.
63. Hotamisligil GS, Ertogan F: The Proteus syndrome: Association with nephrogenic diabetes insipidus. Clin Genet 38:139–144, 1990.
64. Howell M, Ford P: *The True History of the Elephant Man*. Allison & Busby, London, 1980.
65. Jackson bids $1 million for skeleton. Halifax Mail Star, June 17, 1987.
66. Kontras SB: Case report no. 19. Synd Ident 2:1–3, 1974.
67. Kousseff BG: Pleiotropy versus heterogeneity in Proteus syndrome. Pediatrics 78:544–546, 1986.
68. Kreiborg S, Cohen MM Jr, Skovby F: Craniofacial characteristics of Proteus syndrome: Two modes of abnormal growth. Proc Finn Dent Soc 87:183–188, 1991.
69. Krüger G, Pelz L, Wiedemann H-R: Transmission of Proteus syndrome from mother to son? (letter). Am J Med Genet 45:117–118, 1993.
70. Lachman RS, Finklestein J, Mehringer CM, Maenza R: Congenital aggressive lipomatosis. Skeletal Radiol 9:248–254, 1983.
71. Lamireau T, Le Bail B, Sarlangue J, Vergnes P, Lacombe D: Letter to the editor: Rectal polyps in Proteus syndrome. J Pediatr Gastroenterol 17:115, 1993.
72. Legius E, Wu R, Eyssen M, Maryner P, Fryns JP, Cassiman JJ: Encephalocraniocutaneous lipomatosis with a mutation in the *NF1* gene. J Med Genet 32:316–319, 1995.
73. Lessner A, Margo CE: Eyelid tumors in the Proteus syndrome. Am J Ophthalmol 111:521–522, 1991.
74. Maassen D, Voigtländer V: Proteus syndrom. Hautarzt 42:186–188, 1991.
75. Malamitsi-Puchner A, Demetriades D, Bartsocas C, Wiedemann H-R: Proteus syndrome: Course of a severe case. Am J Med Genet 35:283–285, 1990.
76. Malamitsi-Puchner A, Kitsiou S, Bartsocas CS: Proteus syndrome in an 18-month-old boy. Am J Med Genet 27:119–126, 1987.
77. Mason C, Roberts G: Unusual distribution of enamel hypoplasia in an 11-year-old child with Proteus syndrome. Int J Pediatr Dent 5:103–107, 1995.
78. Mayatepek E, Kurczynski TW, Ruppert ES, Hennessy JR, Brinker RA, French BN: Brief clinical report: Expanding the phenotype of the Proteus syndrome: A severely affected patient with new findings. Am J Med Genet 32:402–406, 1989.
79. McCall S, Ramzy MI, Cure JK, Pai GS: Encephalocraniocutaneous lipomatosis and the Proteus syndrome: Distinct entities with overlapping manifestations. Am J Med Genet 43:662–668, 1992.
80. McMullin GP, Super M, Clarke MA: Cranial hemihypertrophy with ipsilateral naevoid streaks, intellectual handicap and epilepsy: A report of two cases. Clin Genet 44:249–253, 1993.
81. Minnesota Dermatological Society Meeting, 1992.
81a. Moore CA, Toriello HV, Abuelo DN, Bull MJ, Curry CJR, Hall BD, Higgins JV, Stevens CA, Twersky S, Weksberg R, Dobyns WB: Macrocephaly-cutis marmorata telangiectatica congenita: a distinct disorder with developmental delay and connective tissue abnormalities. Am J Med Genet 70:67–73, 1997.
82. Montague MFA: *The Elephant Man*. Dutton, New York, 1979.
83. Mulliken JB: Cutaneous vascular anomalies. Semin Vasc Surg 6:204–218, 1993.
84. Mulliken JB, Glowacki J: Hemangiomas and vascular malformations in infants and children: A classification based on endothelial characteristics. Plast Reconstr Surg 69:412–420, 1982.
85. Newman B, Urbach AH, Orenstein D, Dickman PS: Proteus syndrome: emphasis on the pulmonary manifestations. Pediatr Radiol 24:189–193, 1994.
86. Nishimura G, Kozlowski K: Proteus syndrome (report of three cases). Australas Radiol 34:47–52, 1990.
87. Nishimura G, Nishimura J: Multiple juxtasutural, cranial hyphostoses and cardiac tumor: A new hamartomatous syndrome? Am J Med Genet 71:167–171, 1997.
87a. Nowaczyk MJM, Mernagh JR, Bourgeois JM, Thompson PJ, Jurriaans E: Antenatal and post-

natal findings in encephalocraniocutaneous lipomatosis. Am J Med Genet 91:261–266, 2000.
88. Okumura K, Sasaki Y, Ohyama M, Nishi T: Bannayan syndrome—generalized lipomatosis associated with megalencephaly and macrodactyly. Acta Pathol Jpn 36:269–277, 1986.
89. Pathological Society of London: Reports of Societies. Br Med J ii:1135–1143, 1884.
90. Pawlaczyk B, Sioda T: Hypertrophied lumbar and muscular atrophy. Synd Ident IV(1):3–4, 1976.
91. Pearson MA, Hoyme HE: Overlap in the neurofibromatosis and Proteus syndromes may reflect an abnormality of neuroectoderm differentiation. Fourteenth David W. Smith Workshop on Morphogenesis and Malformations, Le Tremblant Club, Quebec, August 12–17, 1993.
91a. Peters KF, Biesecker LG: An opportunity for genetic counseling intervention: Depression in parents of individuals with Proteus syndrome. J Genet Couns 9:161–170, 2000.
92. Rai GS, Coni NK: The 'Elephant Man' of Cambridge. A case report of neurofibromatosis. J Am Geriatr Soc 29:129–130, 1981.
93. Raman R, Kumar V, Arianayagan S, Peh SC: A unilateral mesenchymal disorder of the head. J Cranio-Max-Fac Surg 17:143–145, 1989.
94. Reardon W, Harding B, Winter RM, Baraitser M: Brief clinical report: Hemihypertrophy, hemimegalencephaly, and polydactyly. Am J Med Genet 66:144–149, 1996.
95. Researchers find genetic defect causing elephant man's disease. Halifax Mail Star, September 17, 1987.
96. Riccardi VM: Von Recklinghausen neurofibromatosis. New Engl J Med 305:1617–1627, 1981.
97. Rizzo R, Pavone L, Micali G, Nigro F, Cohen MM Jr: Encephalocraniocutaneous lipomatosis, Proteus syndrome, and somatic mosaicism. Am J Med Genet 47:653–655, 1993.
98. Rizzo R, Pavone L, Sorge G, Parano E, Baraitser M: Proteus syndrome: Report of a case with severe brain impairment and fatal course. J Med Genet 27:399–402, 1990.
99. Rudolph G, Blum WF, Jenne EW, Schöning M, Enders H, Meitinger T, Murken JD, Kampik A: Growth hormone (GH), insulin-like growth factors (IGFs), and IGF-binding protein-3 (IGFBP-3) in a child with Proteus syndrome. Am J Med Genet 50:204–210, 1994.
100. Samlaska CP, Levin SW, James WD, Benson PM, Walker JC, Perlik PC: Proteus syndrome. Arch Dermatol 125:1109–1114, 1989.
100a. Samuel M, Spitz L: Klippel-Trenaunay syndrome: Clinical features, complications and management in children. Br J Surg 82:757–761, 1995.
101. Say B, Carpenter NJ: Report of a case resembling the Proteus syndrome with a chromosome abnormality. Am J Med Genet 31:987–989, 1988.
102. Schoenmakers EFPM, Wanschura S, Mols R, Bullerdiek J, Van den Berghe H, Van de Ven WJM: Recurrent rearrangements in the high mobility group protein gene, HMGI-C, in benign mesenchymal tumours. Nat Genet 10:436–444, 1995.
103. Schwartz CE, Brown AM, Der Kaloustian VM, McGill CC, Saul RA: DNA fingerprinting: The utilization of minisatellite probes to detect a somatic mutation in the Proteus syndrome. In: *DNA Fingerprinting: Approaches and Applications*. T Burke, G Dolf, AJ Jeffreys, and R Wolff, eds. Birkhauser Verlag, Basel, pp. 95–105, 1991.
104. Shaw C, Bourke J, Dixon J: Brief clinical report: Proteus syndrome with cardiomyopathy and a myocardial mass. Am J Med Genet 46:145–148, 1993.
105. Skovby F, Graham JM Jr, Sonne-Holm S, Cohen MM Jr: Compromise of the spinal canal in Proteus syndrome. Am J Med Genet 47:656–659, 1993.
105a. Slavotinek AM, Vacha SJ, Peters KF, Biesecker LG: Sudden death caused by pulmonary thromboembolism in Proteus syndrome. Clin Genet 58:386–389, 2001.
106. Smeets E, Fryns J-P, Cohen MM Jr: Regional Proteus syndrome and somatic mosaicism. Am J Med Genet 51:29–31, 1994.
107. Stephens FE, Isaacson A: Hereditary multiple lipomatosis. J Hered 50:51–53, 1959.
108. Thanos C, Stewart RE, Zonana J: Craniosynostosis, bony exostoses, epibulbar dermoids, epidermal nevus, and slow development. Synd Ident 5:19–21, 1977.
109. Treves F: A case of congenital deformity. Trans Pathol Soc Lond 36:494–498, 1885.
109a. Turner JT, Cohen MM Jr, Biesecker LG: Natural history and complications in Proteus syndrome. American Society of Human Genetics, 51st Annual Meeting, San Diego, October 12–16, 2001.
110. Uitto J: Biochemistry of collagen diseases. Ann Intern Med 105:740–756, 1986.
111. Viljoen DL, Nelson MM, de Jong C, Beighton P: Proteus syndrome in Southern Africa: Natural history and clinical manifestations in six individuals. Am J Med Genet 27:87–98, 1987.
112. Viljoen DL, Saxe N, Temple-Camp C: Cutaneous manifestations of the Proteus syndrome. Pediatr Dermatol 5:14–21, 1988.
113. What the elephant man really had. Newsweek, February 29, 1988, p. 64.
114. Wiedemann H-R, Burgio GR: Letter to the Editor: Encephalocraniocutaneous lipomatosis and Proteus syndrome. Am J Med Genet 25:403–404, 1986.
115. Wiedemann H-R, Burgio GR, Aldenhoff P, Kunze J, Kaufmann HJ, Schirg E: The Proteus

syndrome, partial gigantism of the hands and/or feet, nevi, hemihypertrophy, subcutaneous tumors, macrocephaly, skull anomalies and possible accelerated growth and visceral affections. Eur J Pediatr 140:5–12, 1983.
116. Zachariou Z, Krug G, Benz G, Dawn F: Proteus syndrome associated with a sacrococcygeal teratoma. Eur J Pediatr Surg 6:249–251, 1996.
117. Zhou X-P, Marsh DJ, Hampel H, Mulliken JB, Gimm O, Eng C: Germline and germline mosaic *PTEN* mutations associated with a Proteus-like syndrome of hemihypertrophy, lower limb asymmetry, arteriovenous malformations and lipomatosis. Hum Mol Genet 9:765–768, 2000.
118. Zhu JJ, Maruyama T, Jacoby LB, Herman JG, Gusella JF, Black PM, Wu JK: Clonal analysis of a case of multiple meningiomas using multiple molecular genetic approaches: Pathology case report. Neurosurgery 45:409–416, 1999.

10

Klippel-Trenaunay Syndrome, Parkes Weber Syndrome, and Sturge-Weber Syndrome

This chapter considers Klippel-Trenaunay syndrome (OMIM 149000)[a], Parkes Weber syndrome, and Sturge-Weber syndrome (OMIM 185300)[a] together because all three have various types of vascular malformations and overgrowth involving the limbs in Klippel-Trenaunay and Parkes Weber syndromes and the maxilla in Sturge-Weber syndrome. The three disorders have been said to overlap with each other, but they should be considered separate clinical entities that almost always occur sporadically. In this connection, it is essential to discuss vascular tumors vs. vascular malformations and also the Kasabach-Merritt phenomenon. The analysis here is based on Cohen (10).

KLIPPEL-TRENAUNAY SYNDROME

Klippel-Trenaunay syndrome consists of (a) combined vascular malformations of the capillary, venous, and lymphatic types; (b) varicosities of unusual distribution, in particular the lateral venous anomaly (vide infra), observed during infancy or childhood; and (c) limb enlargement. Males and females are equally affected. The lower limb is involved in almost 95% of patients (Figs. 10–1 and 10–2), the upper limb accounting for almost 5% of patients. Approximately 15% have combined upper and lower limb involvement. Uncommonly, patients may have trunk involvement only (29,46,49,58) (Fig. 10–3).

The original paper of Klippel and Trenaunay (24) shows that "Trenaunay," not "Trénaunay," is correct; there is no accent é, although many articles have added the accent (see 17 for review). Well over 1500 cases have been recorded (29,36,46,49,58). Servelle (49) alone documented 768 operated patients.

Conventional thinking about Klippel-Trenaunay syndrome includes the following: (a) addition of arteriovenous fistulas and renaming the disorder Klippel-Trenaunay-Weber syndrome (3,19,22,25–27,39,48); (b) overlap with Sturge-Weber syndrome (6,15,18,21,44,52); (c) the presence of a bleeding diathesis of the Kasabach-Merritt type (46); and (d) familial aggregation (1,8,12,25,28,29,38) with various genetic interpretations. This conventional thinking can be seriously challenged.

Etiologic Considerations

Koch (25) cited a number of familial cases from the literature. Relatives of probands had isolated varicosities or birthmarks of the posterior neck. Some examples of neurofibromatosis were also included.

[a]On-Line Mendelian Inheritance in Man number.

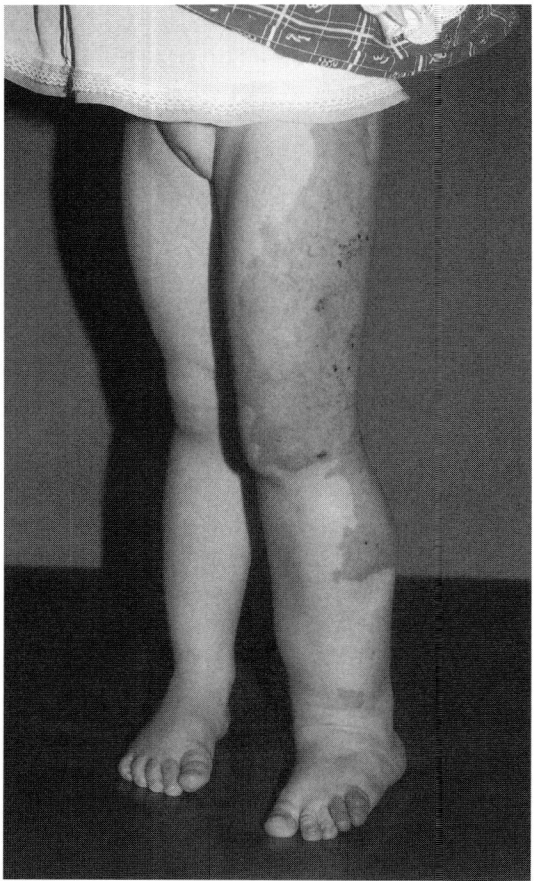

Figure 10–1 Klippel-Trenaunay syndrome. Combined capillary, lymphatic, and venous malformation. Involvement of left leg with extension to buttock and perineum. Note increased girth and axial overgrowth. The cutaneous capillary malformation is studded with lymphatic vesicles. Courtesy of J.B. Mulliken, Boston.

Lian and Alhomme (28) reported congenital varicose veins in three generations of a family in which the propositus had Klippel-Trenaunay syndrome. Norwood and Everett (38) noted an affected propositus whose brother and mother had macular stains scattered over the face and trunk. Lindenauer (29) observed a brother and sister with well-documented Klippel-Trenaunay syndrome. Craven and Wright (12) described a patient with Klippel-Trenaunay syndrome whose grandmother was also said to be affected. Ceballos-Quintal et al. (8) observed a 3-year-old girl with Klippel-Trenaunay syndrome; the mother had a capillary malformation on her back and developed varicose veins in both legs. The maternal grandmother also had varicosities but no vascular malformation.

Aelvoet et al. (1) sent a questionnaire to 114 patients with Klippel-Trenaunay syndrome; results were based on 91 respondents. Klippel-Trenaunay syndrome patients were said to have been found in both a propositus and a second-degree relative in two different families. "Naevi flammei" and "angiomatous naevi" were noted in some relatives of Klippel-Trenaunay syndrome patients. Varicosities were also found in some families. Aelvoet et al. (1) indicated that familial occurrence of Klippel-Trenaunay syndrome was found once in 880 cases.

Happle (20), in reviewing the data provided by Aelvoet et al. (1), suggested that paradominant inheritance could be an explanation of (a) why Klippel-Trenaunay syndrome occurs sporadically, (b) why the lesions of Klippel-Trenaunay syndrome are arranged in mosaic fashion, (c) why relatives with Klippel-Trenaunay syndrome are so rare, and, when recorded, do not exhibit Mendelian inheritance, and (d) why "naevi flammei" show an increased incidence in relatives of Klippel-Trenaunay syndrome patients.

Assuming paradominant inheritance, Klippel-Trenaunay syndrome would be caused by a single gene defect. Heterozygous individuals would almost always be normal and thus the allele would be transmitted imperceptably. The trait would only become expressed if a somatic mutation occurred early during embryonic life. The resultant loss of heterozygosity would result in either homozygosity or hemizygosity for the Klippel-Trenaunay syndrome mutation (20).

Whelan et al. (56) reported a case of Klippel-Trenaunay syndrome associated with a 5:11 balanced translocation. Wexler et al. (55) noted a case with chromosomal mosaicism for a 1:20 translocation.

Careful scrutiny of published "familial cases" indicates one or more of the following problems: (a) inadequate documentation of cases; (b) over-interpretation of minor manifestations in relatives, including "nevus flammeus," hemangiomas, and varicosities,[b] all of which occur

[b] Varicosities in Klippel-Trenaunay syndrome have early onset in infancy or childhood with more extensive distribution than classic varicose veins in the general population.

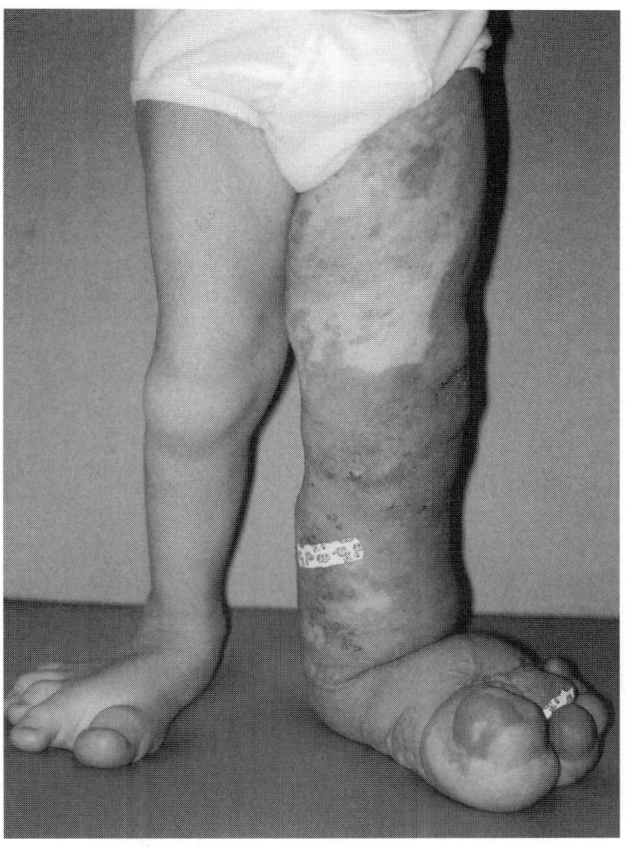

Figure 10–2 Klippel-Trenaunay syndrome. Combined capillary, lymphatic, and venous malformation. Involvement of left leg with an extremely increased girth, axial overgrowth, and macrodactyly. The cutaneous capillary malformation is studded with lymphatic vesicles. Note macrodactyly and gap between great toe and second toe on "unaffected" right leg. Courtesy of J.B. Mulliken, Boston.

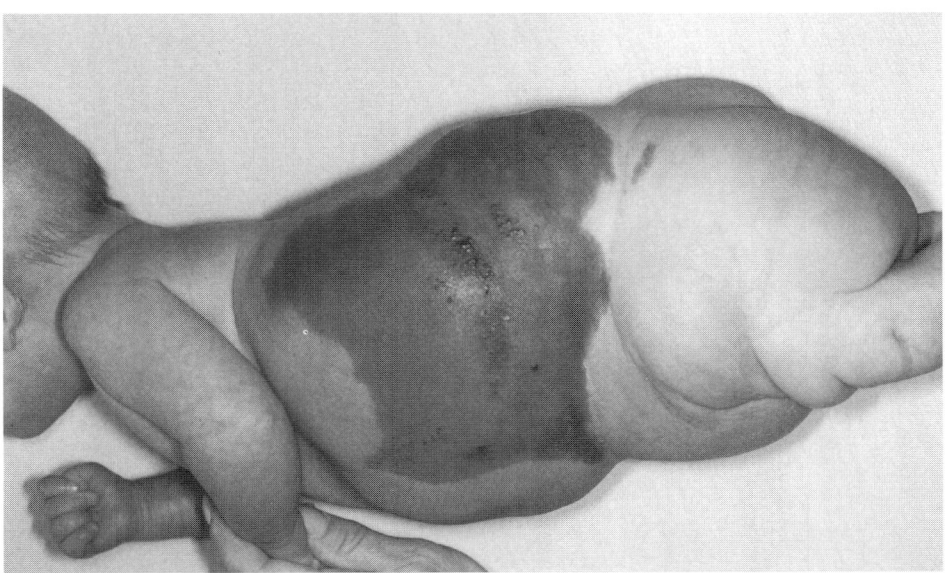

Figure 10–3 Klippel-Trenaunay syndrome with truncal combined capillary, lymphatic, and venous malformation. Note lymphatic vesicles in discolored skin. Soft tissue enlargement is a result of lymphatic macro- and microlymphatic anomalies and excessive fatty tissue. Courtesy of J.B. Mulliken, Boston.

commonly in the general population; and (c) defining Klippel-Trenaunay syndrome is a capillary malformation with or without "hemihypertrophy," with no mention of lymphatic malformations, lateral venous anomaly, lymphatic vesicles or venous flares within the capillary malformation, or macrodactyly; thus, it is uncertain whether these cases represent Klippel-Trenaunay syndrome. Only the affected brother and sister described by Lindenauer (29) are well-documented examples of Klippel-Trenaunay syndrome within a family.

It is possible that when the basic molecular defect becomes known, it may be the same or similar to those of Parkes Weber syndrome and Sturge-Weber syndrome. It is only claimed here that it is useful to distinguish them because their clinical implications are so different. Also, it is not claimed that there is no genetic basis, only that future documentation of families must be much more thorough to prove this.

Capillary Malformations

Capillary malformations of the skin are bluish to purplish in color. Common distribution patterns are shown in Figure 10–4. Most large surgical series of Klippel-Trenaunay syndrome patients do not include patients with capillary malformations involving the face (29,36,46,59).[c] Capillary malformations may be studded with lymphatic vesicles (Figs. 10–1 to 10–3) and venous flares (vide infra).

Varicosities

Varicosities in Klippel-Trenaunay syndrome differ from commonly occurring varicose veins in

[c]Patients with facial involvement in such series are very few in number and no details are given. Samuel and Spitz (46) noted one such patient ($n = 42$). Jacob et al. (22a) noted one patient with "coexisting Sturge-Weber syndrome" ($n = 252$), but also listed Klippel-Trenaunay syndrome patients with "neurofibromatosis" and "Ehlers-Danlos syndrome."

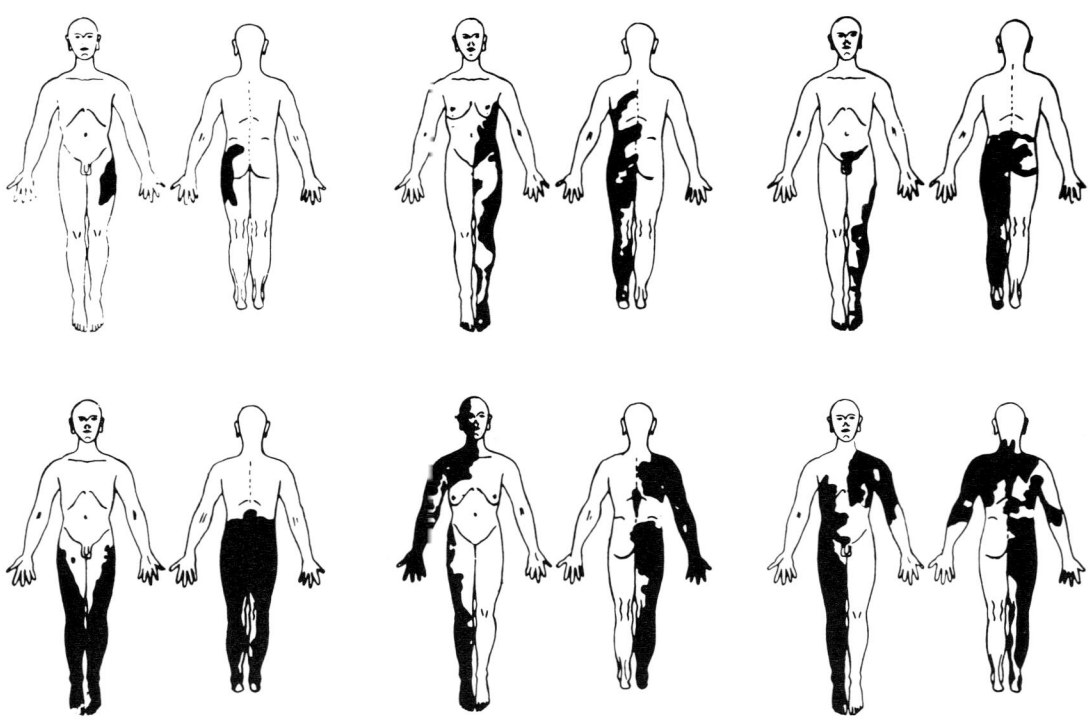

Figure 10–4 Examples of distribution of capillary malformation seen in patients with Klippel-Trenaunay syndrome. From Young (58).

two ways. The distribution is different, being more extensive, and the age of onset is different, first being manifest during infancy or childhood. The classic lesion is the lateral venous anomaly and is known among surgeons as the vein of Servelle (Fig. 10–5); it is found in about 80% of patients. The malformation begins as a plexus of veins on the dorsum and lateral side of the foot and extends superiorly for various distances. Termination occurs in the popliteal vein in 11% of patients, superficial femoral vein in 17%, deep femoral vein in 19%, and external iliac vein in 6%; full leg length distribution is found in 33% of patients (46,59).

Veins may have valves or may be valveless. Ectatic veins may appear as studded venous flares in capillary malformations of the skin. These result from reflex of venous blood secondary to hypertension in the main venous anomaly (59). Intermittent episodes of thrombophlebitis in the affected limb have been reported in about 50% of children ($n = 47$), often associated with pain. Phleboliths result from past thromboses. Pulmonary embolism is found in about 10% of children ($n = 47$) (46) and may be higher in adults (5). The risk is particularly increased postoperatively.

Abnormalities of the deep veins are common in some series but not in others. Defects may include agenesis, atresia, hypoplasia, valvular incompetence, or aneurysmal dilatation (5,29,46, 59). Resection of varicosities in patients with Klippel-Trenaunay syndrome is controversial. Severe vascular reflux and the presence of deep venous anomalies in some cases probably contraindicate excision. Graded elastic compression should be the first line of treatment, with surgical resection being reserved for significant incapacitating problems (46).

Significant arteriovenous communications of the type found in Parkes Weber syndrome are never found in Klippel-Trenaunay syndrome; in many large surgical series (29,46,49,59), clinically significant arteriovenous malformations are not reported (see Parkes Weber syndrome below). In Klippel-Trenaunay syndrome, there are physiologic arteriovenous connections that are always trivial and never clinically important (5,58).

Lymphatic Malformations

Lymphatic abnormalities are very common and are found in more than 70% of patients with Klippel-Trenaunay syndrome (23,59). Cutaneous capillary malformations may be studded with lymphatic vesicles (Figs. 10–1 to 10–3) that leak lymph. Lymphedema of the lower limb is particularly common. When the trunk is involved, lymphatic malformation of the intestine may be associated with a protein-losing enteropathy. Micro- and macrocystic lymphatic malformations often involve the groin, genitalia, and retroperitoneum.

Limb Enlargement

Lower limb enlargement is found in almost all cases. The affected limb may be thicker and longer. Thickness results from soft tissue enlargement and is especially pronounced with lymphatic involvement (Fig. 10–2). Increased adiposity is found in some patients. When the long bones are involved, the affected limb is in-

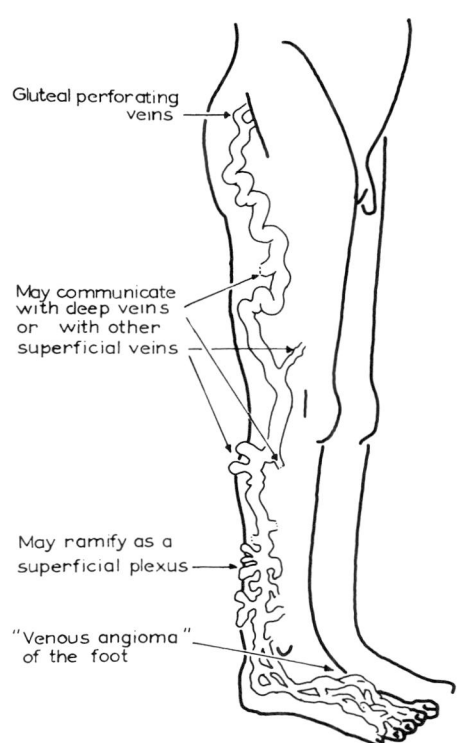

Figure 10–5 Diagram of lateral venous anomaly. See text. From Young (58).

creased in length and bone thickness is also increased. With leg length discrepancy, compensatory scoliosis may result.

Macrodactyly may involve toes on the affected foot but may be present on both feet (Fig. 10–2). Other abnormalities are associated with some cases. Cutaneous syndactyly rarely involves more than two toes. Miscellaneous defects may include polydactyly, clinodactyly, talipes equinovarus, talipes calcaneovarus, and metatarsus varus (33).

Secondary Cutaneous Manifestations

These may include eczema, hyperhidrosis, atrophy, ulceration, and cellulitis (16).

PARKES WEBER SYNDROME

Parkes Weber syndrome, considered a separate entity here, is commonly hyphenated as Parkes-Weber syndrome. In Parkes Weber's own papers (41–43), no hyphen is used. He described patients with enlarged arteries and veins, capillary or venous malformations, and enlargement of a limb. Although Parkes Weber syndrome and Klippel-Trenaunay syndrome are similar, slow-flow venous malformations are predominant in Klippel-Trenaunay syndrome, but arteriovenous (AV) fistulas are always found in Parkes Weber syndrome. Large series of patients are those of Robertson (45) and Young (59). All cases have been sporadic.

The involved limb is warm. The color of the cutaneous vascular malformation is usually more diffuse and pinker than that observed in Klippel-Trenaunay syndrome. Lymphatic malformations do not occur and no lymphatic vesicles are found in the discolored skin. The prognosis in Parkes Weber syndrome is more problematic; cardiac failure may lead to cardiac enlargement and cutaneous ischemia, requiring limb amputation (45,59). Klippel-Trenaunay syndrome and Parkes Weber syndrome are contrasted in Table 10–1.

STURGE-WEBER SYNDROME

Sturge-Weber syndrome, a sporadically occurring disorder, is defined as a capillary malformation of the leptomeninges with or without choroid and facial V_1 or V_1–V_2 involvement

Table 10–1 Comparison of Klippel-Trenaunay Syndrome and Parkes Weber Syndrome

	Klippel-Trenaunay Syndrome	Parkes Weber Syndrome
Types of vascular malformations	Slow flow; capillary, lymphatic, venous	Fast flow; capillary, arterial, venous
Color of cutaneous malformation	Bluish to purplish	Pink and diffuse
Arteriovenous fistulas	Insignificant	Significant
Lateral venous anomaly	Very common	Not found
Lymphatic vesicles[a]	Present	Not found
Venous flares[a]	Present	Not found
Limb affected		
Upper	5%	23%
Lower	95%	77%
Limb enlargement	Usually disproportionate, involving soft and bone; macrodactyly, particularly of toes common	Arm or leg length discrepancy
Prognosis	Usually good; pulmonary embolism encountered occasionally in about 10% of children ($n = 47$). Risk particularly increased postoperatively	More problematic, particularly in those who develop heart failure resulting in cardiac enlargement and cutaneous ischemia, requiring limb amputation

[a]Because Klippel-Trenaunay syndrome has combined capillary, lymphatic, and venous malformations, lymphatic vesicles appear on the surface of the cutaneous capillary malformation and may ooze lymph. The lateral venous anomaly may have protrusions known as venous flares on the surface of the cutaneous capillary malformation.

Source: Data from Young (59), Robertson (45), and Samuel and Spitz (46).

(Table 10–2). The syndrome can be explained by an embryonic defect with secondary consequences. During the sixth week of development, a vascular plexus forms around the cephalic portion of the neural tube and beneath the ectoderm destined to become facial skin. Normally, this vascular plexus regresses during the ninth week, but in Sturge-Weber syndrome, it persists, resulting in a capillary malformation of the leptomeninges overlying the cerebral cortex together with a facial "port-wine" stain on the ipsilateral side. Variation in the persistence or regression of the vascular plexus accounts for cases with unilateral or bilateral involvement (Fig. 10–6) and also for cases with capillary malformation of the leptomeninges with absence of facial involvement (2,11,51).

Capillary malformations of the skin may extend below the head and neck and appear anywhere on the body, including the upper and lower limbs (Fig. 10–7). Limb involvement is different from that found in Klippel-Trenaunay syndrome. The latter has lymphatic malformations, lateral venous anomaly, lymphatic vesicles and venous flares within the capillary malformation, limb enlargement, and macrodactyly, which do not occur in Sturge-Weber syndrome. Only capillary malformations are found in Sturge-Weber syndrome. Hemiparesis, present in some patients, may result in a hypotrophic limb.

Overgrowth may occur in Sturge-Weber syndrome but tends to be minor and is always secondary to the vascular anomaly. Overgrowth of the bony maxilla is common. When the capillary malformation involves the ear, its length may be greater than that of the contralateral ear. Rarely, a digit may be enlarged. In contrast, overgrowth in Klippel-Trenaunay syndrome is striking and macrodactyly may occur in the "uninvolved" limb.

Seizures occur in about 83% of the cases (Table 10–2). These can begin during infancy; seizures are contralateral to the leptomeningeal capillary malformation. Most often seizures are local but generalized seizures may also occur. Hemiparesis is less frequent (2,51).

CT and MRI may demonstrate subtle early leptomeningeal abnormalities. Using SPECT with xenon-133 to evaluate cerebral blood flow, 75% of infants studied prior to the onset of seizures had increased cerebral blood flow in the involved cortex. Patients who had already developed seizures had hypoperfusion of the damaged hemisphere. Thus, rapid cerebral impairment follows seizures in patients with Sturge-Weber syndrome (4,9,13).

Seizures and Cognitive Disability

An alteration in the vascular dynamics of leptomeningeal malformation results in precipitation of calcium deposits in the cerebral cortex underlying the vascular malformation (Fig. 10–8). Seizures and mental deficiency may be secondary to this process. Several other possibilities have been suggested. First, documented microgyria might account for intractable seizures and cognitive deterioration. Second, arterial or venous thrombosis might also explain neurological and neuropsychological deterioration. Third, high seizure rates of discharge from the involved hemisphere might interfere with the function of the normal hemisphere or with its vascular control. Focal hyperperfusion for voluntary and cognitive acts might then be impaired. Fourth, abnormal venous circulation with reduced capacity for venous return might result in venous hypertension and chronic progressive ischemia. Failure to increase cerebral blood flow during seizures might then compromise an already ischemic cortex, resulting in further deficit and more seizures (2,4,30–32,40,50, 53).

Table 10–2 Manifestations of Sturge-Weber Syndrome

Manifestation	Percentage ($n = 52$)
Craniofacial capillary malformation	98
Unilateral	46
Bilateral	54
V_1	100
V_2	76
V_3	60
Extracephalic capillary malformation	52
Seizures	83
Neurologic deficits	65
Headaches	62
Glaucoma	60
Lower limb hemihypoplasia	48

Source: Adapted from Sujansky and Conradi (51).

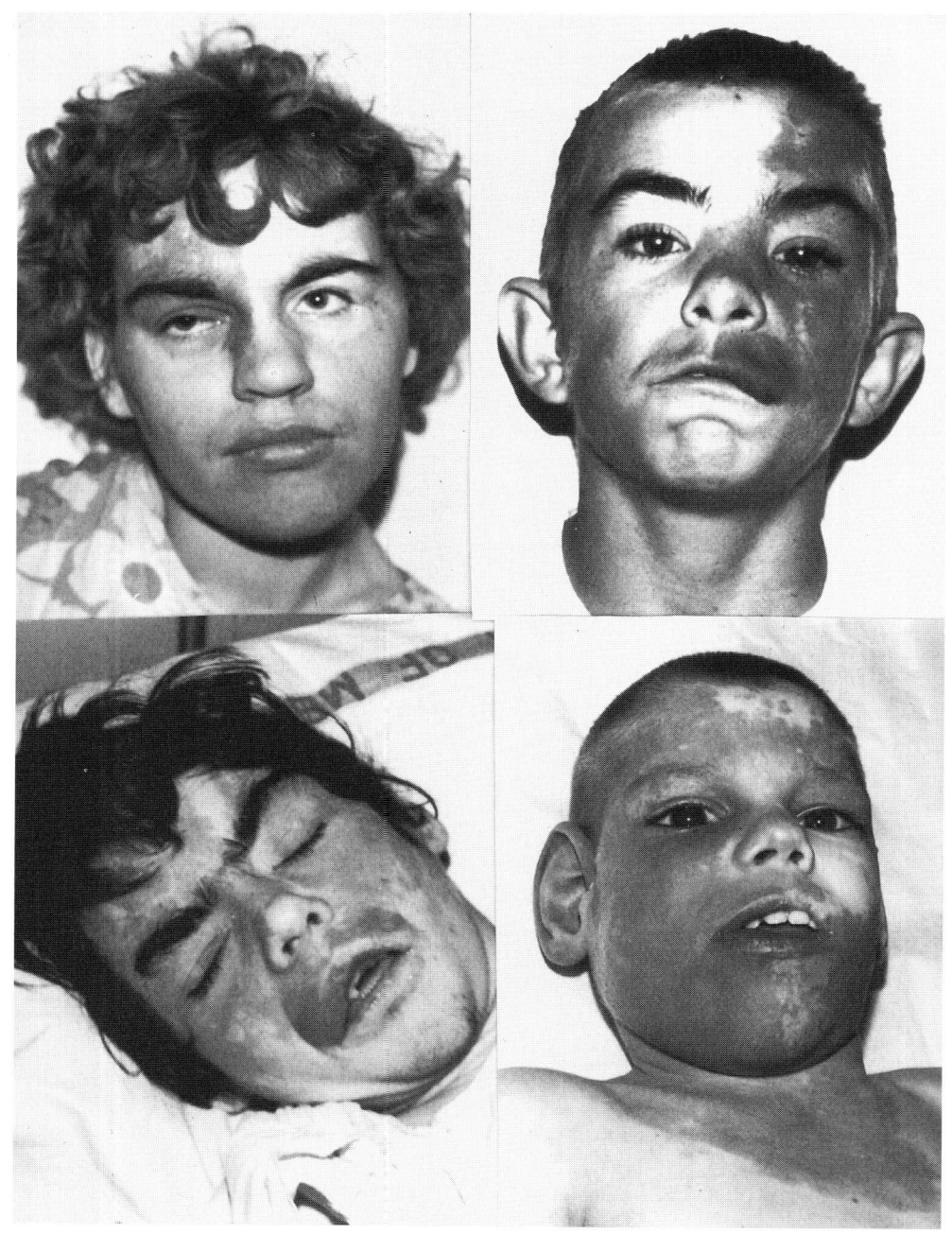

Figure 10–6 Sturge-Weber syndrome. Variation in facial capillary malformation. **Top:** Unilateral involvement. **Bottom:** Bilateral involvement.

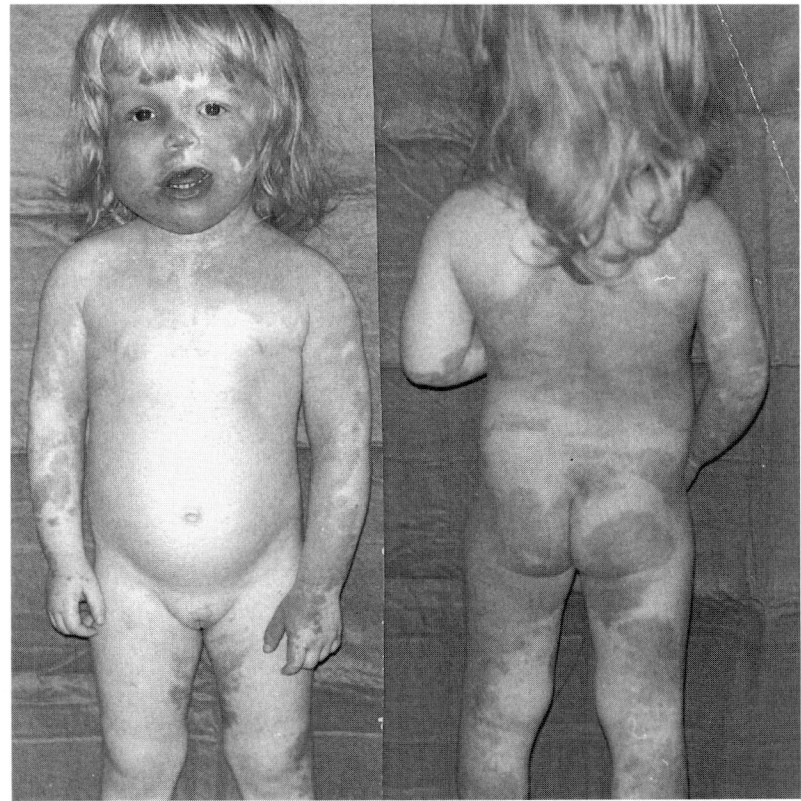

Figure 10–7 Sturge-Weber syndrome. Bilateral facial involvement with extension of capillary malformation to neck, upper chest, back, buttocks, and limbs.

VASCULAR TUMORS AND VASCULAR MALFORMATIONS

Mulliken and Glowacki (37), Mulliken (34), and Burns et al. (7) made a distinction between hemangiomas and vascular malformations based on cellular kinetics and clinical behavior. These differences have been discussed in Chapter 1. Clinical conditions of concern in this chapter—Klippel-Trenaunay syndrome, Parkes Weber syndrome, and Sturge-Weber syndrome—have vascular malformations, not hemangiomas.

KASABACH-MERRITT PHENOMENON

The term "Kasabach-Merritt syndrome" is frequently applied incorrectly to patients with extensive venous or lymphaticovenous malformations who develop a localized intravascular coagulopathy (chronic consumptive coagulopathy) in which the platelet count is minimally depressed, varying from 50,000 to 150,000/mm^3. In contrast, with true Kasabach-Merritt phenomenon, thrombocytopenia is profound, varying from 3000 to 60,000/mm^3 with an average of <25,000/mm^3 (47). The distinction has important treatment implications. For example, heparinization might be indicated in consumptive coagulopathy in vascular malformations, particularly with thrombotic complications, but is contraindicated in Kasabach-Merritt thrombocytopenia found with vascular tumors (47).

Patients with Klippel-Trenaunay syndrome might develop intravascular coagulopathy as a complication, but only two vascular tumors, Kaposiform hemangioendothelioma[d] (Fig. 10–9) and tufted angioma, have been shown to develop Kasabach-Merritt phenomenon as a complication (Table 10–3) (13,14,47,54, 57,60).

---

[d]Kaposiform hemangioendothelioma is not found with AIDS. It is clinically and pathologically distinct from Kaposi sarcoma.

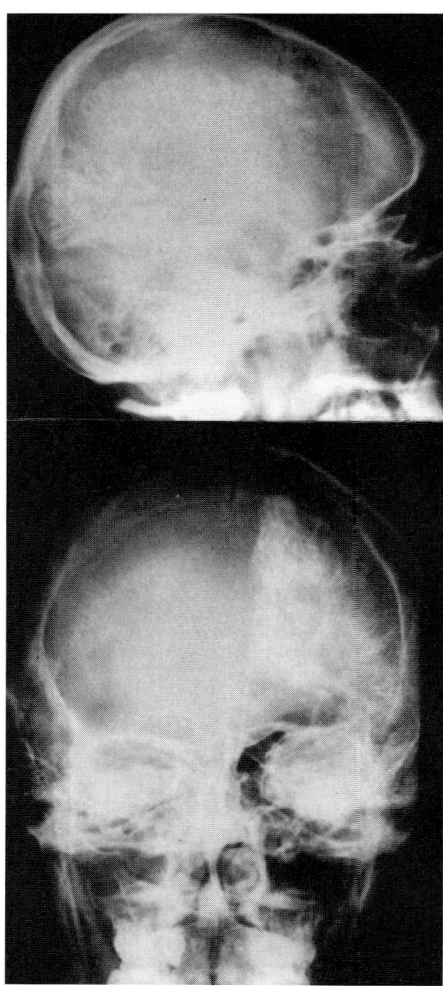

Figure 10–8 Sturge-Weber syndrome. Radiographs showing unilateral distribution of double contoured calcification of cerebral cortex.

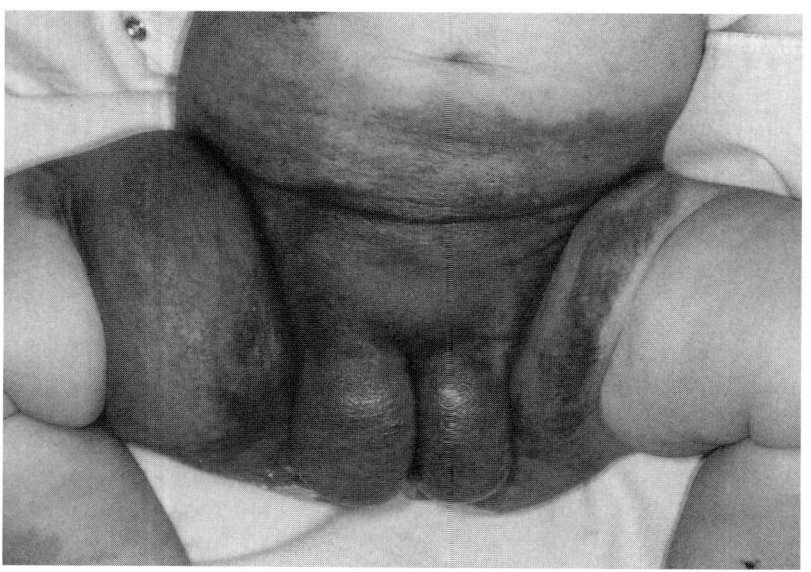

Figure 10–9 Kaposiform hemangioendothelioma in 10-month-old female; histopathologic diagnosis confirmed by biopsy. Tumor appeared at 3 months of age with a platelet count of 16,000/mm^3. Note perineal purpura and edema. Accelerated regression occurred over 3 months after cyclophosphamide for 3 days and interferon alpha-2a for 6 months. From Sarkar et al. (47).

Table 10–3 Comparison of Vascular Lesions in Klippel-Trenaunay Syndrome, Kaposiform Hemangioendothelioma, and Tufted Angioma

	Klippel-Trenaunay Syndrome	Kaposiform Hemangioendothelioma	Tufted Angioma
Clinical appearance	Cutaneous capillary malformation blue to purple in color. Because *combined* vascular malformations occur in Klippel-Trenaunay syndrome, the cutaneous capillary malformation is accompanied by lymphatic and venous malformations that appear on the surface of the capillary malformation as lymphatic vesicles and venous flares.	Cutaneous tumor red to purple in color, centrifugally advancing with rim of ecchymosis	Cutaneous tumor dull red in color that expands slowly at its periphery
Histopathology	Vascular channels lined by single layer of endothelial cells	Tumor with infiltrative growth pattern, spindle-shaped endothelial cells, microthrombi, and hemosiderin	Tumor with discrete vascular tufts in dermis and hypodermis together with peripheral crescent-like slits
Differential diagnosis	Malformation not confused with any other vascular lesion, although sometimes erroneously called "hemangioma"	Can be mistaken for Kaposi sarcoma, but clinical and histopathologic differences. Kaposiform hemangioendothelioma not found with AIDS. HPV-16-like DNA transcripts identified in AIDS and non-AIDS-related Kaposi sarcoma are not found in Kaposiform hemangioendothelioma	Can be mistaken for Kaposi sarcoma or low-grade angiosarcoma, but clinical and histopathologic differences. Tufted angioma not found with AIDS
Kasabach-Merritt phenomenon vs. localized intravascular coagulopathy	Localized intravascular coagulopathy (chronic consumptive coagulopathy). Platelet count minimally depressed, varying from 50,000 to 150,000/mm^3. Found with Klippel-Trenaunay syndrome and non–Klippel-Trenaunay syndrome patients with extensive venous or lymphaticovenous malformations	Kasabach-Merritt phenomenon with profound thrombocytopenia, varying from 3000 to 60,000/mm^3 with an average of <25,000/mm^3	Kasabach-Merritt phenomenon with profound thrombtocytopenia, varying from 3000 to 60,000/mm^3 with an average of <25,000/mm^3

Sources: Sarker et al. (47), Enjolras and Mulliken (13), Enjolras et al. (14), Wilson Jones and Orkin (57), Weiss and Enzinger (54), Zuckerberg et al. (60).

Table 10–4 Criteria for Distinctions Between Klippel-Trenaunay, Parkes Weber, and Sturge-Weber Syndromes

Klippel-Trenaunay syndrome	Slow flow, combined vascular malformation (capillary, lymphatic, and venous) involving limb(s) and/or trunk
Parkes Weber syndrome	Fast flow, combined vascular malformation (capillary, arterial, and venous) involving upper/lower limbs
Sturge-Weber syndrome	Capillary malformation of leptomeninges with or without choroid and facial V_1 or V_1–V_2 involvement. Capillary malformations can occur elsewhere on body

Source: Adapted from Cohen (11).

DIAGNOSIS

Klippel-Trenaunay syndrome should be separated clinically from Parkes Weber syndrome because the prognosis is much more problematic in the latter disorder with its associated AV communications (Table 10–4). Although geneticists, dermatologists, and many other clinicians have merged the two conditions as "Klippel-Trenaunay-Weber syndrome," surgeons who deal with large numbers of Klippel-Trenaunay syndrome patients all separate the two disorders (29,36,46,49,59).

Presumed cases of merged Klippel-Trenaunay syndrome and Sturge-Weber syndrome simply represent Sturge-Weber syndrome with capillary malformations below the head and neck (Table 10–4). None of these presumed "combined cases" have essential manifestations of Klippel-Trenaunay syndrome, such as lymphatic malformations, lateral venous anomaly, lymphatic vesicles and venous flares within the cutaneous capillary malformation, limb enlargement, or macrodactyly.

Documenting the manifestations of Klippel-Trenaunay syndrome more thoroughly is essential in the future. Included should be an MRI with gadolinium to distinguish lymphatic from venous malformations. When this is done, perhaps all or most patients with true Klippel-Trenaunay syndrome will be found to have a lymphatic component. Careful study (magnetic resonance venogram or phlebography/venography) should also document the lateral venous anomaly and any abnormalities that may be present in the deep veins of the leg.

MRI is the most informative modality for studying various vascular malformations and can demonstrate flow characteristics and the extent of involvement within tissue planes. MRI can demonstrate the arteriovenous malformations of Parkes Weber syndrome. Cranial CT and MRI with contrast enhancement can demonstrate early leptomeningeal abnormalities in Sturge-Weber syndrome. Additional single photon emission CT (SPECT) with xenon-133 to evaluate cerebral blood flow is a highly reliable method for diagnosing the CNS abnormalities in Sturge-Weber syndrome. In various conditions, CT may be used to demonstrate intraosseous vascular malformations and also secondary bone changes (13,34,35).

DIFFERENTIAL DIAGNOSIS

Vascular malformations may also occur in Maffucci syndrome (Chapter 11), Bannayan-Riley-Ruvalcaba syndrome (Chapter 8), Proteus syndrome (Chapter 9), and macrocephaly–cutis marmorata syndrome (Chapter 15). Increased limb girth and macrodactyly may be found in hemihyperplasia (Chapter 3).

REFERENCES

1. Aelvoet AE, Jorens PG, Boelen LM: Genetic aspects of the Klippel-Trenaunay syndrome. Br J Dermatol 126:603–607, 1992.
2. Alexander GL, Norman RM: *The Sturge-Weber Syndrome*. Wright and Son, Bristol, pp. 1–5, 55–70, 80–82, 1960.
3. Arrighi F: Hamartose ecto-mesodérmique: Un cas de fusion de maladie de Recklinghausen (avec éléphantiasis nevromateux de Virchow) et de maladie de Klippel-Trénaunay-Parkes Weber. Bull Soc Fr Dermatol Syphiligr 67:564, 1960.
4. Aylett SE, Neville BGR, Cross JH, Boyd S, Chong WK, Kirkham FJ: Sturge-Weber syndrome: cerebral haemodynamics during seizure activity. Dev Med Child Neurol 41:480–485, 1999.

5. Baskerville PA, Ackroyd JS, Browse NL: The etiology of the Klippel-Trenaunay syndrome. Ann Surg 202:624–627, 1985.
6. Bonse G: Röntgenbefunde bei einer Phakomatose (Sturge-Weber kombiniert mit Klippel-Trénaunay). Fortschr Roentgenstr 74:727–729, 1951.
7. Burns AJ, Kaplan LC, Mulliken JB: Is there an association between hemangioma and syndromes with dysmorphic features? Pediatrics 88:1257–1267, 1991.
8. Ceballos-Quintal JM, Pinto-Escalante D, Castillo-Zapata I: A new case of Klippel-Trenaunay-Weber (KTW) syndrome: evidence of autosomal dominant inheritance. Am J Med Genet 63:426–427, 1996.
9. Chiron C, Raynaud C, Tzourio N: Regional cerebral blood flow by SPECT imaging in Sturge-Weber disease: An aid for diagnosis. J Neurol Neurosurg Psychiatry 52:1402–1409, 1989.
10. Cohen MM Jr: Klippel-Trenaunay syndrome: A critical analysis. Am J Med Genet 93:171–175, 2000.
11. Cohen MM Jr: Some neoplasms and some hamartomatous syndrome: Genetic considerations. Int J Oral Maxillofac Surg 27:363–369, 1998.
12. Craven N, Wright AL: Familial Klippel-Trenaunay syndrome. A case report. Clin Exp Dermatol 20:76–79, 1995.
13. Enjolras O, Mulliken JB: Vascular tumors and vascular malformations. Adv Dermatol 13:375–422, 1998.
14. Enjolras O, Wassef M, Mazoyer E, Frieden IJ, Rieu PN, Drouet L, Taïeb A, Stalder J-F, Escande J-P: Infants with Kasabach-Merritt syndrome do not have "true" hemangiomas. J Pediatr 130:631–640, 1997.
15. Furukawa T, Igata A, Toyokura Y, Ikeda S: Sturge-Weber and Klippel-Trenaunay syndrome with nevus of Otta and Ito. Arch Dermatol 102:640–645, 1970.
16. Gloviczki P, Hollier LH, Telander RL: Surgical implications of Klippel-Trénaunay syndrome. Ann Surg 197:353–362, 1983.
17. Gorlin RJ, Cohen MM Jr, Levin LS: *Syndromes of the Head and Neck*, 3rd ed. Oxford University Press, New York, 1990.
18. Gottron HA, Schnyder UW: Vererbung von Hautkrankheiten. In: *Handbuch der Haut-und Geschlechtskrankheiten*, Vol. 7. Springer-Verlag, Berlin, p. 715, 1966.
19. Gourie-Devi M, Prakash B: Vertebral and epidural hemangioma with paraplegia in Klippel-Trénaunay-Weber syndrome. J Neurosurg 48:814–817, 1978.
20. Happle R: Klippel-Trenaunay syndrome: Is it a paradominant trait? Bri J Dermatol 128:465, 1993.
21. Heuser M: De l'entite nosologique des angiomatses neuro-cutanées (Sturge-Weber et Klippel-Trénaunay). Rev Neurol (Paris) 124:213–228, 1971.
22. Inui M, Chiba R, Shike S: An autopsy case of Klippel-Trénaunay-Weber's disease. Acta Pathol Jpn 19:251–263, 1969.
22a. Jacob AG, Driscoll DJ, Shaughnessy WJ, Stanson AW, Clay RP, Gloviczki P: Klippel-Trenaunay syndrome: Spectrum and management. Mayo Clin Proc 73:28–36, 1998.
23. Kinmonth JB, Young AE, Edwards JM et al: Mixed vascular deformities of the lower limbs with particular reference to lymphography and surgical treatment. Brit J Surg 63:899, 1976.
24. Klippel M, Trenaunay P: Du naevus variqueux ostëohypertrophique. Arch Génét Méd Paris 3:611–672, 1900.
25. Koch G: Zur Klinik, Symptomatologie, Pathogenese und Erbpathologie des Klippel-Trenaunay-Weberschen syndroms. Acta Genet Med Gemellol 5:326–370, 1956.
26. Kondo K, Tanaka K, Fujii T, Akita S: Klippel-Trenaunay-Weber syndrome associated with intra-abdominal lymphangioma requiring multiple surgical interventions. Ann Plast Surg 39:435–437, 1997.
27. Kuffer FR, Starzynski TE, Girolami , Murphy L, Grabstald H: Klippel-Trénaunay-Weber syndrome, visceral angiomatosis and thrombocytopenia. J Pediatr Surg 3:65–72, 1968.
28. Lian C, Alhomme P: Les varices congénitale par dysembryoplasie (syndrome de Klippel-Trenaunay). Arch Mal Coeur 38:176, 1945.
29. Lindenauer SM: The Klippel-Trenaunay-Weber syndrome: Varicosity, hypertrophy and hemangioma with no arteriovenous fistula. Ann Surg 162:303–314, 1965.
30. Maria BL, Neufeld JA, Rosainz LC, Ben-David K, Drane WE, Quisling RG, Hamed LM: High prevalence of bihemispheric structural and functional defects in Sturge-Weber syndrome. J Child Neurol 13:595–605, 1998.
31. Maria BL, Neufeld JA, Rosanz LC, Drane WE, Quisling RG, Ben-David K, Hamed LM: Central nervous system structure and function in Sturge-Weber syndrome: Evidence of neurologic and radiologic progression. J Child Neurol 13:606–618, 1998.
32. Marti-Bonmati L, Menor F, Mulas F: The Sturge-Weber syndrome: Correlation between the clinical status and radiological CT and MRI findings. Child Nerv Syst 9:107–109, 1993.
33. McGrory BJ, Amadio PC, Dobyns JH, Stickler GB, Unni KK: Anomalies of the fingers and toes associated with Klippel-Trenaunay syndrome. J Bone Joint Surg 73A:1537–1546, 1991.
34. Mulliken JB: Cutaneous vascular anomalies. Semin Vasc Surg 6:204–218, 1993.
35. Mulliken JB: Vascular Anomalies. In: *Grabb and Smith's Plastic Surgery*, 5th ed. SJ Aston, RW Beasley, CHM Thorne, eds. Lippincott-Raven, Philadelphia, pp. 191–203, 1997.

36. Mulliken JB: Personal communication, 1999.
37. Mulliken JB, Glowacki J: Hemangiomas and vascular malformations in infants and children: A classification based on endothelial characteristics. Plast Reconstr Surg 69:412–420, 1982.
38. Norwood OT, Everett MD: Cardiac failure due to endocrine dependent hemangiomas. Arch Dermatol 89:759–760, 1964.
39. O'Connor PS, Smith JL: Optic nerve variant in the Klippel-Trénaunay-Weber syndrome. Ann Ophthalmol 10:131–137, 1978.
40. Okudaira Y, Arai H, Sato K: Hemodynamic compromise as a factor in clinical progression of Sturge-Weber syndrome. Childs Nerv Syst 13: 214–219, 1997.
41. Parkes Weber F: Angioma formation in connection with hypertrophy of limbs and hemihypertrophy. Br J Dermatol 19:231, 1907.
42. Parkes Weber F: Haemangiectatic hypertrophies of the foot and lower extremity. Med Press (London) 136:261, 1908.
43. Parkes Weber F: Haemangiectatic hypertrophy of the limbs—Congenital phlebarteriectasis and so-called congenital varicose veins. Br J Child Dis 15:13, 1918.
44. Rademacher R: Über einen Fall einer Kombination von Sturge-Weber und Klippel-Trénaunay-Syndrom mit konstitutioneller Neurodermitis. Dermatol Wochenschr 143:381–386, 1961.
45. Robertson DJ: Congenital arteriovenous fistulae of the extremities. Ann R Coll Surg Engl 18:73, 1956.
46. Samuel M, Spitz L: Klippel-Trenaunay syndrome: Clinical features, complications and management in children. Br J Surg 82 757–761, 1995.
47. Sarkar M, Mulliken JB, Kozakewich HPW, Robertson RL, Burrows PE: Thrombocytopenic coagulopathy (Kasabach-Merritt phenomenon) is associated with Kaposiform hemangioendothelioma and not with common infantile hemangioma. Plast Reconstr Surg 100:1377–1386, 1997.
48. Schönenberg H, Redemann M: Klippel-Trénaunay-Weber Syndrom. Klin Pädiatr 184: 449–460, 1972.
49. Servelle M: Klippel and Trenaunay's syndrome. 768 operated cases. Ann Surg 201:365–373, 1985.
50. Simonati A, Colamaria V, Bricolo A, Dalla-Bernardina B, Rizzuto N: Microgyria associated with Sturge-Weber angiomatosis. Child Nerv Syst 10:392–395, 1994.
51. Sujansky E, Conradi S: Outcome of Sturge-Weber syndrome in 52 adults. Am J Med Genet 57:35–45, 1995.
52. Teller H, Lindner B: Über Mischformen der phakomatahosen Syndrome von Sturge-Weber und Klippel-Trénaunay. Z Haut Geschlechtskr 13:113–120, 1952.
53. Vargha-Khadem F, Carr L, Isaacs E, Brett E, Adams C, Mishkin M: Onset of speech after left hemispherectomy in a nine-year-old boy. Brain 120:159–182, 1997.
54. Weiss SW, Enzinger FM: Spindle cell hemangioendothelioma—A low grade angiosarcoma resembling a cavernous hemangioma and Kaposi's sarcoma. Am J Surg Pathol 10:521–530, 1986.
55. Wexler P, McGavran L, Sujansky E: Unilateral chromosomal mosaicism in Klippel-Trenaunay-Weber syndrome with short stature. 13th Annual David W. Smith Workshop on Malformations and Morphogenesis, August 5–9, Wake Forest University, Winston-Salem, North Carolina, 1992.
56. Whelan AJ, Watson MS, Porter FD, Steiner RD: Klippel-Trenaunay-Weber syndrome associated with a 5:11 balanced translocation. Am J Med Genet 59:492–494, 1995.
57. Wilson Jones E, Orkin M: Tufted angioma (angioblastoma). J Am Acad Dermatol 20:214–225, 1989.
58. Young AE: Mixed vascular deformities. M Chir Thesis, University of Cambridge, Cambridge, England, 1978.
59. Young AE: Hemangiomas and malformations. In: *Vascular Birthmarks*. JB Mulliken and AE Young, eds. W.B. Saunders, Philadelphia, 1988.
60. Zuckerberg LR, Nickoloff BJ, Weiss SW: Kaposiform hemangioendothelioma of infancy and childhood: An aggressive neoplasm associated with Kasabach-Merritt syndrome and lymphangiomatosis. Am J Surg Pathol 17: 321–328, 1993.

Maffucci Syndrome

Maffucci syndrome (OMIM 166000)[a] is characterized by multiple enchondromas with bone distortion together with vascular malformations, particularly venous but also capillary and sometimes lymphatic (Figs. 11–1 and 11–2). Early reports are those of Maffucci in 1881 (44) and Kast and von Recklinghausen in 1889 (35). A number of reviews are available (2,9,10,14,34,40). Well over 100 cases have been recorded. To date, the etiology is unknown and all cases have been sporadic.

SKELETAL SYSTEM

Enchondromas are cartilaginous tumors located within bone shafts, often causing bulging of the cortices (31). They are most numerous in the phalanges of the hands and feet, but may involve *any* bone preformed in cartilage. They may occur unilaterally or bilaterally but asymmetrically. Resultant bone abnormalities may include gross bone distortion, limb length discrepancy, bowing of limb bones, scoliosis, short stature, and fractures (2,5,10,12,15,17–19,21,26,29,32,33,37, 38,40,42,45,49,56,60,62).

VASCULAR ABNORMALITIES

Vascular malformations are most commonly venous, but capillary malformations have also been recorded (2,3,13,15,17,19–21,40,43,50,62). Although the hand is a frequent site, any portion of the skin may be involved. Internal sites have also been noted, including the meninges (20), tongue (36–38,41,43,45), buccal mucosa (6,38, 41), palate (3,27,43,56,61), pharynx (41,42,60), esophagus, ileum, and anal mucosa (26,28). Phlebectasia and phlebolithiasis (2,3,7,8,12,21, 29,32,38,40,45,49,57) are common. Lymphatic malformations have been found in some cases (5,38,41,45,58).

NEOPLASMS

Chondrosarcoma may develop in enchondromas and have been reported in a number of cases (2,8,9,19–21,26,32,40,56,57). The incidence of malignant transformation has been estimated as 17.8% (57) and as 30% (34). These figures are clearly inflated because of reporting bias. A variety of other tumors have been noted in association with Maffucci syndrome; these are listed in Table 11–1.

DIFFERENTIAL DIAGNOSIS

Enchondromas differ from osteochondromas, the former occurring within bone, the latter occurring as exostoses at the metaphyses (31). Enchondromas may occur as isolated tumors (31). Multiple enchondromas occur in Ollier enchondromatosis. In this condition, multiple enchondromas are found without vascular malformations. Most cases are sporadic but some familial

[a]On-Line Mendelian Inheritance in Man number.

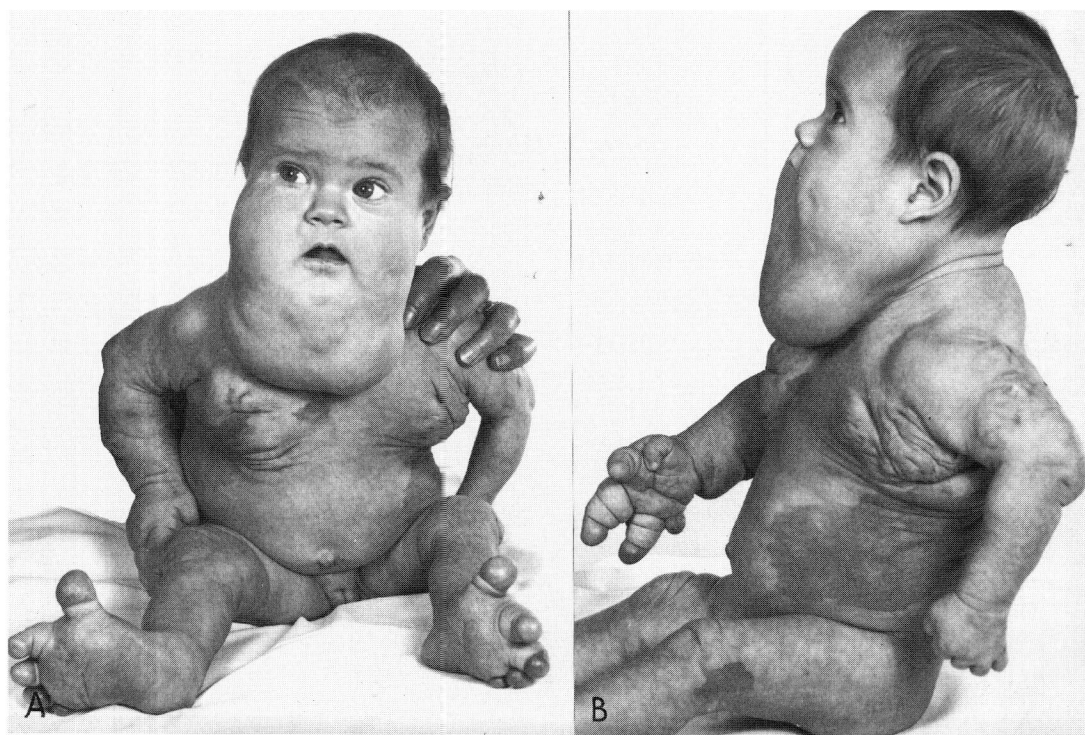

Figure 11–1 **A,B:** Gross distortion of body caused by multiple enchondromas of the hands and feet together with venous, capillary, and lymphatic malformations. From Matthews (47).

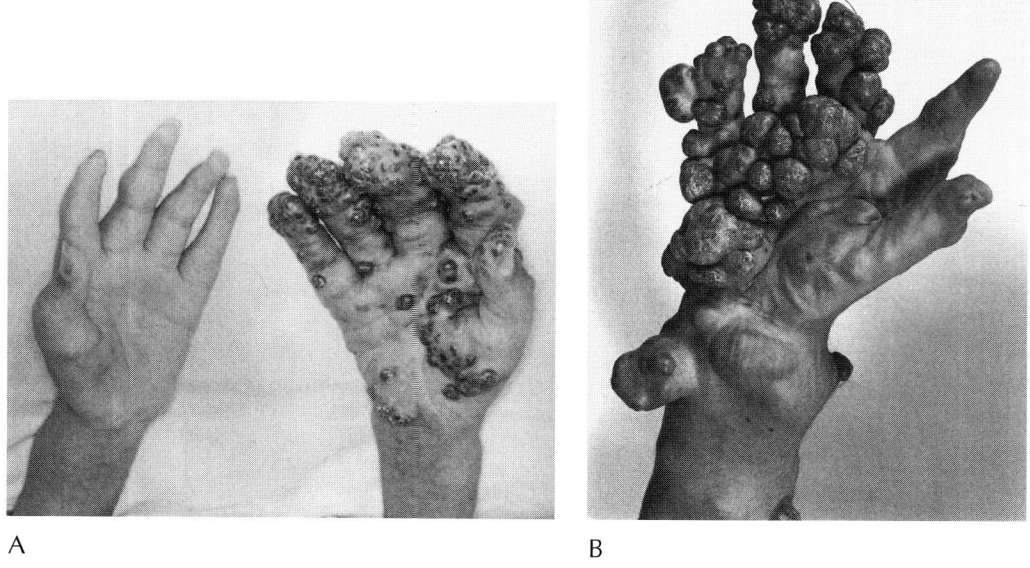

A   B

Figure 11–2 **A:** Vascular malformations and enchondromatous involvement. From Ma and Leung (43). **B:** More severe involvement. From Tilsley and Burden (60). **C:** Distortion from multiple enchondromas. From Bean (9). **D:** Radiograph showing enchondromas of phalanges. From Cauble and Bowman (17).

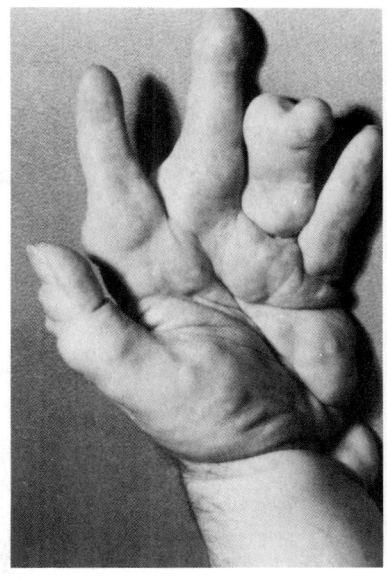
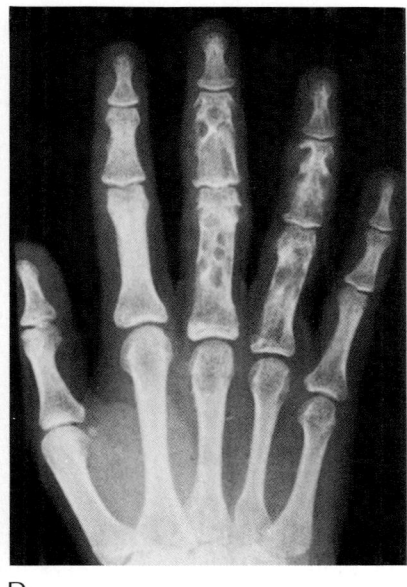

C D

Figure 11–2 (continued).

Table 11–1 Neoplasms Associated with Maffucci Syndrome

Neoplasms	References
Chondrosarcoma	Sun et al. (57), Kaplan et al. (34)
Carotid body tumor	Armstrong et al. (4)
Angiosarcoma	Bean (9)
Fibrosarcoma	Johnson et al. (32)
Pancreatic carcinoma	Johnson et al. (32), Sun et al. (57)
Hepatic adenocarcinoma	Sun et al. (57)
Ovarian teratoma	Kuzma and King (38)
Ovarian cystadenocarcinoma	Lowell and Mathog (42)
Malignant ovarian tumor, mesenchymal origin, otherwise unspecified	Lewis and Ketchan (40)
Glioma	Carleton et al. (14), Cremer et al. (20)
Astrocytoma	Cremer et al. (20)
Pituitary adenoma	Marymount et al. (46)
Brain tumor, unspecified	Sun et al. (57)

Table 11–2 Classification of the Enchondromatoses

Disorders	Mode of Inheritance	OMIM[a]
Isolated enchondroma	Sporadic	—
Ollier enchondromatosis	Sporadic, few familial instances	166000
Maffucci syndrome	Sporadic	166000
Spondyloenchondromatosis	Autosomal recessive	271550
Spondyloenchondromatosis with basal ganglia calcification	Autosomal recessive	—
Dysspondyloenchondromatosis	—	—
Metachondromatosis	Autosomal dominant	156250

[a]On-Line Mendelian Inheritance in Man number, when available.
Source: Adapted from International Working Group on Constitutional Diseases of Bone (30). See also Spranger et al. (54), Frydman et al. (23), Halal and Azouz (25), and Freisinger et al. (22).

instances have been recorded (16,39,51,55). Chondrosarcomas may also occur in Ollier enchondromatosis (48) and two instances of granulosa cell tumor (59,63) have been noted. Enchondromas have been found in several other disorders listed in Table 11–2.

Vascular malformations, limb distortion, and asymmetry occur together with limb enlargement in Klippel-Trenaunay syndrome (Chapter 10). Vascular malformations also occur in the autosomal dominant blue rubber bleb nevus syndrome (11). Gallione et al. (24) suggested that familial venous malformation syndrome that maps to 9p is identical to blue rubber bleb nevus syndrome.

Sakurane et al. (52) reported a patient with Maffucci and blue rubber bleb nevus syndromes. The patient most likely had just Maffucci syndrome. Schnall and Genuth (53) reported a case with enchondromas, vascular malformations, pituitary adenoma, parathyroid adenoma, and neurilemoma that may represent a disorder different from Maffucci syndrome.

REFERENCES

1. Allen BR: Maffucci's syndrome. Br J Dermatol 99(Suppl 16):31–33, 1978.
2. Anderson IF: Maffucci's syndrome: Report of a case with a review of the literature. S Afr Med J 39:1066–1070, 1965.
3. Andrén L, Dymling JF, Elmer A, Hogeman KE: Maffucci's syndrome. Report of four cases. Acta Chir Scand 126:397–405, 1963.
4. Armstrong EA, McLennan JE, Benton C, Chambers AA, Perlman AW, Conners JW: Maffucci's syndrome complicated by an intracranial chondrosarcoma and a carotid body tumor. Case report. J Neurosurg 55:479–483, 1981.
5. Ashenhurst EM: Dyschondroplasia with hemangiomata (Maffucci's syndrome). Arch Neurol 2:552–555, 1960.
6. Bachert C: Ein besonderer Fall von multiplen Hämangiomen im Kopf-Hals-Bereich: Variation des Maffucci-Syndroms? HNO 33:472–474, 1985.
7. Bahk YW: Dyschondroplasia with hemangiomata (Maffucci's syndrome). Radiology 82:407–409, 1964.
8. Banna J, Parwani GS: Multiple sarcomas in Maffucci's syndrome. Br J Radiol 42:304–307, 1969.
9. Bean WB: Dyschondroplasia and hemangiomata (Maffucci's syndrome). Arch Intern Med 95:767–778, 1955.
10. Bean WB: Dyschondroplasia and hemangiomata (Maffucci's syndrome). II. Arch Intern Med 102:544–550, 1958.
11. Bean WB: *Vascular Spiders and Related Lesions of the Skin*. Charles C. Thomas, Springfield, Illinois, 1958, pp 178–185.
12. Beranbaum SL, Tzamouranis G: Maffucci's syndrome. Dyschondroplasia with hemangiomas. Report of a case. Am J Roentgenol 80:479–481, 1958.
13. Berlin R: Maffucci's syndrome. Dyschondroplasia with vascular hamartomas. Acta Med Scand 177:299–307, 1965.
14. Carleton A, Elkington JStC, Greenfield JG, Robb Smith AMT: Maffucci's syndrome (dyschondroplasia with haemangeomata). Q J Med 11:203–228, 1942.
15. Cameron JM: Maffucci's syndrome. Br J Surg 44:596–598, 1957.
16. Carbonell Juanico M, Vineta Teixido J: Otro caso de discondroteosis generalizada congenita, tipo Ollier. Rev Esp Pediatr 18:91–99, 1962.
17. Cauble WG, Bowman HS: Dyschondroplasia and hemangiomas (Maffucci's syndrome). Presentation of one case. Arch Surg 97:678–681, 1968.
18. Chen VT, Harrison DA: Maffucci's syndrome. Hand 10:292–298, 1978.
19. Cook PL, Evans PG: Chondrosarcoma of the skull in Maffucci's syndrome. Br J Radiol 50:833–836, 1977.
20. Cremer H, Gullotta F, Wolf L: The Maffucci-Kast syndrome. Dyschondroplasia with hemangiomas and frontal lobe astrocytoma. J Cancer Res Clin Oncol 101:231–237, 1981.
21. Elmore SM, Cantrell WC: Maffucci's syndrome. Case report with a normal karyotype. J Bone Joint Surg 48A:1607–1613, 1966.
22. Freisinger P, Finidori G, Maroteaux P: Dysspondyloenchondromatosis. Am J Med Genet 45:460–464, 1993.
23. Frydman M, Bar Ziv J, Preminger-Shapiro R, Brezner A, Brand N, Ben-Ami T, Lachman RS, Gruber HE, Rimoin DL: Possible heterogeneity in spondyloenchondrodysplasia, quadriparesis, basal ganglia calcifications. Am J Med Genet 36:279–284, 1990.
24. Gallione CJ, Pasyk KA, Boon LM, Lennon F, Johnson DW, Helmbold EA, Markel DS, Vikkula M, Mulliken JB, Warman ML, Pericak-Vance MA, Marchuk DA: A gene for familial venous malformations maps to chromosome 9p in a second large kindred. J Med Genet 32:197–199, 1995.
25. Halal F, Azouz EM: Generalized enchondromatosis in a boy with only platyspondyly in the father. Am J Med Genet 38:588–592, 1991.
26. Hall BD: Intestinal hemangiomas and Maffucci's syndrome. Arch Dermatol 105:608, 1972.
27. Halper H, Wedlick L: Maffucci's syndrome: With a report of a case. Med J Aust 1:936–939, 1951.
28. Ikram-ul-Haq, Tait GB, Stuart CE: Maffucci's syndrome. J Int Coll Surg 43:133–140, 1965.

29. Indra KG, Bery K, Chawla S: Dyschondroplasia with multiple haemangiomata—Maffucci's syndrome. Br J Radiol 36:697–698, 1963.
30. International Working Group on Constitutional Diseases of Bone: International nomenclature and classification of the osteochondrodysplasias (1997). Am J Med Genet 79:376–382, 1998.
31. Jaffe HL: *Tumors and Tumorous Conditions of the Bones and Joints*. Lea & Febiger, Philadelphia, 1964.
32. Johnson JL, Webster JR Jr, Sippy HI: Maffucci's syndrome (dyschondroplasia with hemangiomas). Am J Med 28:864–866, 1960.
33. Kaibara N, Mitsuyasu M, Katsuki I, Hotokebuchi T, Takagishi K: Generalised enchondromatosis with the unusual complications of soft tissue calcifications and haemangiomas. Follow-up for a twelve year period. Skeletal Radiol 8:43–46, 1982.
34. Kaplan RP, Wang JT, Amron DM, Kaplan L: Maffucci's syndrome: Two case reports with a literature review. J Am Acad Dermatol 29:894–899, 1994.
35. Kast A, von Recklinghausen F: Ein Fall von Enchondrom mit ungewohnlicher Multiplikation. Virchows Arch Pathol Anat 118:1–18, 1889.
36. Kennedy JG: Dyschondroplasia and haemangiomata (Maffucci's syndrome). Report of a case with oral and intracranial lesions. Br Dent J 135:18–21, 1973.
37. Krause GR: Dyschondroplasia with hemangioma (Maffucci's syndrome). Case report. Am J Roentgenol 52:620–623, 1944.
38. Kuzma JF, King JM: Dyschondroplasia with hemangiomatosis (Maffucci's syndrome) and teratoid tumor of the ovary. Arch Pathol 46:74–82, 1948.
39. Lamy M, Aussannaire M, Jammet ML, Nezelof C: Trois cas de maladie d'Ollier dans une fratrie. Bull Mém Soç Méd Hôp Paris 70:62–70, 1954.
40. Lewis RJ, Ketcham AS: Maffucci's syndrome: Functional and neoplastic significance. Case report and review of the literature. J Bone Joint Surg 55A:1465–1479, 1973.
41. Loewinger RJ, Lichtenstein JR, Dodson WE, Eisen AZ: Maffucci's syndrome: A mesenchymal dysplasia and multiple tumour syndrome. Br J Dermatol 96:317–322, 1977.
42. Lowell SH, Mathog RH: Head and neck manifestations of Maffucci's syndrome. Arch Otolaryngol 105:427–430, 1979.
43. Ma GFY, Leung PC: The management of the soft-tissue haemangiomatous manifestations of Maffucci's syndrome. Br J Plast Surg 37:615–618, 1984.
44. Maffucci A: Di un caso di encondroma ed angioma multiple. Contribuzione alla genesi embrionale dei tumor. Mov Med Chir 3:399–412, 565–575, 1881.
45. Marberg K, Dalith F, Bank H: Dyschondroplasia with multiple hemangiomata (Maffucci's syndrome). Ann Intern Med 49:1216–1228, 1958.
46. Marymount JV, Fisher RF, Emde GE, Limbird TJ: Maffucci's syndrome complicated by carcinoma of the breast, pituitary adenoma, and mediastinal hemangioma. South Med J 80:1429–1431, 1987.
47. Matthews D: The congenitally deformed hand. Br J Plast Surg 17:366–375, 1964.
48. Mirra JM, Gold RH, Marcove RC: *Bone Tumors. Diagnosis and Treatment*. J.B. Lippincott, Philadelphia, 1980.
49. Niechajev IA, Hansson LI: Maffucci's syndrome. Case report. Scand J Plast Reconstr Surg 16:215–219, 1982.
50. Phelan EMD, Carty HML, Kalos S: Generalised enchondromatosis associated with haemangiomas, soft-tissue calcifications and hemihypertrophy. Br J Radiol 59:69–74, 1986.
51. Rossberg A: Zur Erblichkeit der Knochenchondromatose. Fortschr Roentgenstr 90:138–139, 1959.
52. Sakurane HF, Sugai T, Saito T: The association of blue rubber bleb nevus and Maffucci's syndrome. Arch Dermatol 95:28–36, 1967.
53. Schnall AM, Genuth SM: Multiple endocrine adenomas in a patient with the Maffucci syndrome. Am J Med 61:952–956, 1976.
54. Spranger J, Kemperdieck H, Bakowski H, Opitz JM: Two peculiar types of enchondromatosis. Pediatr Radiol 7:215–219, 1978.
55. Steudel NI: Multiple Enchondrome der Knochen in Verbindung mit venoesen Angiomen der Weichteile. Bruns Beitr Klin Chir 8:503–521, 1892.
56. Strang C, Rannie I: Dyschondroplasia with haemangiomata (Maffucci's syndrome). Report of a case complicated by intracranial chondrosarcoma. J Bone Joint Surg 32B:376–383, 1950.
57. Sun T-C, Swee RG, Shives TC, Unni KK: Chondrosarcoma in Maffucci's syndrome. J Bone Joint Surg 67A:1214–1219, 1985.
58. Suringa DWR, Ackerman AB: Cutaneous lymphangiomas with dyschondroplasia (Maffucci's syndrome). A unique variant of an unusual syndrome. Arch Dermatol 101:472–474, 1970.
59. Tamimi HK, Bolen JW: Enchondromatosis (Ollier's disease) and ovarian juvenile granulosa cell tumor. Cancer 53:1605–1608, 1984.
60. Tilsley DA, Burden PW: A case of Maffucci's syndrome. Br J Dermatol 105:331–336, 1981.
61. Torri O: Angiome ed encondromi multiple nello istesso individuo. Clin Chir (Milano) 10:81–105, 1902.
62. Umansky AL: Dyschondroplasia with hemangiomata (Maffucci's syndrome). Report of an early case with mild osseous manifestations. Bull Hosp Joint Dis 7:59–68, 1946.
63. Vaz RM, Turner C: Ollier disease (enchondromatosis) associated with ovarian juvenile granulosa cell tumor and precocious pseudopuberty. J Pediatr 108:945–947, 1986.

12

Neurofibromatosis

Although not a classic overgrowth syndrome like Beckwith-Wiedemann syndrome, neurofibromatosis can be regarded as an overgrowth syndrome by virtue of several of its features: macrocephaly, the presence of tumors, and, on occasion, hemihyperplasia of a limb or digit. The text is extensive because neurofibromatosis is common and well known.

Type 1 neurofibromatosis (NF1) (OMIM 162200)[a] is characterized by cutaneous neurofibromas, café-au-lait spots, and Lisch nodules in over 90% of patients at puberty. Other manifestations, such as axillary and inguinal freckling, deeply situated neurofibromas, plexiform neurofibromas, optic gliomas, macrocephaly, learning difficulties, short stature, scoliosis, and pseudoarthrosis, occur less frequently. Inheritance is autosomal dominant with about 50% of cases representing new mutations (32,48,106).

CLASSIFICATION AND TYPES OF NEUROFIBROMATOSIS

Different types of neurofibromatosis have been classified by OMIM, Riccardi (105,106), Cohen (23,24), and Viskochil and Carey (19,132,133). Various forms of neurofibromatosis, using OMIM numbers,[a] are summarized in Table 12–1. The classification of Viskochil and Carey (19,132,133) is based on molecular advances associated with recognized phenotypes (Table 12–2). Their classification includes (*a*) alternative forms of NF1 and NF2 with some classic findings but with incomplete/atypical presentations and (*b*) related forms of NF1 with some classic findings but with additional manifestations.

Segmental Neurofibromatosis (OMIM 152200)[a]

Neurofibromas and café-au-lait spots restricted to one area of the body have been recorded frequently (55,56,86,106,109,110,110a,113). Combemale et al. (28) reviewed 88 cases. Most patients have a segmental distribution of cutaneous neurofibromas; internal manifestations are uncommon. Evidence is consistent with somatic mosaicism for *NF1* mutations. Lázaro et al. (66) reported germline mosaicism in a family with two children who had the same *NF1* deletion found in 10% of the father's sperm.

Neurofibromatosis-Noonan Syndrome (OMIM 601321)[a]

Whether the neurofibromatosis-Noonan syndrome (3,6,8,17,21,57,84,94,112) represents a true syndrome or variable expression of NF1 has been debated. A number of interpretations are possible: (*a*) chance concurrence of Noonan syndrome and neurofibromatosis; (*b*) neurofibromatosis-Noonan syndrome as an unusual variant of Noonan syndrome; (*c*) neurofibromatosis-Noonan syndrome as an unusual type of neurofibromatosis; and (*d*) neurofibromatosis-Noonan syndrome as a newly recognized entity (17). A discrete disorder may occur in a minority of reported patients who lack Lisch nodules, have few neurofibromas of the skin, and lack

[a]On-Line Mendelian Inheritance in Man number.

Table 12–1 Types of Neurofibromatosis

Name (OMIM)[a]	Inheritance Pattern	Chromosome Localization of Gene	Gene	Comments
Neurofibromatosis, type 1 (NF1) (OMIM 162200)	Autosomal dominant	17q11.2	NF1	NF1 most common type. NF1 gene product = neurofibromin. Tumor suppressor gene
Segmental neurofibromatosis, NF1 Riccardi type 5 (OMIM 162200)	Consistent with mosaicism	17q11.2	NF1	Neurofibromas and café-au-lait spots are restricted to one area of the body.
Neurofibromatosis-Noonan syndrome (OMIM 601321)	Autosomal dominant	17q11.2	NF1	In most cases, Noonanoid features represent variable expression of NF1. This is also Riccardi type 9.
Neurofibromatosis, type 2 (NF2) (OMIM 101000)	Autosomal dominant	22q12.2	NF2	NF2 gene product = merlin. Tumor suppressor gene
Segmental neurofibromatosis, NF2 (OMIM 101000)	Consistent with mosaicism	22q12.2	NF2	Likely a common cause of NF2
Neurofibromatosis, type 3, Riccardi type (OMIM 162260)	Sporadic			Combined NF1 and NF2 features with some added distinctive findings: neurofibromas of palms and absent Lisch nodules. CNS tumors in 2nd and 3rd decades usually lead to rapid and fatal course.
Neurofibromatosis, type 3, Intestinal type (OMIM 162220)	Dominant	?	?	Neurofibromas limited to intestine. This is also Riccardi type 8. ?Linkage to 12q13, 14q13. NF1 also postulated.
Neurofibromatosis, type 4 Riccardi type (OMIM 162270)	Autosomal dominant			Variant forms(s) that differ from NF1, NF2, and Riccardi type 3.
Neurofibromatosis, type 6 Café-au-lait type (OMIM114030)	Autosomal dominant	17q11.2	NF1	Familial café-au-lait spots with no other features of NF1. Has been linked to NF1 gene.
Watson syndrome (OMIM 193520)	Autosomal dominant	17q11.2	NF1	Café-au-lait spots, pulmonic stenosis, and mental deficiency. Has been linked to NF1 gene.
Familial spinal neurofibromatosis (OMIM 162210)	Autosomal dominant	17q11.2	NF1	Café-au-lait spots, but usually lack cutaneous neurofibromas and Lisch nodules.
Duodenal carcinoid syndrome (OMIM 162240)	Sporadic	17q11.2	NF1	Combination of duodenal carcinoid tumor, neurofibromatosis, and pheochromocytoma.
Neurofibromatosis, type 7, Riccardi late-onset type	Sporadic	17q11.2	NF1	Neurofibromas become apparent at end of third decade or later. Café-au-lait spots and Lisch nodules absent.

[a]On-Line Mendelian Inheritance in Man number.

Source: Adapted from OMIM, Riccardi (105,106), and Cohen (23,24).

Table 12–2 The Neurofibromatoses

NEUROFIBROMATOSIS TYPE 1 (NF1)
Whole gene deletion phenotype
Alternate forms of NF1 (condition with incomplete/atypical features)
  Mixed
  Localized
    Segmental
    Gastrointestinal[a]
    Familial spinal
    Familial café-au-lait spots
Related forms of NF1 (conditions with additional features)
  NF/Noonan syndrome
  Watson syndrome

NEUROFIBROMATOSIS TYPE 2 (NF2)
Alternate form of NF2
  Schwannomatosis

[a]Carey and Viskochil (19) postulated that gastrointestinal neurofibromatosis represents an alternative form caused by the *NF1* gene but, to date, no mutations have been reported. Reciprocal translocation between chromosomes 12 and 14 has been described in one family and may result by chance or the responsible gene may be linked to one of the breakpoints (12q13 and 14q13) (129).

Source: From Carey and Viskochil (19).

internal neurofibromas; the condition breeds true in affected families. Café-au-lait spots are also known to be a feature of classic Noonan syndrome. In most cases of neurofibromatosis-Noonan syndrome, Noonanoid features represent variable expression of *NF1*. One family has been reported in which Noonan syndrome and NF1 segregated separately (11). Carey et al. (18) reported a two-generation family with neurofibromatosis-Noonan syndrome and a 3 basepair deletion in exon 17 of *NF1*.

Familial Café-au-Lait Spots (OMIM 114030)[a]

Multigenerational families with café-au-lait spots and no other signs of NF1 were first recognized by Riccardi (106). Abeliovich et al. (1) established close linkage to the *NF1* locus. Watson syndrome (OMIM 193520)[a], a combination of café-au-lait spots, pulmonic stenosis, and mental deficiency (64,136) was shown to have linkage to the *NF1* gene by Allanson et al. (7).

Familial Spinal Neurofibromatosis (OMIM 162210)[a]

Several multigenerational families of this alternative form of NF1 have been recorded (9,100,101).

Pulst et al. (101) demonstrated linkage to NF1 and Ars et al. (9) identified a frameshift mutation. In addition to spinal neurofibromas, patients have multiple café-au-lait spots but usually lack cutaneous neurofibromas and Lisch nodules.

Neurofibromatosis, Intestinal Type (OMIM 162220)[a]

In this form, neurofibromatous involvement is limited to the gastrointestinal tract. Onset is delayed until adulthood and some carriers are asymptomatic until their middle or late adult years. Increased risk of intestinal problems include those of bleeding, intussusception, and obstruction (46,71). Inheritance is dominant and most likely autosomal, although no male-to-male transmission has been recorded to date (46). Reciprocal translocation between chromosomes 12 and 14 has been described in one family and may result by chance or the responsible gene may be linked to one of the breakpoints (12q13 and 14q13) (129). Carey and Viskochil (19) postulated that gastrointestinal neurofibromatosis represents an alternative form caused by the *NF1* gene (Table 12–2) but, to date, no mutations have been reported.

Encephalocraniocutaneous Lipomatosis

Legius et al. (67) reported a 2-year-old boy with NF1 and encephalocraniocutaneous lipomatosis. Findings included more than five café-au-lait spots and increased T2-weighted signals in the basal ganglia on MRI scan. An *NF1* mutation was confirmed. The patient also had hemimegalencephaly, regional alopecia, lipomas of the occipital region, and seizures.

Weaver Syndrome–like Phenotype

Asperen et al. (10) reported a mother and son with NF1 and overgrowth with a Weaver syndrome–like phenotype. The proband had more than six café-au-lait spots, Lisch nodules, axillary freckling, and numerous neurofibromas. NF1 was confirmed at the molecular level.

Multiple Lentigines

Wu et al. (142) reported an *NF1* mutation in a patient with multiple lentigines, a feature commonly found in LEOPARD syndrome.

Schwannomatosis

Some patients with NF2 have multiple schwannomas in the absence of acoustic tumors, meningiomas, or ocular pathology (53); Purcell and Dixon (102) reported schwannomatosis with meningiomas, gliomas, and astrocytomas. Gorlin and Koutlas (42) reported a family with multiple schwannomas, nevi, and vaginal leiomyomas but, to date, no NF2 mutations have been identified.

EPIDEMIOLOGY OF NEUROFIBROMATOSIS, TYPE 1[b]

Prevalence estimates have varied from 13/100,000 to 46/100,000 (39). Only one study (99) used NIH diagnostic criteria (44,88), finding a prevalence of 27/100,000; ascertainment was probably incomplete because the study was based on hospital records. The higher prevalence in younger people may reflect earlier death among NF1 patients (39,51).

At least 80,000 individuals in the United States are affected with NF1 (106). Inheritance is autosomal dominant with about 50% of the cases representing new mutations (106). Penetrance is complete with a few anecdotal instances of nonpenetrance. Gonadal mosaicism may explain some families with more than one child affected with NF1 and normal parents (39).

Huson et al. (50) found a birth prevalence of 39/100,000. In Northern Finland, the birth prevalence was estimated to be 27/100,000 (99).

Wolkenstein et al. (139) found that *segmental* NF1 is about 30 times less common than classic NF1. Huson and Ruggieri (52a) estimated a prevalence of about 2.5–2.8/100,000.

Estimates of the rate of new NF1 mutations vary from 1.3×10^{-4} to 4.3×10^{-4} mutations per gene per generation, which is about 10 times higher than the rates for most other diseases (32,50).

Reduced fitness in NF1 means that affected individuals have fewer children, on the average, than other people. Fitness estimates are about half of those found in the general population, and are lower for affected men than for affected women. Diminished reproductive fitness could result from infertility, subfertility, increased morbidity, and increased mortality. The average life span of individuals with NF1 is lower than that observed in the general population (32,50,51).

MOLECULAR BIOLOGY OF THE *NF1* GENE

NF1 is a tumor suppressor gene that maps to 17q11.2. It spans about 355 kilobases of genomic DNA comprising at least 60 exons. The processed transcript is approximately 12 kilobases long and encodes neurofibromin, a 2818 amino acid polypeptide with three alternatively spliced exons: 9a, 23a, and 48a (Fig. 12–1). A central region of about 360 amino acids shows strong homology with mammalian GTPase activating protein (GAP) for members of the $p21^{ras}$ (Ras) family. The GAP-related domain (GRD) is encoded by exons 21–27a (33,69,79,130,131) (Fig. 12–1).

Neurofibromin interacts with Ras as a negative regulator of the Ras/MAPK signaling pathway. Ras proteins play an important role in growth and differentiation. Ras is regulated by cycling between active Ras·GTP and inactive Ras·GDP. Downstream targets of Ras·GTP are shown in Figure 12–2. Analysis of tumors shows evidence of hyperactive Ras as well as frequent loss of the normal *NF1* allele, which is consistent with its role as a tumor suppressor gene (14,137,144).

NF1 transcripts are expressed at low levels in most cells, the highest levels being found in the central nervous system (89). CNS expression is consistent with the problems of cognitive function and with the development of intracranial tumors found in neurofibromatosis. Neurofibromin may also play a role in the embryonic development of congenital skeletal abnormalities.

Many affected animals as well as some animal models have been reported. Mouse models have been used to study the molecular aspects of tumor development in neurofibromatosis (20,134). Bicolor damselfish have been found with neurofi-

---

[b]Prevalence estimates, birth prevalence (so-called "incidence") estimates, and new mutation rates have been converted to a standard epidemiological form. Although incidence and prevalence are different concepts with a mathematical relationship between them, I prefer birth prevalence to incidence because (a) malformations, malformation syndromes, and hamartoneoplastic disorders frequently result in embryonic or fetal death and (b) early pregnancy losses are not ascertainable. Thus, the population represents incomplete ascertainment of only those affected individuals who survive until birth.

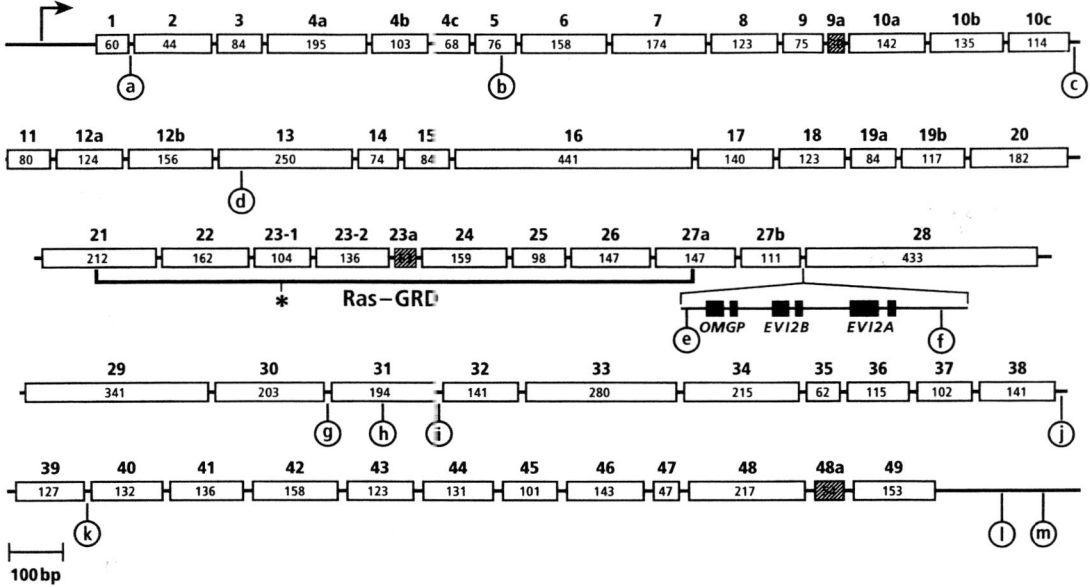

Figure 12–1 Schematic diagram representing the NF1 exons as rectangular boxes and important signposts as lettered circles. Introns are not shown to scale. Scale in lower left corner is for the size of exons. The transcription start site is depicted as a horizontal arrow upstream of exon 1. **a:** *Not*I restriction enzyme site. **b:** Single-nucleotide polymorphism as an *Rsa*I restriction site or adapted as mutagenically separated PCR. **c:** Site of truncation of a cDNA isolated from human placenta cDNA library. **d:** Single-nucleotide polymorphism site adapted for MS-PCR. **e:** Approximate location of the t(1;17) balanced translocation breakpoint and nearby site of GXAlu, a tetranucleotide repeat within an Alu-repetitive element. **f:** Dinucleotide repeat polymorphism. **g:** Insertion/deletion polymorphism of an L1-element. **h:** Site of the most common *NF1* mutation, a C5839T substitution resulting in an Arg1947 to termination. **i:** Site of the t(17;22) translocation breakpoint. **j:** Dinucleotide polymorphism. **k:** Site of a processed AK3 (adenylate kinase 3) pseudogene. **l:** Single-nucleotide polymorphism site adapted for MS-PCR. **m:** Polyadenylation site representing the 3′-end of the *NF1* gene. The GAP-related domain, Ras-GRD, is shown spanning exons 21 to 27a. The asterisk in exon 23–1 represents a site of mRNA processing, C3916U, which leads to premature truncation at codon 1303. The alternative splice forms are in-frame insertions of exons 9a, 23a, and 48a, and they are hash marked. The embedded genes are shown in bold in intron 27b. From Viskochil (131).

bromas, schwannomas, and neurofibrosarcomas (116). Goldfish have been described with multiple schwannomas (neurilemomas), neurofibromas, and malignant nerve sheath tumors (115). Neurofibromas have been observed in various wild and domestic animals including chickens, cows, horses, and dogs (12,15,16,41 77,127). Schwannomas have also been found in dogs (97).

MUTATIONS

Many studies of *NF1* mutations have appeared (35,37,47,54,60,68,74,119,123,125,141). Mutational analysis of the *NF1* gene is a major challenge for two reasons: (*a*) the large size of the gene and (*b*) the presence of many unprocessed *NF1* pseudogenes hampering PRC approaches to the analysis of genomic DNA samples because of co-amplification of *NF1* loci on other chromosomes (37).

More than 80% of new *NF1* gene mutations are of paternal origin (37,65). Fahsold et al. (37) identified 278 mutations. About 80% of these either directly or indirectly yielded premature stop codons; the mutations were evenly distributed over the whole gene from exon 1 to exon 47. About 10% of the mutations were of the missense type or the single amino acid deletion type; these are clustered in the GAP-related domain and in the cysteine/serine-rich domain (exons 11 to 17). Klose et al. (60) noted two independent mutations in the same family.

NEUROFIBROMATOSIS

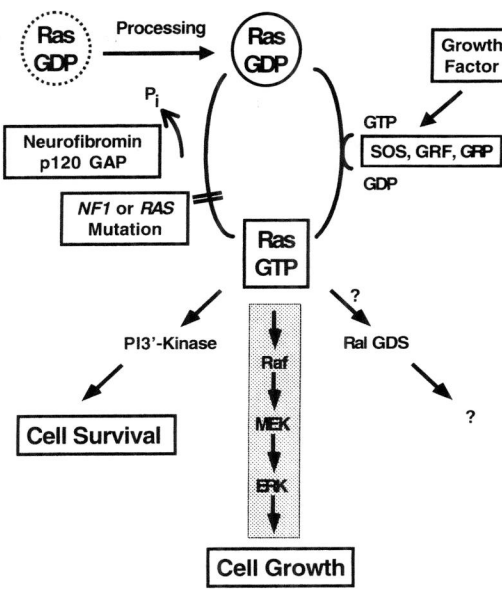

Figure 12–2 Overview of Ras activation by GEFs and signaling through downstream effectors. Ras cycles between an active GTP-bound conformation (Ras·GTP) and an inactive GDP-bound state (Ras·GDP). Growth factors induce cell growth, in part by activating the GEFs Sos, GRF, and GRP that bind Ras and stimulate nucleotide dissociation. Nucleotide exchange increases the percentage of Ras·GTP because the intracellular concentration of free GTP vastly exceeds that of GDP. Signaling terminates when Ras GTP is hydrolyzed to Ras GDP. Neurofibromin and p120 GAP regulate this process by accelerating the conversion of Ras·GTP to Ras·GDP. Oncogenic RAS mutations or inactivation of NF1 perturb Ras signaling by favoring the GTP- bound state. Ras·GTP activation of the Raf/MEK/ERK kinase cascade stimulates proliferation in many cell types, and activation of the PI3K pathway has been shown to promote cellular survival. Ras interacts with other downstream effectors, such as Ral-GDS; all of the components of this pathway remain to be defined. From Weiss et al. (137).

PSEUDOGENES

Many pseudogenes have been identified with NF1-like sequences on chromosomes 2, 12, 14, 15, 18, 20, 21, and 22. It has been hypothesized that gene conversion between nonhomologous pseudogenes and the NF1 gene might produce some mutations that account for the high mutation rate in the NF1 gene. However, only 6 (3.1%) of 196 pseudogene variations were also found among NF1 mutations. Five of the six mutations were typical C → T transitions in a CpG dinucleotide. In fact, of all sequence variants in the NF1 gene itself ($n = 301$), less than 20% represented C → T or G → A transitions within a CpG dinucleotide. Thus, neither frequent deamination of 5-methylcytosine nor interchromosomal gene conversion accounted for the high mutation rate of the NF1 gene (37,58,103).

MICRODELETIONS

Many NF1 microdeletions have been identified. About 5% of patients have large deletions that span most of the gene. Mostly of maternal origin, these deletions are associated with a more severe phenotype, including facial anomalies, developmental delay, mental deficiency, and early onset of cutaneous neurofibromas and plexiform neurofibromas. Dysmorphic facial features consist of downslanting palpebral fissures, large nose with a high nasal bridge, small, pointed chin, low hairline, and broad neck. In some cases, clinical findings indicate a contiguous gene syndrome in which flanking DNA has been included in the deletion. More severe craniofacial anomalies may include microcephaly with a narrow, receding forehead, flat occiput, facial asymmetry, almond-shaped eyes, downslanting palpebral fissures, prominent nose, highly-arched palate, and large, posteriorly angulated ears. Psychomotor retardation, seizures, and spasticity may also occur. Certainly, deletions and their associated clinical findings represent the only clearcut example of a genotype–phenotype correlation known for the NF1 gene to date (5,68, 74,74a,123,124,126,141). Ainsworth et al. (5) and Streubel et al. (123) reported somatic mosaicism for microdeletions. Lázaro et al. (66) noted a 12 kb deletion in a family showing germline mosaicism.

TUMORIGENESIS

Because the NF1 gene is a tumor suppressor, a second inactivating hit is required for tumorigenesis. Loss of heterozygosity (LOH) has been documented for neurofibromas, pheochromocytomas, and malignant myeloid disorders (114,118,143). Analyzing the spectrum of mutations in various neurofibromas of NF1 patients is important because the type and frequency of these mutations could have an impact on the severity of the phenotype (35).

Somatic mutation percentages in the *NF1* gene in neurofibromas have been estimated in different studies: 36% (n = 22) (27), 25% (n = 60) (117), 2.6% (n = 38) (34), and 12% (n = 82) (54). However, Sawada et al. (114) showed that only a subset of cells from the tumor harbored the somatic mutation. Eisenbarth et al. (35) described a systematic approach of searching for somatic NF1 inactivation in neurofibromas; their data supported the hypothesis of Sawada et al. (114). Serra et al. (117a) found that *NF1* mutations were present in Schwann cells but not in fibroblasts; their data also supported the hypothesis of Sawada et al. (114). Horan et al. (49) found that CpG hypermethylation within the *NF1* gene promotor was unlikley to be a common mutational mechanism in the formation of neurofibromas. Happle (45c) discussed the possibility of LOH during early development in the genesis of large plexiform neurofibromas. Serra et al. (116a) identified 45 independent somatic *NF1* mutations, confirming that double inactivation of the *NF1* gene is the general rule in neurofibroma development. Most of the point mutations found produced splicing defects.

EXPRESSIVITY

Within families, both intrafamilial and interfamilial variability is characteristic of NF1. Table 12–3 lists the proposed mechanisms that can be used to explain variable expressivity in NF1 (19).

Allelic heterogeneity explains some of the subtypes, such as neurofibromatosis-Noonan syndrome and familial spinal neurofibromatosis (Tables 12–1, 12–2). The *two-hit hypothesis* applied to NF1 as a tumor suppressor gene has been demonstrated by loss of heterozygosity (LOH) found in neurofibromas and other tumors (see Tumorigenesis above). *Somatic mosaicism* has also been documented in NF1 and may account for later onset or a milder phenotype in some instances (see

Table 12–3 Mechanisms to Explain Variable Expressivity in Neurofibromatosis, Type 1

Allelic heterogeneity
Two-hit hypothesis/tumor suppressor gene
Somatic mosaicism
Contiguous gene deletions
Modifying genes (epistasis)
Epigenetic factors
Environmental factors
Stochastic factors

Source: From Carey and Viskochil (19).

Table 12–4 Features of Neurofibromatosis, Type 1

Features	Percentage
MAJOR DISEASE FEATURES	
>6 café-au-lait spots	>95
Axillary freckling	65–84
Cutaneous neurofibromas	
0–9 years	14
10–19 years	44
20–29 years	85
>30 years	95
Lisch nodules	
0–4 years	22
5–9 years	41
10–19 years	82
>20 years	96
MINOR DISEASE FEATURES	
Short stature (height <3rd centile)	≅30
Macrocephaly (head circumference >97th centile)	≅45
COMPLICATIONS	
Plexiform neurofibromas	
All lesions	25
Large lesions of the head and neck	1–4
Cognitive deficits	
Mental retardation	4–8
Academic learning disability	30–60
Scoliosis	12–20
Optic pathway gliomas	
All lesions	15–20
Symptomatic	5–7
Neurological manifestations	
Headache	10–20
Epilepsy	3–5
Aqueduct stenosis	2.5
Pseudarthrosis of the long bones	3
Sphenoid wing dysplasia	<1
Malignant peripheral nerve sheath tumors	1–4
Renal artery stenosis	1–2
Noonan syndrome–like facies	7
MRI T2 HYPERINTENSITIES[a]	60–70

[a]MRI T2 hyperintensities = magnetic resonance imaging T2 hyperintensities (see text).
Source: Data from Huson and Hughes (52), North (90,92), Riccardi (106), Listernick et al. (73), and Hughes Van Es et al. (128).

Segmental Neurofibromatosis above). *Contiguous gene deletions* that include the *NF1* gene and flanking DNA result in a severe phenotype with facial anomalies (see Microdeletions above). Riccardi (104) suggested roles for *epigenetic factors*, *environmental factors*, and *stochastic factors* in modifying *NF1* gene expression.

Modifying genes explain some of the variable expression in NF1. Easton et al. (34a) found significant familial clustering in four traits, including seizures, optic gliomas, learning disabilities, and scoliosis; such traits exemplify the segregation of epistatic genes unlinked to the *NF1* locus. Furthermore, male predominance has been found with pseudoarthrosis of the tibia (121) and with myelodysplasia (85).

NEUROFIBROMATOSIS, TYPE 1

Major and minor features and complications of neurofibromatosis, type 1 (NF1) (OMIM 162200)[a] are listed in Table 12–4. Riccardi (106) and Huson and Hughes (52) have written extensive monographs on NF1.

Natural History

Over 40% of patients have some manifestations at birth, and over 60% have them by the second year of life. Café-au-lait spots usually develop first, with multiple lesions being present within the first year of life (Fig. 12–3). In over 65% of patients, axillary freckling appears later (Fig. 12–4). Cutaneous neurofibromas appear around the onset of puberty and increase in number throughout life, although about 5% of patients over 40 years of age have no cutaneous tumors (Fig. 12–5). Lisch nodules, best observed in slit lamp examination, begin to appear during early childhood and have been observed in over 95% of all patients (Fig. 12–6). Average height is reduced in about 30% of NF1 patients (40, 106,107).

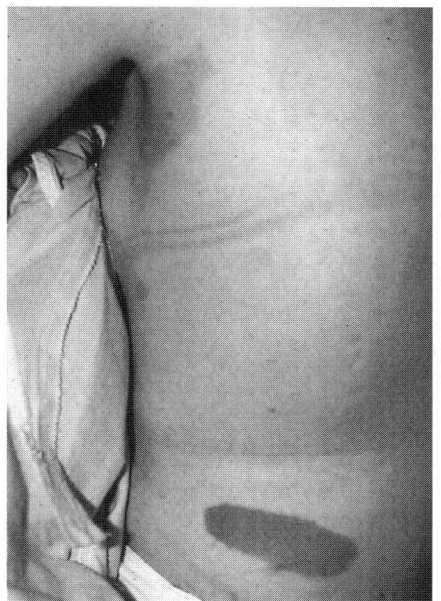

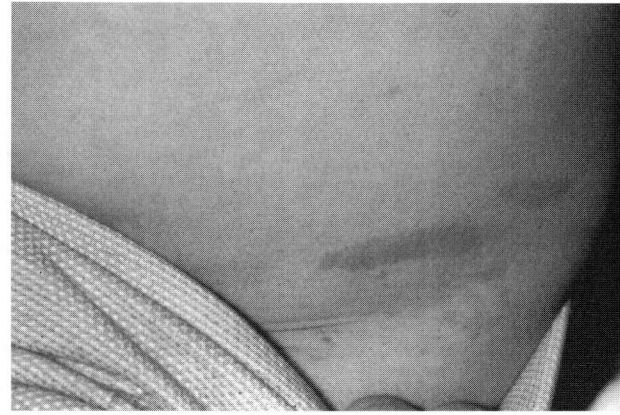

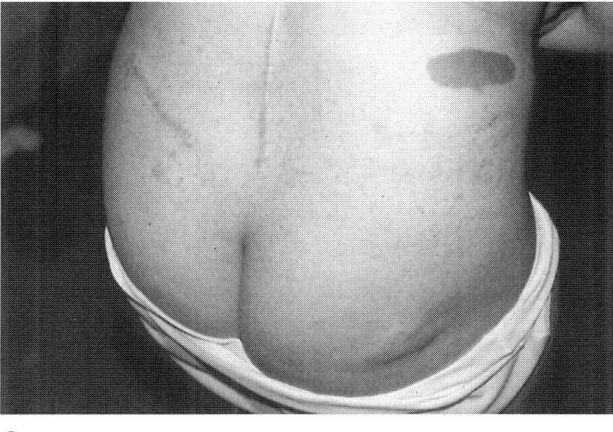

Figure 12–3 Neurofibromatosis, type 1. **A–C:** Café-au-lait spots. Note deeply situated neurofibroma resulting in raised ovoid area on buttock.

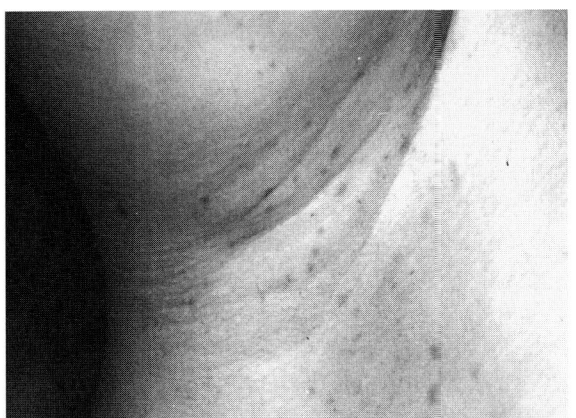

Figure 12–4 Neurofibromatosis, type 1. Axillary freckling.

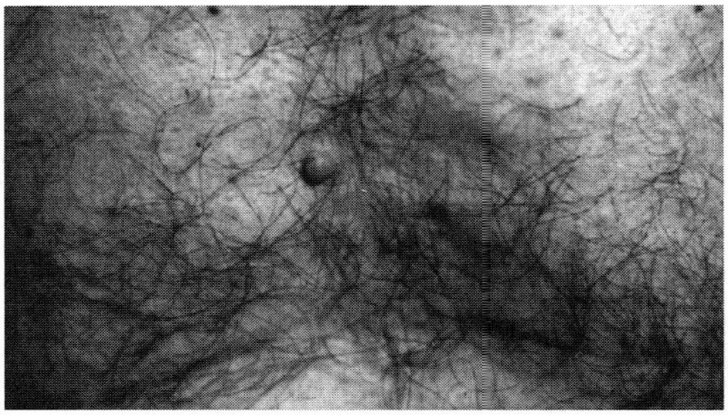

Figure 12–5 Neurofibromatosis, type 1. Neurofibroma. **A:** Small neurofibroma. **B:** Multiple neurofibromas. **C:** Large plexiform neurofibroma.

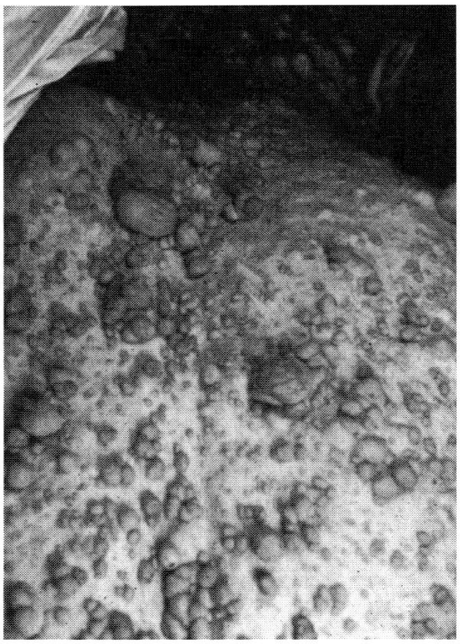

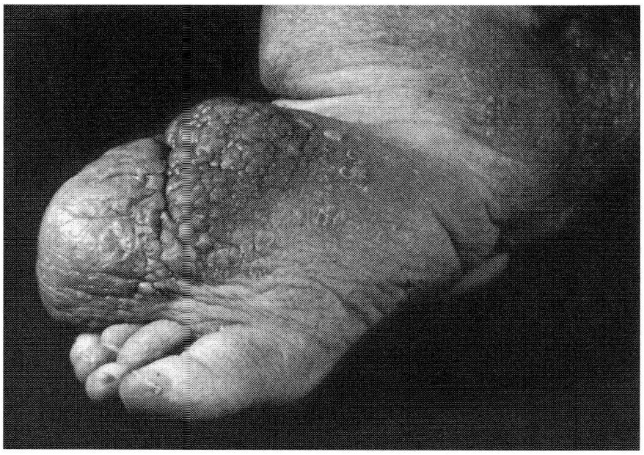

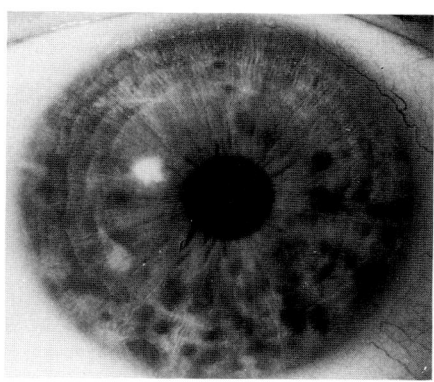

Figure 12–6 Neurofibromatosis, type 1. Lisch nodules. Courtesy of C.G. Summers, Minneapolis.

About 33% of all patients develop one or more complications. Plexiform neurofibromas occur in 30%. About 6% of patients over 18 develop various forms of malignancy. Other important complications include neurological problems in 10% (including seizures, aqueductal stenosis, and spinal neurofibromas), scoliosis in 5%, pseudoarthrosis in 5%, gastrointestinal neurofibromas in 2%, endocrine neoplasms in 2%, and renal artery stenosis in 2% of patients. Approximately 8% of patients have mental retardation, but learning disabilities of various kinds affect 30%–60% (23,40,90,91,106, 107). Autism is found in some cases (82). Sensorineural hearing loss occurs in about 5.5% of NF1 patients (40). Cardiovascular anomalies occur with low frequency (70).

Growth

Clementi et al. (22) studied growth in 528 NF1 patients. Impaired height only affected a subset of subjects and did not seem to be related to disease severity. Although endocrinopathies can also affect growth, only 3.8% of patients were so affected. Slight overweight was found in NF1 adults, particularly males.

Macrocephaly was a feature in most subjects and was not related to hydrocephalus found in 2.3% of patients. OFC velocity in NF1 girls was the same as that of normal girls, but in NF1 boys, the OFC pubertal growth spurt was much more pronounced and delayed than in normal boys. A disproportion between OFC and height in boys was evident and appeared to be related to disease severity (22).

Neoplasia

Neoplasms may be present at birth or appear during childhood or even later. They vary greatly in size, with localized enlargement of many nerve trunks in larger neurofibromas. They are most striking on the skin, with some patients manifesting few, hundreds, or even more neurofibromas and others having large, unilateral pendulous masses (Figs. 12–5 and 12–7A,B). Many organs may be involved, including stomach, intestine, kidney, bladder, larynx, and heart. In the head and neck region, the most commonly affected sites are the scalp, cheek, neck, and oral cavity (23,48,106,107). Neurofibromas of the penis have been reported (63).

Tumors associated with NF1 are listed in Table 12–5. The two main peripheral nerve sheath tumors are neurofibromas and malignant peripheral nerve sheath tumors (MPNSTs). Neurofibromas consist of a mixture of Schwann cells associated with axons in some cases, perineural-like cells, fibroblasts, and cells intermediate between fibroblasts and perineural-like cells (Fig. 12–7A). The tumor expresses S-100 protein but less diffusely than schwannoma (140).

Cutaneous neurofibromas (Figs. 12–5A,B and 12–7A) are the most common tumors, but other forms may also be found: (*a*) intraneural neurofibromas with fusiform enlargement of the affected nerve; (*b*) plexiform neurofibromas (Figs. 12–5C and 12–7B), multinodular growths that form along nerve plexuses or along fascicles of large peripheral nerves; (*c*) diffuse neurofibromas of the skin and subcutaneous tissues; and (*d*) massive soft tissue neurofibromas with frequent hyperpigmentation (140).

With few exceptions, plexiform neurofibromas are associated only with NF1. MPNSTs (Fig. 12–7C) are deep soft tissue tumors that arise from Schwann cells; S-100 protein is commonly found. Most lesions occur in the limbs (53%, $n = 18$) and pain associated with the mass is a risk factor for the development of MPNSTs. Patients with NF1 account for about 60% of all MPNSTs and patients have a 2%–5% overall risk of developing such a malignancy. The capacity

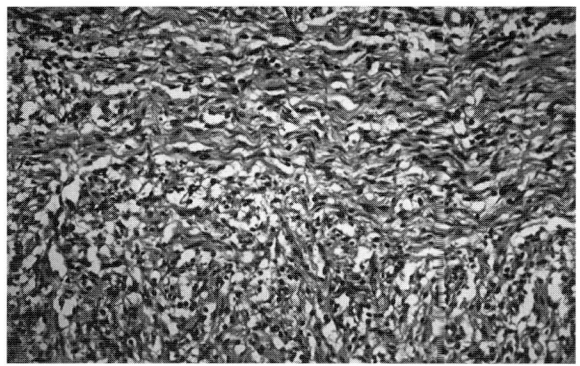

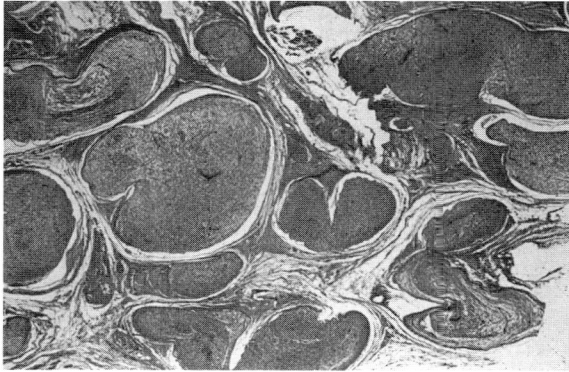

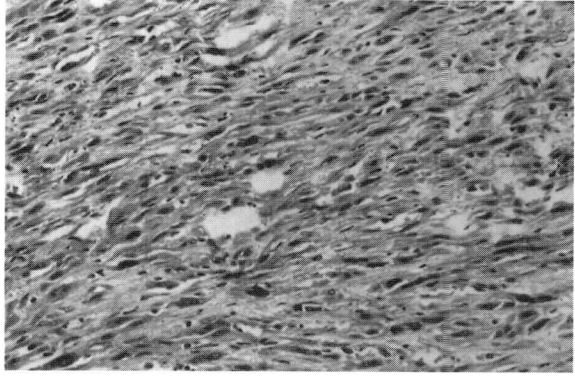

Figure 12–7 Neurofibromatosis, type 1. Histopathology. **A:** Neurofibroma. Note spindle-shaped cells with fusiform or wavy nuclei and delicate connective tissue. **B:** Plexiform neurofibroma. Note tortuous mass of expanded nerve branches cut in various planes of section supported by connective tissue matrix. **C:** Malignant peripheral nerve sheath tumor. Note closely packed hyperchromatic cells.

for malignant transformation is not shared equally by all forms of neurofibromas. Cutaneous neurofibromas do not undergo malignant transformation, but MPNSTs are associated with plexiform neurofibromas or with intraneural tumors involving large or medium-sized nerves or nerve plexuses (59,61,62, 135,140).

Histopathologically, MPNSTs are fasciculated and composed of closely packed hyperchromatic spindle cells, most often with mitotic figures. Low-grade tumors account for only 10%–15% of cases. About 20% of MPNSTs have misleading histologic features, such as epithelioid cells and divergent mesenchymal or glandular differentiation (140).

Table 12–5 Neoplasms in Neurofibromatosis, Type 1

Neurofibroma
Plexiform neurofibroma
Malignant peripheral nerve sheath tumor
Optic glioma
Pheochromocytoma
Leukemia (nonlymphocytic forms)
Angioma
Xanthogranuloma
Carcinoid tumor
Neuroblastoma
Rhabdomyosarcoma
Wilms tumor
Pancreatic adenocarcinoma
Melanoma

Symptomatic optic gliomas are estimated to occur in 1.5%–7% of patients with NF1, predominantly in young children, and often involve the optic chiasm. Reduction in the visual field has been suggested as the most sensitive indicator of gliomas along the optic pathway (120), but this has been challenged (72a). Children are at increased risk for precocious puberty; lesions near the hypothalamus can interfere with tonic central nervous system inhibition of the hypothalamic–pituitary–gonadal axis (38,72,72a,73,120).

Cutaneous angiomas have been found in many cases. They usually develop during early or middle adult life but may occur earlier. Those lesions that are present at birth probably represent capillary malformations, not angiomas (40,106).

Leukemia has been reported with a striking excess of nonlymphocytic forms, particularly juvenile chronic myelogenous leukemia (23,85). Juvenile xanthogranulomas were found in 17 cases of NF1 in the review of Zvulunov et al. (147); they also found 30 cases of the triple association of xanthogranulomas, chronic myelogenous leukemia, and NF1.

A variety of low-frequency tumors have been recorded, including brain tumors other than gliomas, pheochromocytoma, carcinoid tumor, neuroblastoma, rhabdomyosarcoma, Wilms tumor, adenocarcinoma of the pancreas, and melanoma (23,40,48,106,107).

Skin

In addition to nodular tumors of the skin, café-au-lait spots are found in over 95% of NF1 patients. The smooth-edged pigmented macules are usually present at birth, but they may take months, or even a year, to appear (Fig. 12–3). They increase in size during the first decade and vary in size from 1 to 2 mm to over 15 cm. Their distribution is random over the body except for a disproportionately small number on the face. The color varies from yellowish to chocolate brown. The density of melanin macroglobules is significantly higher in biopsies of café-au-lait spots in NF1 patients than in café-au-lait spots found in the general population. The presence of six or more café-au-lait spots >1.5 cm in diameter has come to represent the criterion for diagnosing neurofibromatosis, although fewer are present in some instances. Axillary freckling is present in over 65% of patients and, if present, is a significant diagnostic clue (Fig. 12–4). Inguinal freckling may also be found; pigmented hairy nevi may be noted in some cases. Cutaneous blue–red and pseudoatrophic macules and palmar melanotic macules have been reported as additional cutaneous features (31,32, 40,81,106,138,146).

Central Nervous System

Mental deficiency with an IQ under 70 occurs in about 8% of NF1 patients. Learning disabilities have been reported with frequencies ranging from 30%–60%. There is no characteristic profile; findings have included easy distractibility, impulsiveness, deficient visual–motor coordination, excessive scatter of scores from one set of test items to another, and language and vocabulary deficits. Seizures occur in about 6.5%, and frank hydrocephalus with aqueductal stenosis as well as asymptomatic ventricular dilation have been recorded in about 4% of patients. NF1 is increased about 150-fold in a population of autistic patients. The overall headache frequency of 30% is not significantly different from that found in the general population. Distortion of cortical architecture from glial proliferation and neuronal heterotopias deep in the cerebral white matter have been reported. MRI T2 signal abnormalities occur in 60%–70% of NF1 patients. They are found most often in the basal ganglia, cerebellum, brain stem, and subcortical white matter (4,21a,23,40,82,90–92,95,128).

Skeletal System

Scoliosis, the most common skeletal defect, ranges from mild to severe curvature. Other spinal defects include kyphosis, cervical spine abnormalities, and spondylolisthesis. Pseudoarthroses are found in 5% of NF1 patients. A classic presentation is tibial bowing, resulting in a fracture with nonunion, but the spectrum includes bowing with cortical thickening, hairline fracture, fracture with or without healing, fibular involvement, amputation, bone grafts, and surgeries before fracture. A variety of other anomalies may be observed, including hemihyperplasia of a limb or digit, spina bifida, absent patella, elevated scapulas, congenital dislocations (particularly of the hip, radius, and ulna), and clubfoot (29, 30,121).

Bony defects of the skull, particularly of the posterosuperior orbital wall (11%), overgrowth of cranial bones, and craniofacial asymmetry (8%) have been reported. Intraorbital lesions may produce proptosis and muscle palsies and sphenoid bone dysplasia may produce pulsating exophthalmos (23,106) (Figs. 12–8 and 12–9).

Endocrine System

In childhood, the most common endocrine abnormality is sexual precocity. Other findings have included hypopituitarism, hypogonadism, gigantism, acromegaly, delayed sexual development, obesity, hypoglycemia, diabetes insipidus, goiter, myxedema, and hyperparathyroidism (23, 45a,106).

Eyes

Lisch nodules, appearing in early childhood, are found in most affected adults. Neurofibromas of the eyelids have also been noted in some cases (76,145). Yasunari et al. (145) found bright, patchy choroidal regions under infrared fundus examination in 100% of NF1 patients. They suggested that infrared monochromatic light examination by confocal scanning laser ophthalmoscope should be added as a new screening device.

Cardiovascular System

Lin et al. (70) found that cardiovascular malformations occurred in 2.3% of NF1 patients

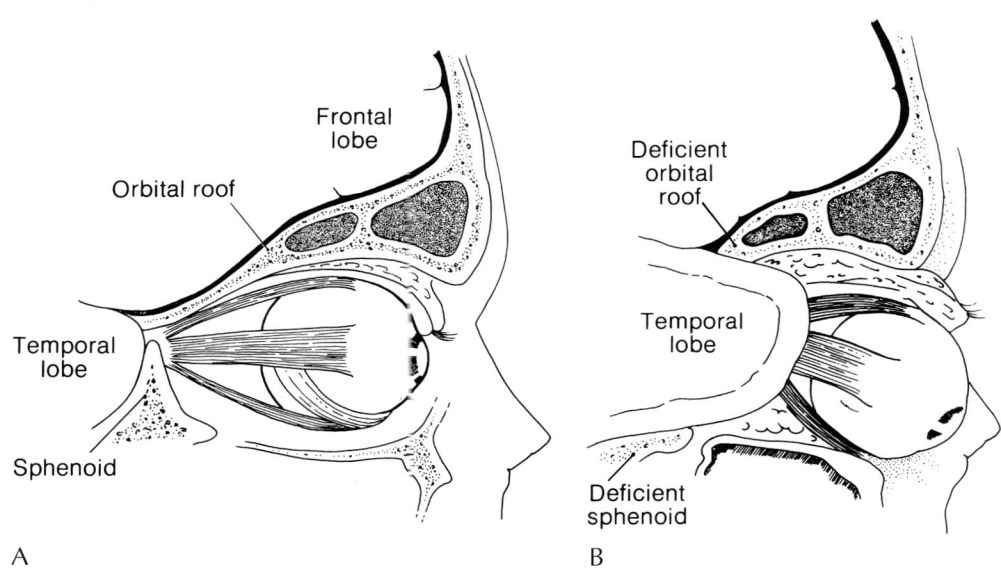

Figure 12–8 Neurofibromatosis, type 1. **A:** Normal anatomy. **B:** Deficient orbital roof and sphenoid wing, allowing prolapse of temporal lobe with exophthalmos. Adapted from Bruwer (13).

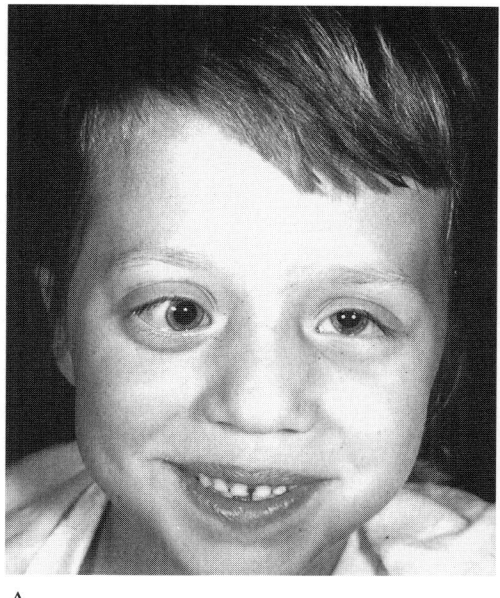
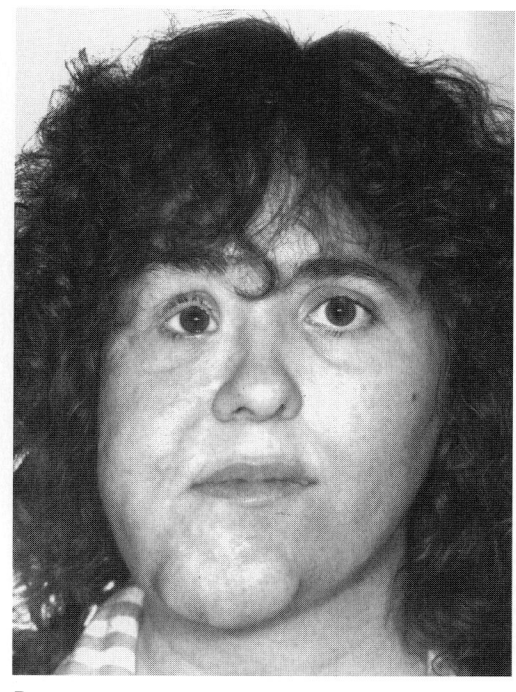

Figure 12–9 Neurofibromatosis, type 1. **A:** Unilateral exophthalmos due to bony defect of posterosuperior orbital wall. **B:** Facial asymmetry.

($n = 2322$). Pulmonic stenosis and coarctation of the aorta make up a higher proportion of all cardiovascular malformations than in the general population. Other abnormalities include cardiac murmur, mitral valve prolapse, electrocardiographic abnormalities, and peripheral vascular abnormalities (70,108). Hamilton et al. (45b) reported a young man, apparently in good health, who died suddenly. Autopsy findings included intramyocardial vasculopathy, nonspecific cardiomyopathic changes, myocardial fibrosis, and a floppy mitral valve.

NEUROFIBROMATOSIS, TYPE 2

Neurofibromatosis, type 2 (NF2) (OMIM 101000)[a], is one-tenth as common as NF1, with a prevalence of 2/100,000 (80). It has autosomal dominant inheritance with >95% penetrance; NF2 it is caused by mutations in a tumor suppressor gene that maps to 22q12.2.

Molecular Biology of the *NF2* Gene

The NF2 protein, merlin, is a member of the protein 4.1 superfamily most closely related to ezrin, radixin, and moesin (ERM), from which its name is derived (merlin = *m*oesin, *e*zrin, *r*adixin-*li*ke protein). It is a 66–69 kDa protein containing 17 exons and 595 amino acids. Members of the protein 4.1 superfamily share a conserved N-terminal region (CNTR). Some family members, including ERM proteins, interact with transmembrane binding partners through the CNTR and localize them to a specific membrane domain via direct interactions between the C-terminal domain and the actin cytoskeleton. The C-terminal portion of merlin contains a coiled-coil domain but lacks the actin-binding domain at the C-terminal end of the ERM proteins. Merlin may function as part of a signal transduction pathway regulating cell–cell and cell–matrix interactions. Increased expression of merlin impairs cell motility, adhesion, and spreading. Although mutant alleles result in loss of function, it has been suggested that some *NF2* mutations closely resemble gain of function in their cellular phenotype. Thus, there may be a spectrum of allelic types with different phenotypic effects (44a,45,85,122).

Mutations

In the development of tumors, a first-hit germline mutation is followed by a second hit. Mutational analysis of the *NF2* gene in schwannomas, meningiomas, and ependymomas has shown inactivation of both copies of the gene In *NF2* truncating mutations of the nonsense and frameshift types, the phenotype tends to be severe. With mutations of the missense and splice site types, the phenotype tends to be mild. However, splice site mutations have a more variable phenotype; patients with 5′ mutations tend to be more severely affected than patients with 3′ mutations. Surprisingly, in some cases, large deletions with complete inactivation of the *NF2* gene have been associated with a mild phenotype. Somatic mosaicism is likely to be a common cause of NF2 in sporadic cases (36,40a,53,75,78,110a, 111). Some milder cases have mosaicism.

Phenotype

Several reviews are available (40a,80,87,96,98). NF2 is characterized by bilateral vestibular schwannomas and, to a lesser extent, schwannomas of other cranial and peripheral nerves and spinal nerve roots; meningiomas; ependymomas; gliomas; cutaneous neurofibromas; and presenile lens opacities or subcapsular cataracts. Bilateral acoustic schwannomas may put pressure on the vestibulocochlear and facial nerve complex, resulting in hearing loss that often begins during the teenage years or early twenties, but on occasion may occur as early as the first decade or as late as the seventh decade. Tumors of the central nervous system such as meningiomas, ependymomas, and gliomas are common; multiple tumors may occur in some patients. In other patients, multiple schwannomas may occur in the absence of acoustic tumors, meningiomas, or ocular pathology. Schwannomatosis has also been noted with meningiomas, gliomas, and astrocytomas. Because NF1 and NF2 may both have central and peripheral manifestations, the previously used terms "peripheral neurofibromatosis" for NF1 and "central neurofibromatosis" for NF2 are outmoded (53,80,87,96,98, 102,141a).

The histopathology of schwannoma (neurilemoma) and neurofibroma differ (Fig. 12-7A,B). Schwannoma has distinctive features that include (*a*) Antoni type A tissue, composed of palisading spindle cells and acellular Verocay bodies, and (*b*) Antoni type B tissue, composed of spindle cells haphazardly distributed in a fibrillar matrix.

Café-au-lait spots and cutaneous neurofibromas occur in NF2, but less commonly than in NF1. Neurofibromas are easy to overlook; they are generally <2 cm in diameter, minimally raised, and often have a roughened surface that may have more prominent hairs than the surrounding skin. Axillary freckling and Lisch nodules are uncommon (80,87,96,98).

DIAGNOSIS

Criteria for the diagnosis of NF1 are listed in Table 12–6. It should be carefully noted that some subtypes of NF1 do not fulfill the criteria set forth in Table 12–6 (see Tables 12–1, 12–2, and Classification and Types of Neurofibromatosis above). Recommended screening studies for children with NF1 are summarized in Table 12–7. Criteria for the diagnosis of NF2 are listed in Table 12–8 and recommended screening studies for children with NF2 are summarized in Table 12–9 (88,98).

Table 12–6 Consensus Criteria for the Diagnosis of Neurofibromatosis, Type 1

The diagnostic criteria are met if a person has two or more of the following:

1. Six or more café-au-lait macules that have a maximum diameter of >5 mm in prepubertal patients and >15 mm in postpubertal patients
2. Two or more neurofibromas of any type, or one plexiform neurofibroma
3. Freckling in the axillary or inguinal regions
4. Optic glioma
5. Two or more Lisch nodules (iris hamartomas)
6. A characteristic osseous lesion, such as sphenoid wing dysplasia or thinning of the long-bone cortex, with or without pseudoarthrosis
7. A first-degree relative (i.e., parent, sibling, or child) with NF1 by the above criteria

Source: From National Institutes of Health Consensus Development Conference on Neurofibromatosis (88) and Pollack and Mulvihill (98).

Table 12–7 Recommended Screening Studies for Children with Proven or Presumptive Neurofibromatosis, Type 1

Annual clinical examination, including neurological assessment and dermatological evaluation
Annual ophthalmologic examination[a]
MR scan examination of the head
   Children diagnosed at younger than 5 years of age
   Children with new neurological deficits, visual loss, or endocrinopathy
MR scan examination of the spine and plain radiographs
   Children with scoliosis
   Children with back pain, radiculopathy, or long-tract signs referable to the spine
Neuropsychological and developmental testing
   Children with learning, speech, or socialization difficulties, or impaired fine motor skills
Genetic counseling should be offered to the family at diagnosis and as needed on an ongoing basis

[a]Because Yasunari et al. (145) found bright, patchy choroidal regions under infrared fundus examination in 100% of NF1 patients, they suggested that infrared monochromatic examination by confocal scanning laser ophthalmoscope should be added as a new screening device.

Source: From Pollack and Mulvihill (98).

Table 12–9 Recommended Screening Studies for Children with Proven or Presumptive Neurofibromatosis, Type 2[a]

Neurological examination
Ophthalmologic examination
Audiogram
MR scan of the head and the spine
Genetic counseling should be offered to the family at diagnosis and as needed on an ongoing basis

[a]The frequency with which these tests are repeated depends on whether or not abnormalities are identified on the initial evaluation. At the least, all tests should be repeated approximately every 3 to 5 years. Annual examinations are recommended for children with known lesions.

Source: From Pollack and Mulvihill (98).

DIFFERENTIAL DIAGNOSIS

Single neurofibromas and single schwannomas (neurilemomas), occurring independently from NF1 and NF2, respectively, are frequently observed by surgeons and pathologists. Multiple isolated neurofibromas have been observed on rare occasions (11a). Plexiform neurofibromas, however, are almost always associated with NF1, only rarely occurring as isolated tumors. Malignant peripheral nerve sheath tumors are most commonly associated with NF1, but they may occur in the general population. Isolated neurofibroma has also been recorded in several confirmed instances of the nevoid basal cell carcinoma syndrome. Similarly, meningiomas, both single and multiple, may occur independently from NF2 (see Chapter 9, Differential Diagnosis). Proteus syndrome has been confused with NF1 in the past (2,23). For example, Joseph Carey Merrick, pejoratively known as the "elephant man," had Proteus syndrome, not neurofibromatosis (23). Meningiomas, both single and multiple, have also been found in several patients with Proteus syndrome (see Chapter 9). Café-au-lait spots in McCune-Albright syndrome have scalloped edges (coast-of-Maine appearance) in contrast to NF1, which has smooth-edged lesions (coast-of-California appearance). Neurofibromatosis, type 1 is easily distinguished from Noonan-like/multiple giant cell lesion syndrome (25), Bannayan-Riley-Ruvalcaba syndrome (Chapter 8), and Klippel-Trenaunay syndrome (Chapter 10).

Lateral meningoceles are protrusions of the arachnoid and dura mater through inter- or intravertebral foramina. Although thoracic lateral meningoceles can be found with NF1, patients with lateral meningocele syndrome (43) do not have either NF1 or Marfan syndrome. Carney syndrome consists of schwannomas, spotty skin pigmentation, myxomas, and endocrine overactivity (93). Gorlin and Koutlas (42) reported a dominantly inherited syndrome of multiple schwannomas, nevi, and vaginal leiomyomas. Al-Sannaa et al. (8a) reported café-au-lait spots associated with trigonomicrocephaly, severe micrognathia, large ears, atrioventricular septal defect, and symmetrical cutaneous syndactyly.

Table 12–8 Consensus Criteria for the Diagnosis of Neurofibromatosis, Type 2

The diagnostic criteria are met if a person has either of the following:

1. Bilateral eighth nerve masses seen with appropriate scanning techniques, such as MR or CT
2. A first-degree relative with NF2, and either unilateral eighth nerve mass or two of the following:
    A. Neurofibroma
    B. Meningioma
    C. Glioma
    D. Schwannoma
    E. Juvenile posterior subcapsular cataract

Source: From National Institutes of Health Consensus Development Conference on Neurofibromatosis (88) and Pollack and Mulvihill (98).

REFERENCES

1. Abeliovich D, Gelman-Kohan Z, Silverstein S, Lerer I, Chemke J, Merin S, Zlotogora J: Familial café-au-lait spots: A variant of neurofibromatosis type I. J Med Genet 32:985–986, 1995.
2. Ablon J: Parents' responses to their child's diagnosis of neurofibromatosis 1. Am J Med Genet 93:136–142, 2000.
3. Abuelo DN, Meryash DL: Neurofibromatosis with fully expressed Noonan syndrome. Am J Med Genet 29:937–941, 1988
4. Afifi AK, Dolan KD, Van Gilder JC, Fincham RW: Ventriculomegaly in neurofibromatosis—1. Neurofibromatosis 1:299–305, 1988.
5. Ainsworth PJ, Chakraborty PK, Weksberg R: Examples of somatic mosaicism in a series of de novo neurofibromatosis type 1 cases due to a maternally derived deletion. Hum Mutat 9:452–457, 1997.
6. Allanson JE, Hall JG, Van Allen MI: Noonan phenotype associated with neurofibromatosis. Am J Med Genet 21:457–462, 1985.
7. Allanson JE, Upadhyaya M, Watson GH, Partington M, MacKenzie A, Lahey D, MacLeod H, Sarfaranzi M, Broadhead W, Harper PS, Huson SM: Watson syndrome—Is it a subtype of type 1 neurofibromatosis? J Med Genet 28:752–756, 1991.
8. Allanson JE, Watson GH: Watson syndrome—nineteen years on. Proc Greenwood Genet Ctr 6:173, 1987.
8a. Al-Sannaa N, Forrest CR, Teebi AS. New syndrome? Trigonomicrocephaly, severe micrognathia, large ears, atrioventricular septal defect, symmetrical cutaneous syndactyly of hands and feet, multiple café-au-lait spots: New acrocraniofacial dysostosis syndrome? Am J Med Genet 101:279–282, 2001.
9. Ars E, Kruyer H, Gaona A, Casquero P, Rosell J, Volpini V, Serra E, Lázaro C, Estivill X: A clinical variant of neurofibromatosis type 1: Familial spinal neurofibromatosis with a frameshift mutation in the *NF1* gene. Am J Hum Genet 62:834–841, 1998.
10. Asperen CJ van, Overweg-Plandsoen WCG, Cnossen MH, van Tijn DA, Hennekam RCM: Familial neurofibromatosis type 1 associated with an overgrowth syndrome resembling Weaver syndrome. J Med Genet 35:323–327, 1998.
11. Bahuau M, Houdayer C, Assouline B, Blanchet-Bardon C, Le Merrer M, Lyonnet S, Giraud S, Récan D, Lakhdar H, Vidaud M, Vidaud D: Novel recurrent nonsense mutation causing neurofibromatosis type 1 (NF1) in a family segregating both NF1 and Noonan syndrome. Am J Med Genet 75:265–272, 1998.
11a. Blakley P, Louis DN, Short MP, MacCollin M: A clinical study of patients with multiple isolated neurofibromas. J Med Genet 38:485–488, 2001.
12. Bossart GD: Neurofibromas in a Macaw (*Ara chloroptera*): Morphologic and immunocytochemical diagnosis. Vet Pathol 20:773–76, 1983.
13. Bruwer A: Neurofibromatosis and congenital unilateral pulsating and nonpulsating exophthalmos. Arch Ophthalmol 53:2–12, 1955.
14. Buchberg A, Cleveland E, Jenkins N: Sequence homology shared by neurofibromatosis type-1 gene and IRA-1 and IRA-2 negative regulators of the RAS cyclic AMP pathway. Nature 347:291–294, 1990.
15. Canfield P: A light microscopic study of bovine peripheral nerve sheath tumours. Vet Pathol 15:283–291, 1978.
16. Canfield P: The ultrastructure of bovine peripheral nerve sheath tumors. Vet Pathol 15:291–300, 1978.
17. Carey JC: Neurofibromatosis-Noonan syndrome. Am J Med Genet 75:263–264, 1998.
18. Carey JC, Stevenson DA, Ota M, Neil S, Viskochil DH: Is there a NF/Noonan syndrome? II. Documentation of the clinical and molecular aspects of an important family. Proc Greenwood Genet Ctr 17:52–53, 1998.
19. Carey JC, Viskochil DH: Neurofibromatosis type 1: A model condition for the study of the molecular basis of variable expressivity in human disorders. Am J Med Genet 89:7–13, 1999.
20. Cichowski K, Shih TS, Schmitt E, Santiago S, Reilly K, McLaughlin ME, Bronson RT, Jacks T: Mouse models of tumor development in neurofibromatosis type 1. Science 286:2172–2176, 1999.
21. Clayton-Smith J, Donnai D: Neurofibromatosis-Noonan syndrome—Independent segregation of the two conditions within a family. Third Manchester Birth Defects Conference, Manchester, UK, October 25–28, 1988.
21a. Clementi M, Battistella PA, Rizzi L, Boni S, Tenconi R: Headache in patients with neurofibromatosis type 1. Headache J 36:10–13, 1996.
22. Clementi M, Milani S, Mammi I, Boni S, Monciotti C, Tenconi R: Neurofibromatosis type 1 growth charts. Am J Med Genet 87:317–323, 1999.
23. Cohen MM Jr: Overgrowth syndromes: An update. Adv Pediatr, 46: 441–491, 1999.
24. Cohen MM Jr: Some neoplasms and some hamartomatous syndromes: genetic considerations. Int J Oral Maxillofac Surg 27:363–369, 1998.
25. Cohen MM Jr, Gorlin RJ: Noonan-like/multiple giant cell lesion syndrome. Am J Med Genet 40:159–166, 1991.
26. Colman SD, Rasmussen SA, Ho VT, Abernathy CR, Wallace MR: Somatic mosaicism in a patient with neurofibromatosis type 1. Am J Hum Genet 58:484–490, 1996.
27. Colman SD, Williams CA, Wallace MR: Benign neurofibromas in type 1 neurofibromatosis (NF1) show somatic deletion of the *NF1* gene. Nat Genet 11:90–92, 1995.
28. Combemale P, Abitan R, Kanitakis J: Segmental neurofibromatosis: Report of two cases and

critical review of the literature. Eur J Dermatol 4:194–201, 1994.
29. Crawford AH: Neurofibromatosis in children. Acta Orthoped Scand 57:1–60, 1986.
30. Crawford AH, Bagamery N: Osseous manifestations of neurofibromatosis in childhood. J Pediatr Orthoped 6:72–88, 1986.
31. Crowe FW, Schull WJ: Diagnostic importance of café-au-lait spot in neurofibromatosis. Arch Intern Med 91:758–766, 1953.
32. Crowe FW, Schull WJ, Neel JV: *A Clinical, Pathological and Genetic Study of Multiple Neurofibromatosis*. Charles C. Thomas, Springfield, IL, 1956.
33. Danglot G, Regnier V, Fauvet D, Vassal G, Kujas M, Bernheim A: Neurofibromatosis 1 (NF1) mRNAs expressed in the central nervous system are differentially spliced in the 5′ part of the gene. Hum Mol Genet 4:915–920, 1995.
34. Däschner K, Assum G, Eisenbath I: Clonal origin of tumour cells in a plexiform neurofibroma with LOH in intron 38 and in dermal neurofibromas without LOH of the *NF1* gene. Biochem Biophys Res Commun 234:346–350, 1997.
34a. Easton DF, Ponder MA, Huson SM, Ponder BAJ: An analysis of variation in expression of neurofibromatosis (NF) type 1 (NF1): Evidence for modifying genes. Am J Hum Genet 53:305–313, 1993.
35. Eisenbarth I, Beyer K, Krone W, Assum G: Toward a survey of somatic mutation of the *NF1* gene in benign neurofibromas of patients with neurofibromatosis type 1. Am J Hum Genet 66:393–401, 2000.
36. Evans DGR, Wallace AJ, Wu CL, Trueman L, Ramsden RT, Strachan T: Somatic mosaicism: A common cause of classic disease in tumor-prone syndromes? Lessons from type 2 neurofibromatosis. Am J Hum Genet 63:727–736, 1998.
37. Fahsold R, Hoffmeyer S, Mischung C, Gille C, Ehlers C, Kücükceylan N, Abdel-Nourm M, Gewies A, Peters H, Kaufmann D, Buske A, Tinschert S, Nürnberg P: Minor lesion mutational spectrum of the entire *NF1* gene does not explain its high mutability but points to a functional domain upstream of the GAP-related domain. Am J Hum Genet 66:790–818, 2000.
38. Faravelli F, Upadhyaya M, Osborn M, Huson SM, Hayward R, Winter R: Unusual clustering of brain tumours in a family with NF1 and variable expression of cutaneous features. J Med Genet 36:893–896, 1999.
39. Friedman JM: Epidemiology of neurofibromatosis type 1. Am J Med Genet 89:1–6, 1999.
40. Friedman JM, Birch PH: Type 1 neurofibromatosis: A descriptive analysis of the disorder in 1,728 patients. Am J Med Genet 70:138–143, 1997.
40a. Gareth D, Evans R, Sainio M, Baser ME: Neurofibromatosis type 2. J Med Genet 37:897–904, 2000.
41. Goedegebuure SA: A case of neurofibromatosis in the dog. J Small Animal Pract 16:329–335, 1975.
42. Gorlin RJ, Koutlas IG: Multiple schwannomas, multiple nevi, and multiple vaginal leiomyomas: A new dominant syndrome. Am J Med Genet 78:76–81, 1998.
43. Gripp KW, Scott CI Jr, Hughes HE, Wallerstein R, Nicholson L, States L, Bason LD, Kaplan P, Zderic SA, Duhaime A-C, Miller F, Magnusson MR, Zackai EH: Lateral meningocele syndrome: Three new patients and review of the literature. Am J Med Genet 70:229–239, 1997.
44. Gutmann DH, Aylsworth A, Carey JC, Korf B, Marks J, Pyeritz RE, Rubenstein A, Viskochil D: The diagnostic evaluation and multidisciplinary management of neurofibromatosis 1 and neurofibromatosis 2. JAMA 278:51–57, 1997.
44a. Gutmann DH, Haipek CA, Burke SP, Sun C-X, Scoles DR, Pulst SM: The *NF2* interactor, hepatocyte growth factor-regulated tyrosine kinase substrate (HRS), associates with merlin in the 'open' conformation and suppresses cell growth and motility. Hum Mol Genet 10:825–834, 2001.
45. Gutmann DH, Sherman L, Seftor L, Haipek C, Lu KH, Hendrix M: Increased expression of the NF2 tumor suppressor gene product, merlin, impairs cell motility, adhesion and spreading. Hum Molec Genet 8:267–275, 1999.
45a. Habiby R, Silverman B, Listernick R, Charrow J: Precocious puberty in children with neurofibromatosis type 1. J Pediatr 126:364–367, 1995.
45b. Hamilton SJ, Allard MF, Friedman JM: Cardiac findings in an individual with neurofibromatosis 1 and sudden death. Am J Med Genet 100:95–99, 2001.
45c. Happle R: Letter to the editor: Large plexiform neurofibromas may be explained as a Type 2 segmental manifestation of neurofibromatosis 1. Am J Med Genet 98:363–364, 2001.
46. Heimann R, Verhest A, Verschraegen J, Grosjean W, Draps JP, Hecht F: Hereditary intestinal neurofibromatosis. I. A distinctive genetic disease. Neurofibromatosis 1:26–32, 1988.
47. Hoffmeyer S, Nürnberg P, Ritter H, Fahsold R, Leistner W, Kaufmann D, Krone W: Nearby stop codons in exons of the neurofibromatosis type 1 gene are disparate splice effectors. Am J Hum Genet 62:269–277, 1998.
48. Hope DG, Mulvihill JJ: Malignancy in neurofibromatosis. Adv Neurol 29:33–56, 1981.
49. Horan MP, Cooper DN, Upadhyaya M: Hypermethylation of the neurofibromatosis type 1 (NF1) gene promoter is not a common event in the inactivation of the *NF1* gene in NF1-specific tumours. Hum Genet 107:33–39, 2000.
50. Huson SM, Compston DAS, Clark P, Harper PS: A genetic study of von Recklinghausen neurofibromatosis in southeast Wales. 1. Preva-

lence, fitness, mutation rate, and effect of parental transmission on severity. J Med Genet 26:704–711, 1989.
51. Huson SM, Harper PS, Compston DAS: Von Recklinghausen neurofibromatosis: A clinical and population study in south east Wales. Brain 111:1355–1381, 1988.
52. Huson SM, Hughes RAC: *The Neurofibromatoses: A Pathogenetic and Clinical Overview*. London: Chapman and Hall Medical, 1994.
52a. Huson SM, Ruggieri M: The neurofibromatoses. In: Harper J, Oranje JM, Rose M, editors. Textbook of Pediatric Dermatology. Vol. 2, Oxford: Blackwell Science Publishers, p. 1204–1224, 2000.
53. Jacoby LB, Jones D, Davis K, Kronn D, Short MP, Gusella J, MacCollin M: Molecular analysis of *NF2* tumor-suppressor gene in schwannomatosis. Am J Hum Genet 61:1293–1302, 1997.
54. John AM, Ruggieri M, Ferner R, Upadhyaya M: A search for evidence of somatic mutations in the *NF1* gene. J Med Genet 37:44–49, 2000.
55. Jung EG: Segmental neurofibromatosis (NF-5). Neurofibromatosis 1:306–311, 1988.
56. Kaplan DL, Pestana A: Cutaneous segmental neurofibromatosis. South Med J 82:516–517, 1989.
57. Kaplan P, Rosenblatt B: A distinctive facial appearance in neurofibromatosis von Recklinghausen. Am J Med Genet 21:463–470, 1985.
58. Kehrer-Sawatzki, Schwickardt T, Assum G, Rocchi M, Krone W: A third neurofibromatosis type 1 (*NF1*) pseudogene at chromosome 15q11.2. Hum Genet 100:595–600, 1997.
59. King AA, DeBaun MR, Riccardi VM, Gutmann DH: Malignant peripheral nerve sheath tumors in neurofibromatosis 1. Am J Med Genet 93:388–392, 2000.
60. Klose A, Peters H, Hoffmeyer S, Buske A, Lüder A, Hess D, Lehmann R, Nürnberg P, Tinschert S: Two independent mutations in a family with neurofibromatosis type 1 (NF1). Am J Med Genet 83:6–12, 1999.
61. Korf BR: Plexiform neurofibromas. Am J Med Genet 89:31–37, 1999.
62. Korf BR: The *NF1* genetic analysis consortium. In: *Neurofibromatosis, Type 1: From Genotype to Phenotype*. M Upadhyaya and DN Cooper, eds. BIOS Scientific Publisher, Oxford, pp. 57–63, 1998.
63. Kousseff BG, Hoover DL: Penile neurofibromas. Am J Med Genet 87:1–5, 1999.
64. Kumar BB: Watson's syndrome. Am J Dis Child 123:612, 1972.
65. Lázaro C, Gaona A, Ainsworth P, Tenconi R, Vidaud D, Kruyer H, Ars E, Volpini V, Estivill X: Sex differences in mutational rate and mutational mechanism in the *NF1* gene in neurofibromatosis type 1 patients. Hum Genet 98:696–699, 1996.
66. Lázaro C, Gaona A, Lynch M, Kruyer H, Ravella A, Estivill X: Molecular characterization of the breakpoints of a 12-kb deletion in the *NF1* gene

in a family showing germline mosaicism. Am J Hum Genet 57:1044–1049, 1995.
67. Legius E, Wu R, Eyssen M, Marynen P, Frijns JP, Cassiman JJ: Encephalocraniocutaneous lipomatosis with a mutation in the *NF1* gene. J Med Genet 32:316–319, 1995.
68. Leppig KA, Kaplan P, Viskochil D, Weaver M, Ortenberg J, Stephens K: Familial neurofibromatosis 1 microdeletions: Cosegregation with distinct facial phenotype and early onset of cutaneous neurofibromata. Am J Med Genet 73:197–204, 1997.
69. Li Y, O'Connell P, Huntsman Breidenbach H, Cawthon R, Stevens J, Xu G, Neil S, Robertson M, White R, Viskochil D: Genomic organization of the neurofibromatosis 1 gene (*NF1*). Genomics 25:9–18, 1995.
70. Lin AE, Birch PH, Korf BR, Tenconi R, Niimura M, Poyhonen M, Uhas KA, Sigorini M, Virdis R, Romano C, Bonioli E, Wolkenstein P, Pivnick EK, Lawrence M, Friedman JM, and the NNFF International Database Participants: Cardiovascular malformations and other cardiovascular abnormalities in neurofibromatosis 1. Am J Med Genet 95:108–117, 2000.
71. Lipton S, Zuckerbrod M: Familial enteric neurofibromatosis. Med Times 94:544–548, 1966.
72. Listernick R, Charrow J, Gutmann DH: Intracranial gliomas in neurofibromatosis type 1. Am J Med Genet 89:38–44, 1999.
72a. Listernick R, Charrow J, Gutmann DH. Letter to the editor. Comments on neurofibromatosis 1 and optic pathway tumors. Am J Med Genet 102:105, 2001.
73. Listernick R, Darling C, Greenwald M, Strauss L, Charrow J: Optic pathway tumors in children: The effect of neurofibromatosis type 1 on clinical manifestations and natural history. J Pediatr 127:718–722, 1995.
74. López-Correa C, Brems H, Lázaro C, Estivill X, Clementi M, Mason S, Rutkowski JL, Marynen P, Legius E: Molecular studies in 20 submicroscopic neurofibromatosis type 1 gene deletions. Hum Mutat 14:387–393, 1999.
74a. López-Correa C, Dorschner M, Brems H, Lázaro C, Clementi M, Upadhyaya M, Dooijes D, Moog U, Kehrer-Sawatzki H, Rutkowski JL, Fryns J-P, Marynen P, Stephens K, Legius E: Recombination hotspot in *NF1* microdeletion patients. Hum Mol Genet 10:1387–1392, 2001.
75. López-Correa C, Zucman-Rossi J, Brems H, Thomas G, Legius E: *NF2* gene deletion in a family with a mild phenotype. J Med Genet 37:75–77, 2000.
76. Lubinsky MS: Patterns and pathogenesis in neurofibromatosis type 1 (NF1): A "new" NF1 association and evidence for independent constitutional determinants. 21st David W. Smith Workshop on Malformations and Morphogenesis, La Jolla, California, August 2–5, 2000.
77. Luginbuhl H, Frankhauser R, McGrath JT:

Spontaneous neoplasms of the nervous system in animals. Prog Neurol Surg 2:85–164, 1968.
78. MacCollin M, Ramesh V, Jacoby LB, Louis DN, Rubio M-P, Pulaski K, Trofatter J: Mutational analysis of patients with neurofibromatosis 2. Am J Hum Genet 55:314–320, 1994.
79. Marchuk D, Saulino A, Tavkkol R, Swaroop M, Wallace M, Andersen L, Mitchell A, Gutmann D, Boguski M, Collins F: cDNA cloning of the type 1 neurofibromatosis gene: Complete sequence of the NF1 gene product. Genomics 11:931–940, 1991.
80. Martuza RL, Eldridge R: Neurofibromatosis 2 (bilateral acoustic neurofibromatosis). N Engl J Med 318:684–688, 1988.
81. Martuza RL, Phillippe I, Fitzpatrick TB, Zwaan J, Seki Y, Lederman J: Melanin macroglobules as a cellular marker of neurofibromatosis: A quantitative study. J Invest Dermatol 85:347–350, 1985.
82. Mbarek O, Marouillat S, Martineau J, Barthélémy C, Müh J-P, Andres C: Association study of the NF1 gene and autistic disorder. Am J Med Genet 88:729–732, 1999.
83. McCartney BM, Kulikauskas RM, LaJeunesse DR, Fehon RG: The *neurofibromatosis-2* homologue, *Merlin*, and the tumor suppressor expanded function together in *Drosophila* to regulate cell proliferation and differentiation. Development 127:1315–1324, 2000.
84. Mendez HMM: The neurofibromatosis-Noonan syndrome. Am J Med Genet 21:471–476, 1985.
85. Miles DK, Freedman MH, Stephens K, Pallavicini M, Sievers E, Weaver M, Grunberger T, Thompson P, Shannon KM: Patterns of hematopoietic lineage involvement in children with neurofibromatsis, type 1, and malignant myeloid disorders. Blood 88:4314–4320.
86. Miller RM, Sparkes RS: Segmental neurofibromatosis. Arch Dermatol 113:837–838, 1977.
87. Mulvihill JJ, Parry DM, Sherman JL, Pikus A, Kaiser-Kupfer MI, Eldridge R: Neurofibromatosis 1 (Recklinghausen disease) and neurofibromatosis 2 (bilateral acoustic neurofibromatosis). An update. Ann Intern Med 113:39–52, 1990.
88. National Institutes of Health Consensus Development Conference on Neurofibromatosis. Neurofibromatosis: Conference statement. Arch Neurol 45:575–578, 1988.
89. Nordlund M, Gu X, Shipley M, Ratner N: Neurofibromin is enriched in the endoplasmic reticulum of CNS neurons. J Neurosci 13:1588–1600, 1993.
90. North K: Neurofibromatosis type 1: Am J Med Genet 97:119–127, 2000.
91. North KN: Cognitive function and academic performance. In: *Neurofibromatosis: Phenotype, Natural History and Pathogenesis*, 3rd ed. JM Friedman, DH Gutmann, M MacCollin, VM Riccardi, eds. Johns Hopkins University Press, Baltimore, 1999.
92. North KN: Neurofibromatosis type 1: Establishment of a clinic and review of the first 200 patients. J Child Neurol 8:395–403, 1993.
93. Nwokoro NA, Korytkowski MT, Rose S, Gorin MB, Stadler MP, Witchel SF, Mulvihill JJ: Spectrum of malignancy and premalignancy in Carney syndrome. Am J Med Genet 73:369–377, 1997.
94. Opitz JM, Weaver DD: The neurofibromatosis-Noonan syndrome. Am J Med Genet 21:477–490, 1985.
95. Ozonoff S: Cognitive impairment in neurofibromatosis type 1. Am J Med Genet 89:45–52, 1999.
96. Parry DM, Eldridge R, Kaiser-Kupfer MI, Bouzas E, Pikus A, Patronas N: Neurofibromatosis 2 (NF2): Clinical characteristics of 63 affected individuals and clinical evidence for heterogeneity. Am J Med Genet 52:450–461, 1994.
97. Patnaik AK, Erlandson RA, Lieberman PH: Canine malignant melanotic schwannomas: A light and electron microscopic study of two cases. Vet Pathol 21:483–488, 1984.
98. Pollack IF, Mulvihill JJ: Neurofibromatosis. In: *Principles and Practice of Pediatric Neurosurgery*. L Albright, I Pollack, D Adelson, eds. chapter 40, pp. 719–740, 1999.
99. Poyhonen M, Kytölä S, Leisti J: Epidemiology of neurofibromatosis type 1 (NF1) in Northern Finland. J Med Genet 37:632–636, 2000.
100. Poyhonen M, Niemela S, Herva R: Risk of malignancy and death in neurofibromatosis. Arch Pathol Lab Med 121:139–143, 1997.
101. Pulst SM, Riccardi VM, Fain P, Korenberg JR: Familial spinal neurofibromatosis: Clinical and DNA linkage analysis. Neurology 41:1923–1925, 1991.
102. Purcell SM, Dixon SL: Schwannomatosis. An usual variant of neurofibromatosis or a distinct clinical entity. Arch Dermatol 125:390–393, 1989.
103. Régnier V, Meddeb M, Lecointre G, Richard F, Duverger A, Nguyen VC, Dutrillaux B, Bernheim A, Danglot G: Emergence and scattering of multiple neurofibromatosis (NF1)-related sequences during hominoid evolution suggest a process of pericentromeric interchromosomal transposition. Hum Mol Genet 6:9–16, 1997.
104. Riccardi VM: Genotype, malleotype, phenotype, and randomness: lessons from neurofibromatosis-1 (NF-1). Am J Hum Genet 53:301–304, 1993.
105. Riccardi VM: Neurofibromatosis: Clinical heterogeneity. Curr Probl Cancer 7:1–34, 1982.
106. Riccardi VM: *Neurofibromatosis. Phenotype, Natural History and Pathogenesis*, 2nd ed. Johns Hopkins University Press, Baltimore, 1992.
107. Riccardi VM, Mulvihill JJ, eds: *Advances in Neurology*, Vol. 29, *Neurofibromatosis (von Recklinghausen Disease)*. Raven Press, New York, 1981.
108. Rosenquist GC, Krovetz LJ, Haller JA Jr, Simon AL, Bannayan GA: Acquired right ventricular outflow obstruction in a child with neurofibromatosis. Am Heart J 79:103–108, 1970.

109. Rothe RR, Martines R, James WD: Segmental neurofibromatosis. Arch Dermatol 123:917–920, 1987.
110. Rubinstein AE, Bader JL, Aron AA, Wallace S: Familial transmission of segmental neurofibromatosis. Neurology 33(Suppl):76, 1983.
110a. Ruggieri M: Letter to the editor: Mosaic (segmental) neurofibromatosis type 1 (NF1) and type 2 (NF2): No longer neurofibromatosis type 5 (NF5). Am J Med Genet 101:178–180, 2001.
111. Ruttledge MH, Andermann AA, Phelan CM, Claudio JO, Han F-Y, Cretien N, Rangaratnam S, MacCollin M, Short P, Parry D, Michels V, Riccardi VM, Weksberg R, Kitamura K, Bradburn JM, Hall BD, Propping P, Rouleau GA: Type of mutation in the neurofibromatosis type 2 gene (NF2) frequently determines severity of disease. Am J Hum Genet 59:331–342, 1996.
112. Saul RA: Letter to the editor: Noonan syndrome in a patient with hyperplasia of the myenteric plexuses and neurofibromatosis. Am J Med Genet 21:491–492, 1985.
113. Saul RA, Stevenson RE: Segmental neurofibromatosis: A distinct type of neurofibromatosis? Proc Greenwood Genet Ctr 3:3–6, 1984.
114. Sawada S, Florell S, Purandare S, Ota M, Stephens K, Viskochil D: Identification of NF1 mutations in both alleles of a dermal neurofibroma. Nat Genet 14:110–112, 1996.
115. Schlumberger HG: Nerve sheath tumors in an isolated goldfish population. Cancer Res 12:890–899, 1952.
116. Schmale MC, Hensley G, Udey LR: Multiple schwannomas in the bicolor damselfish, *Pomacentrus partitus*: A possible model of von Recklinghausen neurofibromatosis. Am J Pathol 112:238–241, 1983.
116a. Serra E, Ars E, Ravella A, Sánchez A, Puig S, Rosenbaum T, Estivill X, Lázaro C. Somatic NF1 mutational spectrum in benign neurofibromas: mRNA splice defects are common among point mutations. Hum Genet 108:416–429, 2001.
117. Serra E, Puig S, Otero D: Confirmation of the double-hit model for the NF1 gene in benign neurofibromas. Am J Hum Genet 61:512–519, 1997.
117a. Serra E, Rosenbaum T, Winner U, Aledo R, Ars E, Estivill X, Lenard H-G, Lázaro C: Schwann cells harbor the somatic NF1 mutation in neurofibromas: Evidence of two different Schwann cell subpopulations. Hum Mol Genet 9:3055–3064, 2000.
118. Shannon KM, O'Connell P, Math GA, Paderanga D, Olson K, Dindorf P, McCormick F: Loss of the normal NF1 allele from the bone marrow of children with type 1 neurofibromatosis and malignant myeloid disorders. N Engl J Med 330:597–601, 1994.
119. Shen MH, Harper PS, Upadhyaya M: Molecular genetics of neurofibromatosis type 1 (NF1). J Med Genet 33:2–17, 1996.
120. Sigorini M, Zuccoli G, Ferrozzi F, Bacchini E, Street ME, Piazza P, Rossi M, Virdis R: Magnetic resonance findings and ophthalmologic abnormalities are correlated in patients with neurofibromatosis type 1 (NF1). Am J Med Genet 93:269–272, 2000.
121. Stevenson DA, Birch PH, Friedman JM, Viskochil DH, Balestrazzi P, Boni S, Buske A, Korf BR, Niimura M, Pivnick EK, Schorry EK, Short MP, Tenconi R, Tonsgard JH, Carey JC: Descriptive analysis of tibial pseudarthrosis in patients with neurofibromatosis 1. Am J Med Genet 84:413–419, 1999.
122. Stokowski RP, Cox DR: Functional analysis of the neurofibromatosis type 2 protein by means of disease-causing point mutations. Am J Hum Genet 66:873–891, 2000.
123. Streubel B, Latta E, Kehrer-Sawatzki H, Hoffmann GF, Fonatsch C, Rehder H: Somatic mosaicism of a greater than 1.7-Mb deletion of genomic DNA involving the entire NF1 gene as verified by FISH: Further evidence for a contiguous gene syndrome in 17q11.2. Am J Med Genet 87:12–16, 1999.
124. Tonsgard JH, Yelavarthi KK, Cushner S, Short MP, Lindgren V: Do NF1 gene deletions result in a characteristic phenotype? Am J Med Genet 73:80–86, 1997.
125. Upadhyaya M, Cooper DN: The mutation spectrum in neurofibromatosis type 1 and its underlying mechanism. In: *Neurofibromatosis Type 1: From Genotype to Phenotype*. M Upadhyaya and DN Cooper, eds. BIOS Scientific Publisher, Oxford, pp. 65–68, 1998.
126. Upadhyaya M, Ruggieri M, Maynard J, Osborn M, Hartog C, Mudd S, Penttinen M, Cordeiro I, Ponder M, Ponder BAJ, Krawczak M, Cooper DN: Gross deletions of the neurofibromatosis type 1 (NF1) gene are predominantly of maternal origin and commonly associated with a learning disability, dysmorphic features and developmental delay. Hum Genet 102:591–597.
127. Vandevelde M, Braund KG, Hoff EJ: Central neurofibromas in two dogs. Vet Pathol 14:470–478, 1977.
128. Van Es S, North K, McHugh K, de Silva M: MRI abnormalities in children with NF1. Paediatr Radiol 26:478–487, 1996.
129. Verhest A, Verschraegen J, Grosjean W, Draps JP, Vamos E, Heimann R, Hecht F: Hereditary intestinal neurofibromatosis. II. Translocation between chromosomes 12 and 14. Neurofibromatosis 1:33–36, 1988.
130. Viskochil D: Gene structure and expression. In: *Neurofibromatosis Type 1: From Genotype to Phenotype*. M Upadhyaya and DN Cooper, eds. BIOS Scientific Publishers, Oxford, pp. 1998.

131. Viskochil D: Neurofibromatosis 1. Am J Med Genet 89:v–viii, 1999.
132. Viskochil D, Carey JC: Nosological considerations of the neurofibromatoses. J Dermatol 19:873–880, 1992.
133. Viskochil D, Carey JC: The Neurofibromatoses: A Pathogenetic and Clinical Overview. Alternate and Related Forms of the Neurofibromatoses. Chapman and Hall Medical, New York, pp. 445–474, 1994.
134. Vogel KS, Klesse LJ, Velasco-Miguel S, Meyers K, Rushing EJ, Parada LF: Mouse tumor model for neurofibromatosis type 1. Science 286:2176–2179, 1999.
135. Waggoner DJ, Towbin J, Gottesman G, Gutmann DH: Clinic-based study of plexiform neurofibromas in neurofibromatosis 1. Am J Med Genet 92:132–135, 2000.
136. Watson GH: Pulmonary stenosis, café-au-lait spots and dull intelligence. Arch Dis Child 42:303–307, 1967.
137. Weiss B, Bollag G, Shannon K: Hyperactive Ras as a therapeutic target in neurofibromatosis type 1. Am J Med Genet 89:14–22, 1999.
138. Westerhof W, Konrad K: Blue-red macules and pseudoatrophic macules: Additional cutaneous signs in neurofibromatosis. Arch Dermatol 118:577–581, 1982.
139. Wolkenstein P, Mahmoudi A, Zeller J, Revuz J: More on the frequency of segmental neurofibromatosis [letter]. Arch Dermatol 131:1466, 1995.
140. Woodruff JM: Pathology of tumors of the peripheral nerve sheath in type 1 neurofibromatosis. Am J Med Genet 89:23–30, 1999
141. Wu B-L, Schneider GH, Korf BR: Deletion of the entire *NF1* gene causing distinct manifestations in a family. Am J Med Genet 69:98–101, 1997.
141a. Wu CL, Thakker N, Neary W, Black G, Lye R, Ramsden RT, Read AP, Evans DGR: Differential diagnosis of type 2 neurofibromatosis: Molecular discrimination of NF2 and sporadic vestibular schwannomas. J Med Genet 35:973–977, 1998.
142. Wu R, Legius E, Robberecht W, Dumoulin M, Cassiman J-J, Fryns J-P: Neurofibromatosis type 1 gene mutation in a patient with features of LEOPARD syndrome. Hum Mutat 8:51–56, 1996.
143. Wu W, Mulligan L, Ponder MA, Liu L, Smith BA, Mathew CG, Ponder BA: Loss of alleles in pheochromocytomas from patients with type 1 neurofibromatosis. Genes Chromosom Cancer 4:337–341, 1992.
144. Xu G, O'Connell P, Viskochil D, Cawthon R, Robertson M, Culver M, Dunn D, Stevens J, Gesteland R, White R, Weiss R: The neurofibromatosis type 1 gene encodes a protein related to GAP. Cell 62:599–608, 1990.
145. Yasunari T, Shiraki K, Hatton H, Miki T: Frequency of choroidal abnormalities in neurofibromatosis type 1. Lancet 356:988–992, 2000.
146. Yesudian P, Premalatha S, Thambiah AS: Palmar melanotic macules. A sign of neurofibromatosis. Int J Dermatol 23:468–471, 1984.
147. Zvulunov A, Barak Y, Metzker A: Juvenile xanthogranuloma, neurofibromatosis, and juvenile chronic myelogenous leukemia. Arch Dermatol 131:904–908, 1995.

13

Fragile X Syndrome

More than 125 X-linked mental retardation (XLMR) syndromes have been identified, and of these, fragile X syndrome is the most common (43,59). The syndrome is the prototype of an ever growing list of disorders with dynamic mutations that result from instability of triplet repeats. The mutant gene in fragile X syndrome is *FMR1* (OMIM 309550)[a] and the repeated triplet is CGG (68). Several excellent reviews are available, the one by Nussbaum and Ledbetter (44) being particularly exhaustive, and many international fragile X workshops have been held (21).

PREVALENCE

Prevalence estimates are summarized in Table 13–1. Fragile X syndrome is not as prevalent as initially estimated. The discrepancy can be explained by the use of a molecular diagnosis, which is more accurate than the cytogenetic test previously employed.

Prevalence estimates of healthy female carriers are also summarized in Table 13–1. The higher estimate in the study of Falik-Zaccai et al. (16) is partially attributable to the current lack of an accurate definition of a premutation (meiotically unstable allele). Further studies are needed to establish whether this unexpectedly high prevalence of premutation carriers is unique to the specific populations studied or whether it applies to other populations, which is probable (54). Evidence that expansion to full mutation on transmission from a premutated mother is more likely to occur in male fetuses than in female fetuses (34) and may explain a relative lack of premutated males in the general population (50). Large population studies on an unselected series of newborns would be useful in settling the true prevalence of affected (fully mutated) males, normal transmitting (premutated) males, and fully mutated and premutated female carriers. Caution must be exercised in planning such studies to avoid untoward effects on the screened subjects (42).

GENETICS

Many genetic and molecular papers have appeared (1,3,6,11,28,31,36,49,56,57,61,62). This section considers (a) gene structure and protein isoforms and (b) the origin and effects of full mutations.

Gene Structure and Protein Isoforms

The *FMR1* gene maps to Xq27.3 and has 17 exons spanning 38 kb of genomic DNA. The polymorphic CGG repeat is located in the 5′ untranslated region of exon 1 and is included in all *FMR1* transcripts (3). *FMR1* was shown to be ubiquitously transcribed during murine and human embryogenesis with the highest levels of differentiated neurons in the hippocampus and basal ganglia (1); in adult mice, it is expressed only in neurons and spermatogonia. The 4.4 kb full-length mRNA encodes a protein with a max-

[a]On-Line Mendelian Inheritance in Man number.

Table 13–1 Prevalence Estimates[a] of Fragile X Syndrome and Healthy Female Carriers

Estimates	Reference
FRAGILE X SYNDROME	
67/100,000	Webb et al. (69)
25/100,000[b]	Morton et al. (40)
17/100,000[b]	de Vries et al. (14)
HEALTHY FEMALE CARRIERS	
386/100,000	Rousseau et al. (51)
407/100,000[c]	Ryynänen et al. (52)
1176/100,000[c]	Falik-Zaccai et al. (16)

[a]Estimates have been converted to standard epidemiologic form. With a standardized denominator, numerators can be compared more effectively.

[b]More realistic estimates by the use of molecular diagnosis, which is more accurate than the cytogenetic test previously employed.

[c]Difference probably reflects current lack of an accurate definition of a premutation.

imum size of 632 amino acids and a molecular weight of 70–80 kDa (15). Although 20 different transcripts can be produced by alternative splicing (3), only 4 or 5 of them and their corresponding protein products are actually detected in various tissues. Isoform 7 (ISO7), which lacks only the 21 amino acids of exon 12, makes almost all the FMR1 protein and corresponds to the highest band on Western blotting with an approximate molecular weight of 80 kDa (57).

Two KH domains (KH1 and KH2) and one RGG box, common to several RNA-binding proteins, have been identified in exons 8, 10, and 15, respectively (56). It has been shown that FMR1 can bind synthetic RNAs in vitro, and the importance of KH domains was underscored by the description of a severely retarded fragile X patient with a point mutation change in a highly conserved KH2 isoleucine to asparagine (Ile304Asn) (11), which impaired the RNA binding activity of FMR1. It has also been shown that ISO7 is localized in the cytoplasm (15). In contrast, minor isoforms are lacking exon 14 and, with a different C-terminus (ISO6 or ISO12), are confined to the nucleus (57). Although no specific nuclear localization signal (NLS) is present in the first half of FMR1, studies with deletion constructs indicate that the N-terminus of the protein (exons 1–5) can direct the protein to the nucleus; sequences in exon 14 are essential for its subsequent export to the cytoplasm (57).

Origin and Effects of Full Mutations

In more than 95% of cases, fragile X syndrome is caused by a single type of mutation—expansion and hypermethylation of a potentially unstable CGG trinucleotide repeat in the 5′ UTR of the *FMR1* gene (full mutation). This causes transcriptional silencing of the gene and absence of the FMR1 protein. A full mutation appears to be generated by a lengthy multistep process requiring sequential action by a different mechanism (6). To date, no direct conversion of a wild-type to a fully mutated allele has been observed in fragile X families in which mothers of affected individuals were found to be carriers of an already expanded CGG triplet.

Different alleles at the CGG repeat are generally included in one of three classes depending on their total length: wild-type (6–50 repeats), premutation (50–200 repeats), and full mutation (200–1000 hypermethylated repeats). However, it has been shown that the boundaries between these classes are not absolute and that the initial instability depends not only on the total length but also on the repeat configuration. Detailed analysis of over 400 wild-type alleles has shown that the CGG repeat stretch is commonly interrupted by AGG triplets, mainly two, at intervals of 9–10 CGG units, which apparently have a stabilizing effect by preventing replication slippage.

The secondary structures formed by the full mutation and/or the increased number of CpG dinucleotide targets presumably favor the hypermethylation of the *FMR1* gene harboring a full mutation (28).

The question of when and in which cells the pre-to-full expansion takes place is still debated. It was initially proposed that expansion to full mutation was postzygotic because sperm cells obtained from male patients were shown to harbor only premutations (49). However, recent evidence demonstrates the presence of full mutations in the oogonia and spermatogonia of female fetuses and male fetuses, respectively (36), supporting the hypothesis of a selection process that favors premutations in the male germline.

CLINICAL PHENOTYPE

General Features and Variability

The phenotype is variable. In newborns, the birthweight may be elevated, relative macrocephaly may be found, and the anterior fontanelle may be large. Typical adult males have tall stature, large testes, relative macrocephaly, prominent forehead, hypoteloric sunken eyes, long narrow face, midface hypoplasia, prominent mandible, and large ears (Figs. 13–1 to 13–3). The phenotype tends to change with age. In infants and adolescents, the phenotype is milder and, often, macrocephaly, increased height, and hypotonia are the only findings. Hypotonia is virtually a constant feature and is usually accompanied by joint laxity. Mitral valve prolapse is frequently observed in hemizygotes after 18 years of age. On occasion,

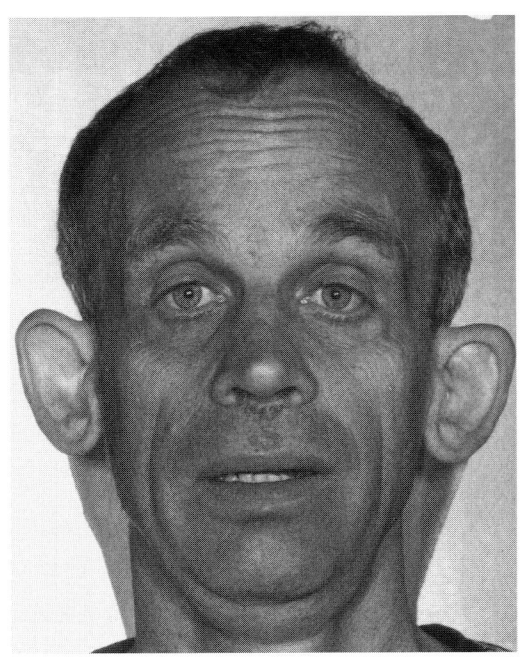

Figure 13–2 Fragile X syndrome. Narrow face and prominent ears. From McDermott et al. (39).

a small child may have the same phenotype as that found in typical adults.[b] A subgroup of patients have been noted to have short stature and obesity. Infrequently, hemizygotes have been noted to appear entirely normal. About one-third of female carriers with the full mutation have a behavioral phenotype that includes mild mental retardation, shyness, poor eye contact, and learning disabilities. Some, particularly the more retarded ones, have the typical long face, mandibular prognathism, and large everted ears (10,19,20,22,30,33,39,58,59a).

Typical Craniofacial Appearance

In typical adult males, an increased head circumference and dolichocephaly are found together with a high quadrangular forehead, prominent supraorbital ridges, and a long narrow face. Puffiness under the eyes occurs in

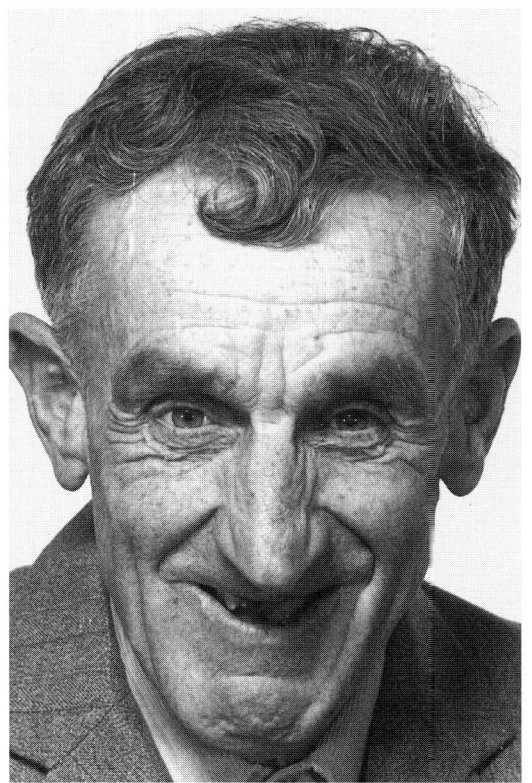

Figure 13–1 Fragile X syndrome. Long face, prominent forehead, sunken eyes, broad based nose, prominent chin, and prominent ears. From McDermott et al. (39).

[b]Parvari et al. (45) reported an 8.5 Mb deletion, including the *FMR1* gene, in a 4-year-old boy with a facial appearance consistent with fragile X syndrome and a height and weight above the 97th centile.

FRAGILE X SYNDROME

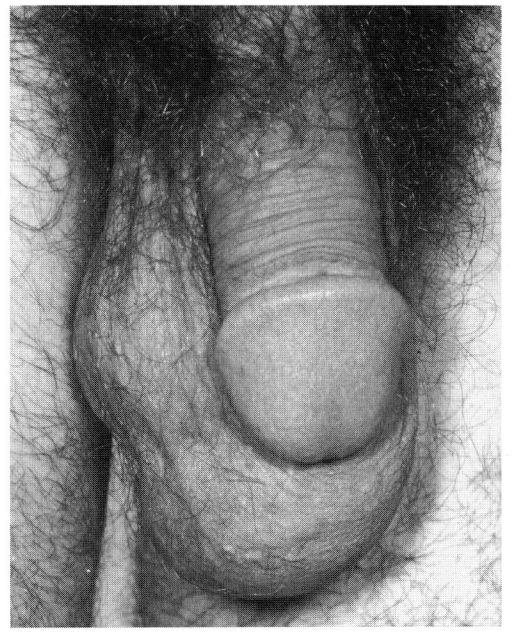

Figure 13–3 Fragile X syndrome. Macroorchidism. From McDermott et al. (39).

some cases. The palpebral fissure length is increased and the inter-inner canthal distance is decreased. Strabismus and refractive errors may be present. The nose often appears broadly based and midface hypoplasia is found (Figs. 13–1 and 13–2). The chin becomes long and prominent during adolescence. The ears are large, outstanding, and may be somewhat soft. The helices may be simple and the lobules may be absent. Otitis media is common and the palate is highly arched (20,39).

Central Nervous System and Performance

Central nervous system findings and performance have been discussed by many authors (9,10,19,20,22,30,33,41,46–48,53,59a,63,67,75). IQs in hemizygotes have been reported to range from 20–70. IQs in females with the full mutation range from 50–107. Delayed speech is very common. Retardation seems to increase with age. Those with higher IQs exhibit dysfluencies and stuttering and, frequently, a characteristic intonation. With lower IQs, less verbal ability is found together with repetitive phrases. Females who carry the full mutation may have learning disabilities. Even psychosis has been noted in some cases (9,19,20,22,53,63,75).

Neuropsychiatric evaluation shows delayed milestones, hypotonia, increased deep tendon reflexes, emotional instability, and automutilation, particularly handbiting. An adverse response to touch on the skin is found. Aggressive behavior occurs in about 50%. Seizures may be found during infancy; a characteristic EEG pattern has been reported as trains of medium-high voltage spikes discharging from the temporal region during sleep. A cognitive profile has been reported to consist of attention deficit hyperactivity disorder, oppositional defiant disorder, enuresis, and encopresis. Fragile X boys show greater variability in total sleep time than normal and difficulty in sleep maintenance compared with controls. In some cases, autism is found, characterized by avoidance of eye contact, hand flapping, or other stereotypic movements, perseverative speech, and echolalia (4,19,20,22,23,30,41,67).

MRI of the brain shows volume conservation of tissue, diminished white-to-gray matter ratio, relatively enlarged caudate nucleus and hippocampus, and increased cerebrospinal fluid, particularly in the lateral ventricles. In males, a relative decrease in the size of the superior temporal gyrus and cerebellar vermis occurs with a relative increase in the size of the fourth ventricle. Likewise, in young females, a relative decrease in the size of the cerebellar vermis is found together with an increase in the size of the fourth ventricle. Neuropathologic studies have demonstrated more long dendritic spines and fewer shorter ones than normal with significant immature morphology in both temporal and visual cortical areas (29,46–48).

Connective Tissue Findings

Joint laxity involves particularly the thumbs but also the fingers, metacarpophalangeal joints, knees, and ankles. The skin feels velvety and soft over the dorsa of the hands. Single palmar creases are found in about one-fourth of the cases. Flat feet are common. Mitral valve prolapse, encountered in approximately 80% of hemizygotes after 18 years of age, is accompanied by aortic dilatation in about 15% of the cases (27).

Genitourinary System

Macro-orchidism, either unilateral or bilateral, is easier to detect in postpubertal males (Fig. 13–3). The testes tend to be softer than normal and the scrotum may be hyperpigmented. There is increased seminiferous tubule length and interstitial edema. The penis is often enlarged (9,14,20,32).

Early menopause and an increased rate of twinning, both reported in premutation carriers, are indications of ovarian failure, which has been found in about 20% of carriers. The data supporting increased twinning conflict and need to be resolved (19,33,55).

DIAGNOSIS

Molecular diagnosis of the CGG amplification is available since the cloning of the *FMR1* gene in 1991; it relies on Southern blotting and hybridization of specific probes, while PCR is employed to detect repeat lengths in the premutation range. The cytogenetic test in low-folate media is obsolete and has been abandoned. A rapid method based on antibody detection of the FMR1 protein in the cells of blood smears is useful for screening affected males (73,74) and has been adapted for uncultured amniotic cells (72) and hair roots (65,71,74).

Prenatal diagnosis depends on the availability of sufficient DNA to perform Southern blotting after double digestion including a methylation-sensitive enzyme (usually EagI or BssHII), while the sex of the fetus can be determined by standard karyotype or Y-specific PCR analysis. False positives, due to suboptimal amplification, and false negatives, due to the possible presence of reverted alleles in the wild-type range, can occur when performing PCR alone on a sample from a male fetus. Furthermore, only direct DNA analysis after digestion with methylation-sensitive enzymes can demonstrate the methylation status of the *FMR1* CpG island, especially in the presence of a full mutation (58). Given that in extra-embryonic tissues, such as chorionic villi, a full mutation may remain largely undermethylated until 10–11 weeks of gestation (5,35,60), chorionic villus sampling might not reveal the hypermethylation already present in the embryonic tissues and may need confirmation by amniocentesis.

DIFFERENTIAL DIAGNOSIS

A subgroup of fragile X patients have short stature and obesity with a superficial resemblance to Prader-Willi syndrome (12). Several patients initially thought to have Sotos syndrome were diagnosed as having fragile X syndrome. Pitfalls in clinical diagnosis justify the view that every mentally retarded patient should be tested for fragile X syndrome in the absence of another reasonable diagnosis. Difficulties in the diagnosis of fragile X syndrome in young children have been discussed by Stoll (59a).

GUIDELINES FOR HEALTH SUPERVISION

Useful guidelines for health supervision of fragile X children have been published by the American Academy of Pediatrics (2) and include advice for both physical and behavioral aspects of the syndrome. After confirming the diagnosis with molecular testing and appropriate parental counseling for recurrence risk for subsequent pregnancies, a series of medical examinations can be envisioned depending on the age of the child. Development during the first year of life can be normal, although hypotonia and irritability may be apparent. In early childhood, the following examinations are important: ophthalmologic examination (strabismus, myopia), echocardiogram if a murmur or click is present (mitral valve prolapse), and orthopedic examination (flat feet, scoliosis, and loose joints). Inguinal hernias should also be excluded. A history of seizures or startle episodes should be reviewed; performing an EEG may be appropriate, although antiepileptic medication after a single seizure is not advisable, given the self-limited course of epileptic manifestations in adolescence (41). Hyperactive behavior and severe attention deficit, which are a major concern during school age, can be treated pharmacologically (24). Torrioli et al. (64) reported the results of a preliminary clinical trial, suggesting that L-acetylcarnitine might be beneficial in ameliorating the hyperactive behavior of affected children. However, socialization and school integration, possibly within a mainstream program with individual support, are important in helping to overcome these problems. Sports and regular physical activity are important to counteract hypotonic posture and to improve motor coordination. Speech, language, and occupational therapy should be goal oriented to help adolescents and young adults attain as much autonomy as possible. Support from family organizations is important, especially for parents and sibs.

Treatments aimed at recovering the function of the *FMR1* gene have been attempted with folic acid because of its action on cytogenetic expression of the fragile site. Although some reports indicated some beneficial effects on behavior (15), others have not confirmed these observations (18,70). Folate supplementation has no efficacy for the treatment of fragile X syndrome patients. Observations on intellectually normal (58) or minimally affected (25,37) males with an unmethylated full mutation confirm that the abnormally amplified CGG tract per se can still be transcribed and translated. Even if translation may not be completely efficient (17), lymphoblastoid cell lines containing only unmethylated full mutations of two such males have shown the presence of FMR1 protein in every cell, but at reduced levels (58). Given the observations of these exceptional individuals and knowing that the coding sequence of the mutated *FMR1* gene is intact, Chiurazzi et al. (7) tested the possibility of restoring its activity in vitro, employing a DNA demethylation protocol. These authors obtained in vitro reactivation of FMR1 expression after inducing DNA demethylation with 5-azadeoxycytidine in lymphoblastoid cell lines from patients.

Given that the effect of DNA hypermethylation in silencing the *FMR1* gene seems to be potentiated by deacetylation of histones, Chiurazzi et al. (8) performed another set of experiments with phenylbutyrate, an inhibitor of histone deacetylase, and showed that treatment of fragile X cell lines restores FMR1 transcription. Although the effect was weak, it appeared to be synergistic with that of 5-azadeoxycytidine. Phenylbutyrate is structurally similar to L-acetylcarnitine, used in vivo by Torrioli et al. (64) in the clinical trial discussed above.

McConkie-Rosell et al. (38) carried out a longitudinal study of women-at-risk for inheriting the fragile X mutation. Problems addressed were (a) how upsetting the women perceived their information to be, (b) how serious a problem they perceived fragile X syndrome to be, and (c) their feelings about the carrier testing process. Such information is useful for counseling purposes.

REFERENCES

1. Abitbol M, Menini C, Delezoide AL, Rhyner T, Vekemans M, Mallet J: Nucleus basalis magnocellularis and hippocampus are the major sites of FMR1 expression in the human fetal brain. Nat Genet 4:147–153, 1993.
2. American Academy of Pediatrics, Committee on Genetics: Health supervision for children with fragile X syndrome. Pediatrics 98:297–300, 1996.
3. Ashley CT, Sutcliffe JS, Kunst CB, Leiner HA, Eichler EE, Nelson DL, Warren ST: Human and murine *FMR1*: alternative splicing and translational initiation downstream of the CGG repeat. Nat Genet 4:244–251, 1993.
4. Backes M, Genç B, Schreck J, Doerfler W, Lehmkuhl G, von Gontard A: Cognitive and behavioral profile of fragile X boys: Correlations to molecular data. Am J Med Genet 95:150–156, 2000.
5. Castellvi-Bel S, Mila M, Soler A, Carrio A, Sanchez A, Villa M, Jimenez MD, Estivill X: Prenatal diagnosis of fragile X syndrome: $(CGG)_n$ expansion and methylation of chorionic villus samples. Prenatal Diagn 15:801–807, 1995.
6. Chiurazzi P, Macpherson J, Sherman S, Neri G: Editorial Comment: Significance of linkage disequilibrium between the fragile X locus and its flanking markers. Am J Med Genet 64:203–208, 1996.
7. Chiurazzi P, Pomponi MG, Willemsen R, Oostra BA, Neri G: In vitro reactivation of the *FMR1* gene involved in fragile X syndrome. Hum Molec Genet 7:109–113, 1998.
8. Chiurazzi P, Pomponi MG, Pietrobono R, Bakker CE, Neri G, Oostra B: Synergistic effect of histone hyperacetylation and DNA demethylation in the reactivation of the *FMR1* gene. Hum Molec Genet 8:2317–2323, 1999.
9. Chudley AE, Hagerman RJ: Fragile X syndrome. J Pediatr 110:821–831, 1987.
10. Cianchetti C, Sannio-Fancello G, Fratta A-L, Manconi F, Orano A, Pischedda M-P, Pruna D, Spinicci G, Archidiacono N, Filippi G: Neuropsychological, psychiatric, and physical manifestations in 149 members from 18 fragile X families. Am J Med Genet 40:234–243, 1991.

11. De Boulle K, Verkerk AJMH, Reyniers E, Vits L, Hendrickx J, Van Ro B, van den Bos F, de Graaff E, Oostra BA, Willems PJ: A point mutation in the *FMR1* gene associated with fragile X mental retardation. Nat Genet 3:31–35, 1993.
12. de Vries BB, Fryns JP, Butler MG, Canziani F, Wesby-van-Swaay E, van-Hemel JO, Oostra BA, Halley DJ, Niermeijer MF: Clinical and molecular studies in fragile X patients with a Prader-Willi-like phenotype. J Med Genet 30:761–766, 1993.
13. de Vries BBA, Robinson H, Stolte-Dijkstra F, Tjon Pian Gi CV, Dijkstra PF, van Doorn J, Halley DJ, Oostra BA, Turner G, Niermeijer MF: General overgrowth in the fragile X syndrome: Variability in the phenotype expression of the *FMR1* gene mutation. J Med Genet 32:764–769, 1995.
14. de Vries BBA, van den Ouweland AMW, Mohkamsing S, Duivenvoorden HJ, Moi E, Gelsema K, van Rijn M, Halley DJ, Sandkuijl LA, Oostra BA, Tibben A, Niermeijer MF: Screening and diagnosis of the fragile X syndrome among the mentally retarded: An epidemiological and psychological survey. Am J Hum Genet 61:660–667, 1997.
15. Devys D, Lutz Y, Rouyer N, Bellocq JP, Mandel JL: The FMR1 protein is cytoplasmic, most abundant in neurons and appears normal in carriers of a fragile X premutation. Nat Genet 4:335–340, 1993.
16. Falik-Zaccai TC, Shachak E, Borochowits Z, Magal N, Zatz S, Schochat M, Ziu H, Navon R, Legum C, Shomrat R: Fragile X syndrome: Population carrier screening and implication for prenatal diagnosis. Am J Hum Genet 65:A214, 1999.
17. Feng Y, Zhang F, Lokey LR, Chastain JL, Lakkis L, Eberhart D, Warren ST: Translational suppression by trinucleotide repeat expansion at FMR1. Science 268:731–734, 1995.
18. Froster-Iskenius U, Bodeker R, Oepen T, Matthes R, Piper U, Schwinger E: Folic acid treatment in males and females with fragile-(X)-syndrome. Am J Med Genet 23:273–239, 1986.
19. Fryns J-P: The female and the fragile X: A study of 144 obligate female carriers. Am J Med Genet 23:157–169, 1986.
20. Fryns J-P: The fragile X syndrome: A study of 83 families. Clin Genet 26:497–528, 1984.
21. Fryns J-P, Borghgraef M, Brown TW, Chelly J, Fisch GS, Hamel B, Hanauer A, Lacombe D, Luo L, MacPherson JN, Mandel J-L, Moraine C, Mulley J, Nelson D, Oostra B, Partington M, Ramakers GJA, Ropers H-H, Rousseau F, Schwartz C, Steinbach P, Stoll C, Tranebjaerg L, Turner G, Van Bokhoven H, Vian na-Morgante A, Villard L, Warren ST: 9th international workshop on fragile X syndrome and X-linked mental retardation. Am J Med Genet 94:345–360, 2000.
22. Fryns J-P, Jacobs J, Kleczkowska A, van den Berghe H: The psychological profile of the fragile X syndrome. Clin Genet 25:131–134, 1984.
23. Gould EL, Loesch DZ, Martin MJ, Hagerman RJ, Armstrong SM, Huggins RM: Melatonin profiles and sleep characteristics in boys with fragile X syndrome: A preliminary study. Am J Med Genet 95:307–315, 2000.
24. Hagerman R: Fragile X: treatment of hyperactivity. Pediatr 99:753, 1997.
25. Hagerman RJ, Hull CE, Safanda JF, Carpenter L, Staley LW, O'Connor RA, Seydel C, Mazzocco M, Snow K, Thibodeau SN, Kuhl D, Nelson DL, Caskey CT, Taylor AK: High functioning fragile X males: Demonstration of an unmethylated fully expanded *FMR1* mutation associated with protein expression. Am J Med Genet 51:298–308, 1994.
26. Hagerman RJ, Jackson AW, Levitas A, Braden M, McBogg P, Kemper M, McGavran L, Berry R, Matus I, Hagerman PJ: Oral folic acid versus placebo in the treatment of males with the fragile X syndrome. Am J Med Genet 23:241–262, 1986.
27. Hagerman RJ, Van Housen K, Smith ACM, McGavran L: Consideration of connective tissue dysfunction in the fragile X syndrome. Am J Med Genet 17:111–121, 1984.
28. Hansen RS, Canfield TK, Lamb MM, Gartler SM, Laird CD: Association of fragile X syndrome with delayed replication of the *FMR1* gene. Cell 73:1403–1409, 1993.
29. Irwin SA, Patel B, Idupulapati M, Harris JB, Crisostomo RA, Larsen BP, Kooy F, Willems PJ, Cras P, Kozlowski PB, Swain RA, Weiler IJ, Greenough WT: Abnormal dendritic spine characteristics in the temporal and visual cortices of patients with fragile-X syndrome: A quantitative examination. Am J Med Genet 98:161–167, 2001.
30. Lachiewicz AM, Dawson DV, Spiridigliozzi GA: Physical characteristics of young boys with fragile X syndrome: Reasons for difficulties in making a diagnosis in young males. Am J Med Genet 92:229–236, 2000.
31. Laggerbauer B, Ostareck D, Keidel E-M, Ostareck-Lederer A, Fischer U: Evidence that fragile X mental retardation protein is a negative regulator of translation. Hum Mol Genet 10:329–338, 2001.
32. Limprasert P, Jarvratanasirikul S, Vasikhanonte P: Letter to the Editor: Unilateral macroorchidism in fragile X syndrome. Am J Med Genet 95:516–517, 2000.
33. Loesch DZ, Hay DA: Clinical features and reproductive patterns in fragile X female heterozygotes. J Med Genet 25:407–414, 1988.
34. Loesch DZ, Huggins R, Petrovic L, Slater H: Expansion of the CGG repeat in fragile X in the *FMR1* gene depends on the sex of the offspring. Am J Hum Genet 57:1408–1413, 1995.

35. Luo S, Courtland Robinson J, Reiss AL, Migeon BR: DNA methylation of the fragile X locus in somatic and germ cells during fetal development: Relevance to the fragile X syndrome and X inactivation. Somat Cell Molec Genet 19:393–404, 1993.
36. Malter HE, Iberr C, Willemsen R, de Graaff E, Tarleton JC, Leisti J, Warren ST, Oostra BA: Characterization of the full fragile X syndrome mutation in fetal gametes. Nat Genet 15:165–169, 1997.
37. McConkie-Rosell A, Lachiewicz AM, Spiridigliozzi GA, Tarleton J, Schoenwald S, Phelan MC, Goonewardena P, Ding X, Brown WT: Evidence that methylation of the FMR-1 locus is responsible for variable phenotypic expression of the fragile X syndrome. Am J Hum Genet 53:800–809, 1993.
38. McConkie-Rosell A, Spiridigliozzi GA, Sullivan JA, Dawson DV, Lachiewicz AM: Longitudinal study of the carrier testing process for fragile X syndrome: Perceptions and coping. Am J Med Genet 98:37–45, 2001.
39. McDermott A: Fragile X chromosome: Clinical and cytogenetic studies from seven families. J Med Genet 20:169–171, 1983.
40. Morton JE, Bundey S, Webb TP, MacDonald F, Rinde PM, Bullock S: Fragile X syndrome is less common than previously estimated. J Med Genet 34:1–5, 1997.
41. Musumeci SA, Ferri R, Elia M, Colognola RM, Bergonzi P, Tassinari CA: Epilepsy and fragile X syndrome: a follow-up study. Am J Med Genet 38:511–513, 1991.
42. Neri G, Chiurazzi P: Fragile X syndrome screening: A current opinion. Commun Genet 3:38–40, 2000.
43. Neri G, Opitz JM: Sixty years of X-linked mental retardation: A historical footnote. Am J Med Genet 97:228–233, 2000.
44. Nussbaum RL, Ledbetter DH: The fragile X syndrome. In *The Metabolic and Molecular Bases of Inherited Disease*. CR Scriver, AL Beaudet, WS Sly, D. Valle D, eds., Chapter 19, pp. 795–810, 1995.
45. Parvari R, Mumm S, Galil A, Manor E, Bar-David Y, Carmi R: Deletion of 8.5 Mb, including the *FMR1* gene, in a male with the fragile X syndrome phenotype and overgrowth. Am J Med Genet 83:302–307, 1999.
46. Reiss AL, Abrams MT, Greenlaw R, Freund L, Denckla MB: Neurodevelopmental effects of the *FMR1* full mutation in humans. Nat Med 1:159–167, 1995.
47. Reiss AL, Aylward E, Freund LS, Joshi PK, Bryan RN: Neuroanatomy of fragile X syndrome: The posterior fossa. Ann Neurol 29:26–32, 1991.
48. Reiss AL, Lee J, Freund L: Neuroanatomy of fragile X syndrome: The temporal lobe. Neurology 44:1317–1324, 1994.
49. Reyniers E, Vits L, De Boulle K, van Velzen D, de Graaff E, Verkerk AJMH, Jorens HZ, Darby JK, Oostra BA, Willems PJ: The full mutation in the *FMR1* gene of male fragile X patients is absent in their sperm. Nat Genet 4:143–146, 1993.
50. Rousseau F, Morel ML, Rouillard P, Khandjian EW, Morgan K: Surprisingly low prevalence of the FMR1 premutations among males from the general population. Am J Hum Genet 59 (Suppl): A188, 1996.
51. Rousseau F, Rouillard P, Morel ML, Khandjian EW, Morgan K: Prevalence of carriers of premutation-size alleles of the *FMR1* gene and implications for the population genetics of the fragile X syndrome. Am J Hum Genet 57:1006–1018, 1995.
52. Ryynänen M, Heinonen S, Makkonen M, Kajanoja E, Mannermaa A, Pertti K: Feasibility and acceptance of screening for fragile X mutations in low-risk pregnancies. Eur J Hum Genet 7:212–216, 1999.
53. Schapiro MB, Murphy DGM, Hagerman RJ, Azari NP, Alexander GE, Miezejeski CM, Hinton VJ, Horwitz B, Haxby JV, Kumar A, White B, Grady CL: Adult fragile X syndrome: Neuropsychology, brain anatomy, and metabolism. Am J Med Genet 60:480–493, 1995.
54. Sherman SL: The high prevalence of fragile X premutation carrier females: is this frequency unique to the French Canadian population? Am J Hum Genet 57:991–993, 1995.
55. Sherman SL: Premature ovarian failure in the fragile X syndrome. Am J Med Genet 97:189–194, 2000.
56. Siomi H, Siomi MC, Nussbaum RL, Dreyfuss G: The protein product of the fragile X gene, *FMR1*, has characteristics of an RNA-binding protein. Cell 74:291–298, 1993.
57. Sittler A, Devys D, Weber C, Mandel JL: Alternative splicing of exon 14 determines nuclear or cytoplasmic localisation of FMR1 protein isoforms. Hum Molec Genet 5:95–102, 1996.
58. Smeets HJM, Smits APT, Verheij C, Theelen JPG, van de Burgt I, Hoogeven AT, Oosterwijk JC, Oostra BA: Normal phenotype in two brothers with a full FMR1 mutation. Hum Mol Genet 4:2103–2108, 1995.
59. Stevenson RE: Splitting and lumping in the nosology of XLMR. Am J Med Genet 97:174–182, 2000.
59a. Stoll C: Problems in the diagnosis of fragile X syndrome in young children are still present. Am J Med Genet 100:110–115, 2001.
60. Sutcliffe JS, Nelson DL, Zhang F, Pieretti M, Caskey CT, Saxe D, Warren ST: DNA methylation represses FMR-1 transcription in fragile X syndrome. Hum Mol Genet 1:397–400, 1992.
61. Tassone F, Hagerman RJ, Chamberlain WD, Hagerman PJ: Transcription of the *FMR1* gene in individuals with fragile X syndrome. Am J Med Genet 97:195–203, 2000.

62. Tassone F, Hagerman RJ, Loesch DZ, Lachiewicz A, Taylor AK, Hagerman PJ: Fragile X males with unmethylated, full mutation trinucleotide repeat expansions have elevated levels of FMR1 messenger RNA. Am J Med Genet 94:232–236, 2000.
63. Theobald TM, Hay DA, Judge C: Individual variation and specific cognitive deficits in the fra(X) syndrome. Am J Med Genet 28:1–11, 1987.
64. Torrioli MG, Vernacotola S, Mariotti P, Bianchi E, De Gaetano A, Calvani M, Chiurazzi P, Neri G: Double-blind, placebo-controlled study of L-acetylcarnitine for the treatment of hyperactive behavior in fragile X syndrome. Am J Med Genet 87:366–368, 1999.
65. Tunçbilek E, Alikasifoglu M, Aktas D, Duman F, Yanik H, Anar B, Oostra B, Willemsen R: Screening for the fragile X syndrome among mentally retarded males by hair root analysis. Am J Med Genet 95:105–107, 2000.
66. Van Roy BC, De Smedt MC, Raes RA, Dumon JE, Leroy JG: Fragile X trait in a large kindred: Transmission also through normal males. J Med Genet 20:286–289, 1983.
67. Veenema H, Veenema T, Geraedts J: The fragile X syndrome in a large family II. Psychological investigation. J Med Genet 24:32–38, 1987.
68. Verkerk AJMH, Pieretti M, Sutcliffe JS, Su YH, Kuhl DPA, Pizzuti A, Reiner O, Richards S, Victoria MF, Zhang F, Eussen BE, van Ommen GJB, Blonden LAJ, Riggins GJ, Chastain JL, Kunst CB, Galjaard H, Caskey CT, Nelson DL, Oostra BA, Warren ST: Identification of a gene (*FMR-1*) containing a CGG repeat coincident with a breakpoint cluster region exhibiting length variation in fragile X syndrome. Cell 65:905–914, 1991.
69. Webb TP, Bundey SE, Thake AI, Todd J: Population incidence and segregation ratios in the Martin-Bell syndrome. Am J Med Genet 23:573–580, 1986.
70. Webb T, Crawley P, Bundey S: Folate treatment of a boy with fragile-X syndrome. J Ment Defic Res 34:67–73, 1990.
71. Willemsen R, Anar B, de Diego Otero Y, de Vries BB, Hilhorst-Hofstee Y, Smits A, van Looveren E, Willems PJ, Galjaardt H, Oostra BA: Non invasive test for fragile X syndrome, using hair root analysis. Am J Hum Genet 65:98–103, 1999.
72. Willemsen R, Los F, Mohkamssing S, Van den Ouweland A, Deelen W, Galjaard H, Oostra BA: Rapid antibody test for prenatal diagnosis of fragile X syndrome on amniotic fluid cells: A new appraisal. J Med Genet 34:250–251, 1997.
73. Willemsen R, Mohkamsing S, De Vries B, Devys D, van den Ouweland A, Mandel JL, Galjaard H, Oostra BA: Rapid antibody test for fragile X syndrome. Lancet 345:1147–1148, 1995.
74. Willemsen R, Oostra BA: FMRP detection assay for the diagnosis of the fragile X syndrome. Am J Med Genet 97:183–188, 2000.
75. Wisniewski KE, Segan SM, Miezejeski CM, Sersen EA, Rudelli RD: The fra(X)syndrome: Neurological, electrophysiological, and neuropathological abnormalities. Am J Med Genet 38:476–480, 1991.

14

Chromosomal Disorders with Overgrowth

Chromosomal aneuploidy is commonly associated with intrauterine growth retardation. However, several chromosomal duplications and deletions are associated with fetal overgrowth (Table 14–1).

dup(4)(p16.3)

Partington et al. (10a) reported translocations involving 4p16.3 in three families; deletion resulted in Pitt-Rogers-Danks syndrome that includes growth deficiency, and duplication that resulted in an overgrowth syndrome. Features of the overgrowth syndrome included mental deficiency, coarse facial appearance, abundant head hair with bushy eyebrows and synophrys, prominent supraorbital ridges, square jaw, small upturned nose, and large hands and feet. Stature was above average and head circumference was large. The suggestion of Partington et al. (10a) that duplication of FGFR3, located at 4p16, might produce a dosage effect resulting in overgrowth is not tenable (4a).

dup(5p)

Reichenbach et al. (13) reported complete duplication of 5p and reviewed six other cases. Macrocephaly was present in 7/7 cases. A tendency toward increased birth length (4/7:1 >97th centile, 1 >90th centile, 2 >75th centile) and increased birth weight (2/7: 75th–90th centile) has been evident. Patients have had generalized hypotonia, psychomotor retardation, seizures, and hydrocephalus. Recurrent respiratory infections and failure to thrive have also been recorded. Other abnormalities have included ocular hypertelorism, epicanthic folds, low nasal bridge, midface deficiency, micrognathia, abnormal ears, congenital heart defects, tracheobronchial abnormalities, and clubfeet. Avansino et al. (2) tabulated 10 cases and further defined the critical region to proximal 5p (band 5p13).

dup(12p)

Rauch et al. (12) reviewed 10 cases of dup(12p), including 3 of their own. Another case was reported by Allen et al. (1). Of 11 cases, birth weight was >4000 g in 3 cases and >3600 g in 6. Head circumference was ≥97th centile in 4 patients.

In addition to large birth weight and macrocephaly, common features include mental deficiency, muscular hypotonia, short neck, high forehead, broad nasal bridge, prominent cheeks, large philtrum, short nose, anteverted nostrils, broad everted lower lip, and foot deformities. Polydactyly and accessory nipples are only found with almost complete duplication of 12p (12).

Table 14–1 Chromosomal Disorders with Overgrowth

---
dup(4)(p16.3)
dup(5p)
dup(12p)
i(12p) mosaicism
　(mosaic tetrasomy 12p, Pallister-Killian syndrome)
dup(12)(q11 → q15)
dup(15)(q25–qter)
del(15)(q12)
del(22)(q13 → qter)

Pallister-Killian Syndrome
[Mosaic i(12p), Mosaic Tetrasomy 12p]

To date, over 60 cases of Pallister-Killian syndrome have been recorded (3), which have been reviewed by several authors (3,10,14). The condition is caused by mosaic 12p tetrasomy. Chromosome analysis of peripheral lymphocytes is commonly normal. Diagnosis is based on characteristic phenotypic features and isochromosome 12p can be demonstrated in skin fibroblasts or bone marrow cells (6). Bielanska et al. (3) reported a mild case diagnosed by FISH. Struthers et al. (17) observed that i(12p) was maternally inherited in their case and in their review found that six of seven cases were of maternal origin. They suggested that premeiotic mitotic error is the most likely mechanism. Cormier-Daire et al. (5), using microsatellite DNA markers of chromosome 12p, detected three alleles including two different alleles of maternal origin in cultured skin fibroblasts, and suggested that tetrasomy 12p results from a prezygotic event with nondisjunction occurring during maternal meiosis. Zollino et al. (21) noted that unexplained fetal overgrowth can be regarded as an indicator of fetal chromosome pathology. They reported mitotic instability of the i(12p) clones in their case and cautioned that it was likely responsible for failing to establish a prenatal cytogenetic diagnosis.

In Pallister-Killian syndrome, the average birth weight adjusted for term is about 3600 g, with patients varying from the 75th to the 90th centiles. Postnatal growth deficiency has also been reported (14). Clinical features are summarized in Table 14–2 and illustrated in Figures 14–1 and 14–2; a number of other abnormalities have also been noted, including polyhydramnios, diaphragmatic hernia, congenital heart defects, optic hypoplasia, and cataracts (10,14). Bielanska et al. (3) reported a case with hemihyperplasia.

dup(12)(q11 → q15)

Wajntal et al. (20) reported dup(12)(q11 → q15) in an infant with overgrowth. Birthweight was 6200 g. At 9–10 months, length was >97th centile. Clinical findings included hypotonia, psychomotor retardation, asymmetric craniofacial appearance, ptosis of the eyelids, nystagmus, highly arched palate, large ears, preauricular pit, short neck, umbilical hernia, small hands, clinodactyly of the fifth fingers, and talipes equinovarus.

Table 14–2 Abnormalities in i(12p) Mosaicism (Mosaic Tetrasomy 12p, Pallister-Killian Syndrome)

PERFORMANCE
Hypotonia
Mental deficiency
Seizures

SKIN AND HAIR
Pigmentary dysplasia
Bitemporal alopecia
Sparse hair
Sparse eyebrows

CRANIOFACIAL
Coarse face
Broad, high forehead
Ocular hypertelorism
Epicanthic folds
Broad nasal bridge
Small, upturned nose
Prominent upper lip
Macrostomia
Macroglossia
Abnormal ears

OTHER
Accessory nipples
Short neck
Webbed neck
Short limbs
Distal digital hypoplasia
Anal abnormalities
Abnormal genitalia
Hearing deficit
Various other anomalies

Source: Adapted from Reynolds et al. (14), Bielanska et al. (3), and Mathieu et al. (10).

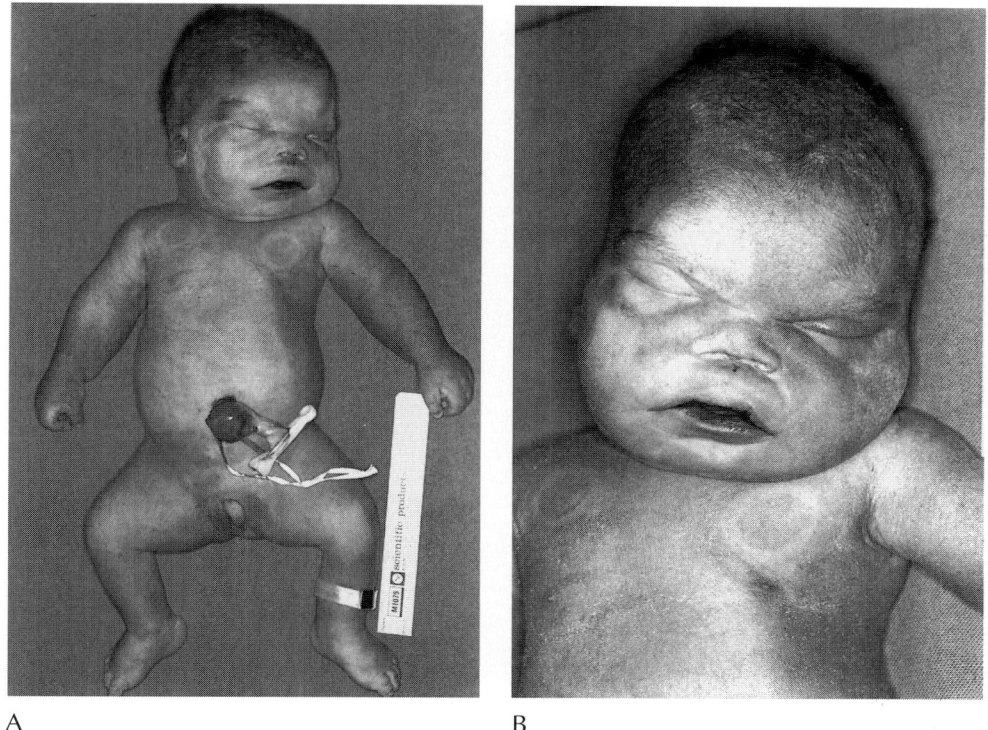

Figure 14–1 Pallister-Killian syndrome. Tetrasomy i(12p). **A:** Note altered body proportions and multiple depigmented areas. **B:** Short nose, low nasal bridge, prominent premaxilla, and large mouth. From Shivashanker et al. (16).

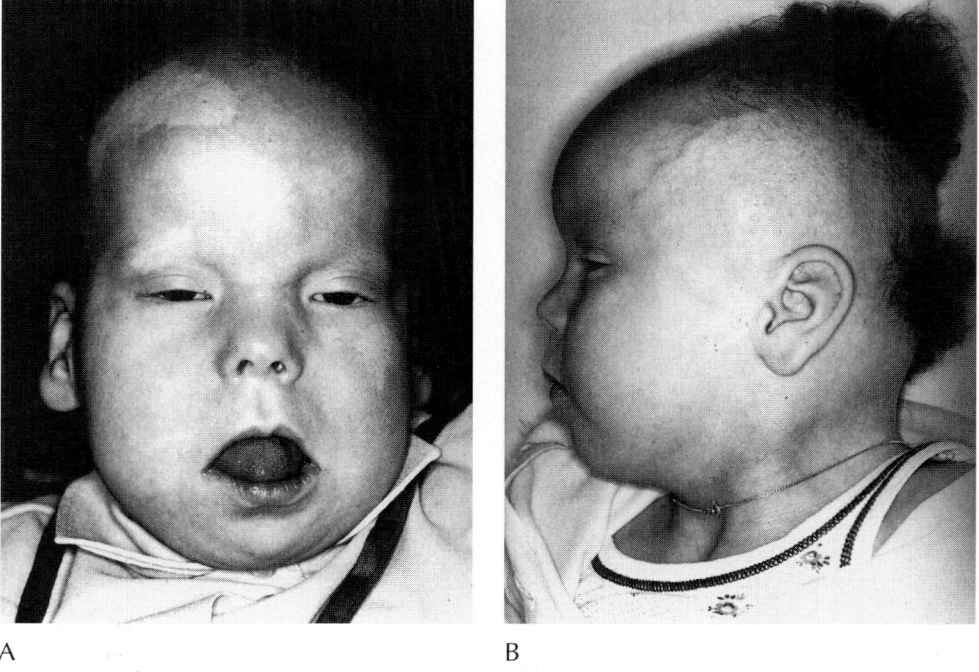

Figure 14–2 Pallister-Killian syndrome. **A,B:** Fine, sparse hair, particularly on frontal and temporal areas. Course face. Note hypopigmented area of scalp, high forehead, medially sparse eyelashes, short nose with flat bridge, anteverted nostrils, downturned mouth, and thin upper lip. From Killian et al. (8).

Table 14–3 Comparison of dup(15)(q21–qter) and dup(15)(q25–qter)

SHARED CLINICAL SIGNS
GROWTH
Postnatal growth retardation

PERFORMANCE
Hypotonia
Mental deficiency
Seizures

FACE
Facial asymmetry
Downslanting palpebral fissures
Pointed chin/micrognathia

OTHER
Congenital heart defects
Scoliosis, chest deformity

CLINICAL SIGNS SPECIFIC TO dup(15)(q21–qter)
GROWTH
Normal birthweight
Microcephaly

CLINICAL SIGNS SPECIFIC TO dup(15)(q25–qter)
GROWTH
Large birthweight
Tall stature
Macrocephaly

OTHER
Craniosynostosis
Broad thumbs/halluces

Source: Adapted from Zollino et al. (22).

dup(15)(q25–qter)

Zollino et al. (22) reported two patients with partial duplication of distal 15q and reviewed the literature. They were able to define two clinical subtypes, depending on where the duplication occurs: dup(15)(q21–qter) and dup(15)(q25–qter). Although they share some clinical features, overgrowth characterizes the latter subtype and craniosynostosis has been reported in several instances (9,11,18,22) (Table 14–3).

del(15)(q12)

Wajntal et al. (20) reported del(15)(q12) in a patient with overgrowth. Birth weight, birth length, and OFC were >97th centile. Clinical findings included psychomotor retardation, broad forehead, ocular hypertelorism, large ears, hypoplastic antihelices, and fifth finger clinodactyly.

The deleted region in the patient of Wajnatal et al. (20) overlaps the Prader-Willi/Angelman region (4). The patient did have mild oculocutaneous albinoidism, macrostomia, and a tendency to obesity, but with a fat distribution different from that found in Prader-Willi syndrome. The patient had no other features suggestive of either syndrome.

The deleted region also shows overlap with the chromosomal findings in the cases of Sotos syndrome reported by Wajntal and Koiffman (19). Two cases had deletion of 15q12 or 13 and one patient had a 15q;15q Robertsonian translocation.

del(22)(q13 → qter)

Romain et al. (15) reported an 18-month-old girl whose length was at the 97th centile, although her birth weight had been only 3600 g. Cytogenetic study showed del(22)(q13 → qter). Clinical features included a low-pitched, growling cry, hypotonia, developmental delay, fullness of the cheeks, eyebrows, and eyelids, epicanthic folds, wide nasal bridge, long philtrum, and thick lower lip.

Fujita et al. (6) reported a patient with accelerated growth, hearing loss, inner ear anomalies, and delayed myelinization of the brain, and tabulated 18 cases from the literature. Common findings included hypotonia, developmental delay, accelerated growth, ptosis of the eyelids, epicanthic folds, long philtrum, high-arched palate, dysplastic ears, hearing loss, and dolichocephaly.

REFERENCES

1. Allen TL, Brothman AR, Carey JC, Chance PF: Cytogenetic and molecular analysis in trisomy 12p. Am J Med Genet 63:250–256, 1996.
2. Avansino JR, Dennis TR, Spallone P, Stock AD, Levin ML: Proximal 5p trisomy resulting from a marker chromosome implicates band 5p13 in 5p trisomy syndrome. Am J Med Genet 87:6–11, 1999.
3. Bielanska MM, Khalifa MM, Duncan AMV: Brief clinical report: Pallister-Killian syndrome: A mild case diagnosed by fluorescence in situ hybridization. Review of the literature and expansion of the phenotype. Am J Med Genet 65: 104–108, 1996.

4. Cassidy SB, Schwartz S: Prader-Willi and Angelman syndrome: Disorders of genomic imprinting. Medicine 77:140–151, 1998.

4a. Cohen MM Jr, Neri G: New overgrowth syndrome and FGFR3 dosage effect. J Med Genet 35:348–349, 1998.

5. Cormier-Daire V, Le Merrer M, Gigarel N, Morichon N, Prieur M, Lyonnet S, Vekemans M, Munnich A: Prezygotic origin of the isochromosome 12p in Pallister-Killian syndrome. Am J Med Genet 69:166–168, 1979.

6. Fujita Y, Mochizuki D, Mori Y, Nakamoto N, Kobayashi M, Omi K, Kodama H, Yanagawa Y, Abe T, Tsuzuku T, Yamanouchi Y, Takano T: Girl with accelerated growth, hearing loss, inner ear anomalies, delayed myelination of the brain, and del(22) (q13.1q13.2). Am J Med Genet 92:195–199, 2000.

7. Horn D, Majewski F, Hildebrandt B, Körner H: Pallister-Killian syndrome: Normal karyotype in prenatal chorionic villi, in postnatal lymphocytes, and in slowly growing epidermal cells, but mosaic tetrasomy 12p in skin fibroblasts. J Med Genet 32:68–71, 1995.

8. Killian W, Zonana J, Schroer R: Abnormal hair, craniofacial dysmorphism and severe mental retardation—a new syndrome? J Clin Dysmorphol 1:6–13, 1983.

9. Kristoffersson U, Bergwall B: Partial trisomy 15(q25qter) in two brothers. Hereditas 100:7–10, 1984.

10. Mathieu M, Piussan Ch, Thepot F, Gouget A, Lacombe D, Pedespan JM, Serville F, Fontan D, Ruffie M, Nivelon-Chevallier A, Amblard F, Chauveau P, Moirot H, Chabrolle JP, Croquette MF, Teyssier M, Plauchu H, Pelissier MC, Gilgenkrantz S, Turc-Carel C, Turleau C, Prieur M, Le Merrer M, Gonzales M, Joye N, Taillemite JL, Bouillie J, Eschard C, Motte J, Journel H: Collaborative study of mosaic tetrasomy 12p or Pallister-Killian syndrome (nineteen fetuses or children). Ann Génét 40:45–54, 1997.

10a. Partington MW, Fagan K, Soubjaki V, Turner G: Translocations involving 4p16.3 in three families: Deletion causing the Pitt-Rogers-Danks syndrome and duplication resulting in a new overgrowth syndrome. J Med Genet 34:719–728, 1997.

11. Pedersen C: Partial trisomy 15 as a result of an unbalanced 12/15 translocation in a patient with cloverleaf skull anomaly. Clin Genet 9:378–380, 1976.

12. Rauch A, Trautmann U, Pfeiffer RA: Clinical and molecular cytogenetic observations in three cases of "trisomy 12 p syndrome." Am J Med Genet 63:243–249, 1996.

13. Reichenbach H, Holland H, Dalitz E, Demandt C, Meiner A, Chudoba I, Lemke J, Claussen U, Froster UG: De novo complete trisomy 5p: Clinical report and FISH studies. Am J Med Genet 85:447–451, 1999.

14. Reynolds JF, Daniel A, Kelly TE, Gollin SM, Stephan MJ, Carey J, Adkins WN, Webb MJ, Char F, Jimenez JF, Opitz JM: Isochromosome 12p mosaicism (Pallister mosaic aneuploidy or Pallister-Killian syndrome): Report of 11 cases. Am J Med Genet 27:257–274, 1987.

15. Romain DR, Goldsmith J, Cairney H, Columbano-Green LM, Smythe RH, Parfitt RG: Partial monosomy for chromosome 22 in a patient with del(22)(pter → q13.1::q13.33 → qter). J Med Genet 27:588–589, 1990.

16. Shivashanker L, Whitney E, Colmorgen G, Young T, Munshi G, Wilmouth D, Byrne K, Reeves G, Borgaonkar D, Picciano S, Martin-Deleon P: Prenatal diagnosis of tetrasomy 47,XY,+i(12p) confirmed by in situ hybridization. Prenat Diagn 8:85–91, 1988.

17. Struthers JL, Cuthbert CD, Khalifa MM: Parental origin of the isochromosome 12p in Pallister-Killian syndrome: Molecular analysis of one patient and review of the reported cases. Am J Med Genet 84:111–115, 1999.

18. Van Allen MI, Siegel-Bartelt J, Feigenbaum A, Teshima IE: Craniosynostosis associated with partial duplication of 15q and deletion of 2q. Am J Med Genet 43:688–692, 1992.

19. Wajntal A, Koiffman CP: Chromosome aberrations in Sotos syndrome [letter, comment]. Clin Genet 40:472, 1991.

20. Wajntal A, Moretti-Ferreira D, De Souza DH, Koiffmann CP: Cytogenetic evidence of involvement of chromosome regions 15q12 and 12q15 in conditions with associated overgrowth. DNA Cell Biol 12:227–231, 1993.

21. Zollino M, Bajer J, Neri G: Chromosome instability limited to the aneuploid clone in the Pallister-Killian syndrome: A pitfall in prenatal diagnosis. Prenat Diagn 19:178–185, 1999.

22. Zollino M, Tiziano F, Di Stefano C, Neri G: Partial duplication of the long arm of chromosome 15q: Confirmation of a causative role in craniosynostosis and definition of a 15q25–qter trisomy syndrome. Am J Med Genet 87:391–394, 1999.

15

Other Syndromes

In this chapter, five syndromes with overgrowth are discussed: Costello syndrome, macrocephaly–cutis marmorata syndrome, Cantú syndrome, Nevo syndrome, and Elejalde syndrome.

COSTELLO SYNDROME

The syndrome (OMIM 218040)[a] was first described by Costello (13–15) in two children with psychomotor retardation, postnatal growth deficiency, macrocephaly, coarse facial features, curly hair, nasal papillomas, short neck, and dark skin (Figs. 15–1 to 15–4). Der Kaloustian et al. (17) named the disorder "Costello syndrome." Several reviews are available (29,37,38,45,46). Van Eeghen et al. (45) tabulated 39 cases and reported 1 of their own (Table 15–1).

In most cases, pregnancy has been complicated by polyhydramnios. Birth weight is normal or relatively high and macrocephaly is constant. Poor feeding and swallowing difficulties are common during the neonatal period (≤5). Patients generally go through two clinical phases: marasmic and pseudothesaurismic. The latter phase is characterized by macrocephaly, full cheeks, a large mouth with thick lips, a large tongue, and gingival hyperplasia (46).

Postnatal growth deficiency occurs in 97% of patients. Although macrocephaly has been observed in all cases, head circumference has normalized at an older age in some patients (15,17).

Growth and development data are shown in Table 15–2.

Legault et al. (28a) found growth hormone deficiency in one case and Okamoto et al. (36a) reported partial growth hormone deficiency. Perhaps growth hormone deficiency might explain the short stature in at least some Costello syndrome patients and should be sought when auxologic criteria dictate.

Van Eeghen et al. (45) found cardiac abnormalities in 75% of patients ($n = 39$). Lin (29) tabulated 62 cases from the literature and found right-sided obstruction in 9 cases, ventricular/atrial septal defects in 7 cases, hypertrophic cardiomyopathy in 34% ($n = 62$), and rhythm disturbance in 31% ($n = 62$).

Papillomas may occur at various ages and are particularly common in the perioral and perianal regions, but they may also be found at a number of other sites. In addition, some malignant neoplasms have been reported (Table 15–3).

At this writing, the genetics of Costello syndrome is unresolved. Affected sibs have been reported by Zampino et al. (46), Johnson et al. (26), and Berberich et al. (3). Consanguinity has been noted in two of the five families described by Borochowitz et al. (4). A 1;22 translocation has been recorded (16). Lurie (30) analyzed 20 families in which all sibs of Costello syndrome probands were normal. On the basis of increased paternal age (38 years) and paternal-maternal age difference (7.36 years), Lurie (30) suggested autosomal dominant inheritance with most patients representing de novo mutations. Sporadic dominant mutations with gonadal mosaicism or

---

[a]On-Line Mendelian Inheritance in Man number.

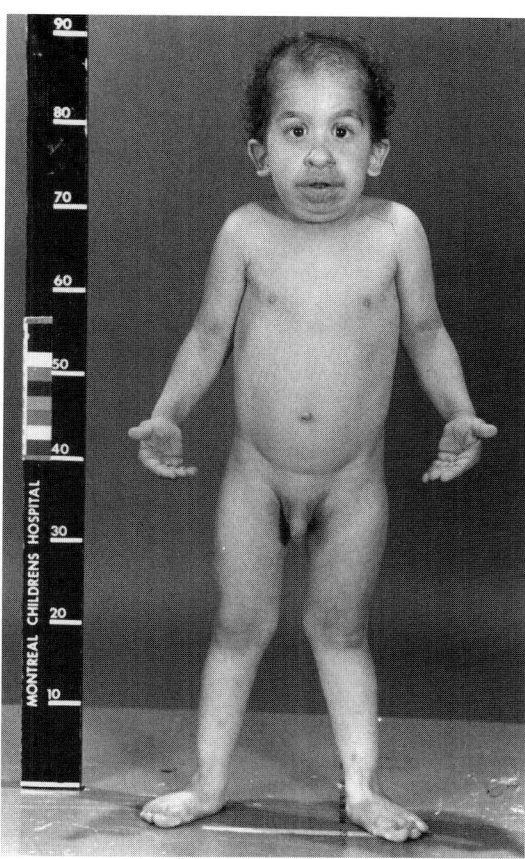

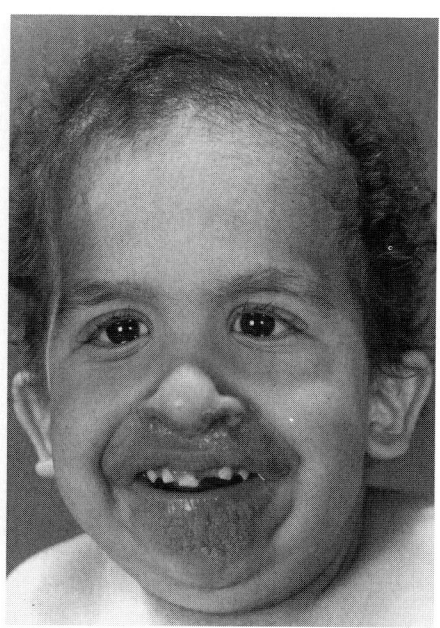

Figure 15–2 Costello syndrome. Curly hair, coarse face, downslanting palpebral fissures, bulbous nose, thick lips, papillomas, and low-set, malformed ears. Courtesy of V.M. Der Kaloustian, Montreal, Quebec.

Figure 15–1 Costello syndrome. Short stature, sparse hair, coarse face, bulbous nose, thick lips, and short neck. Courtesy of V.M. Der Kaloustian, Montreal, Quebec.

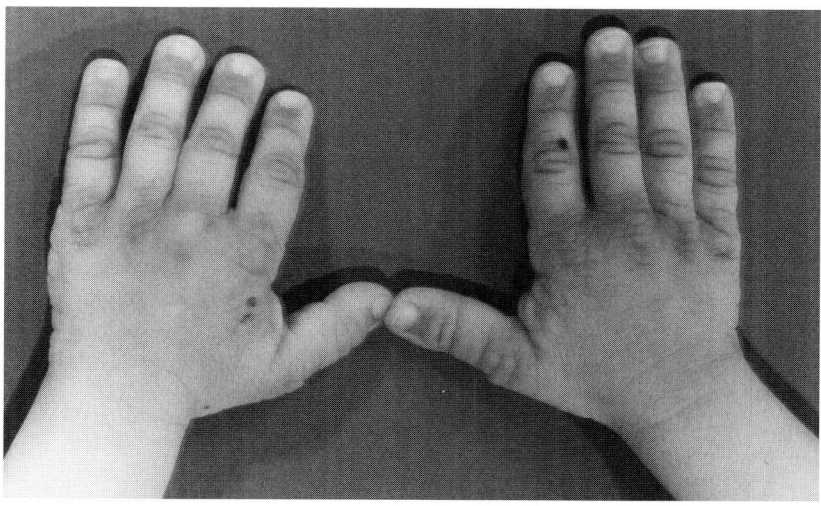

Figure 15–3 Costello syndrome. Hands with loose skin and short, broad fingers. Courtesy of V.M. Der Kaloustian, Montreal, Quebec.

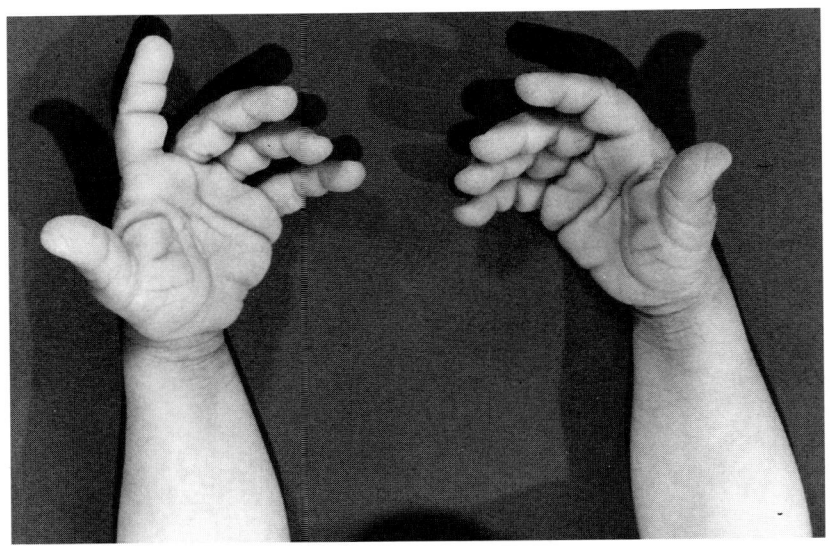

Figure 15–4 Costello syndrome. Deep palmar creases. Courtesy of V.M. Der Kaloustian, Montreal, Quebec.

Table 15–1 Features of Costello Syndrome

Features	Percentages (n = 39)	Features	Percentages (n = 39)
GROWTH		Highly arched palate	67
		Dental abnormalities	59
Postnatal growth deficiency	97	Malformed ears	90
CENTRAL NERVOUS SYSTEM		Low-set ears	78
		Short neck	93
Mental deficiency	100	Hoarse voice	88
EEG abnormalities	75		
Hypotonia	64	MUSCULOSKELETAL SYSTEM	
CRANIOFACIAL ANOMALIES		Limited elbow extension	70
Macrocephaly	98	Hyperextensible fingers	89
Sparse/curly hair	96	Broad distal phalanges	100
Coarse facial appearance	95	Tight achilles tendons	72
Downslanting palpebral fissures	100	Delayed bone age	78
Epicanthic folds	94	SKIN	
Strabismus	61		
Full cheeks	93	Loose skin, hands and feet	100
Low nasal bridge	97	Deep palmar/plantar creases	100
Short bulbous nose	97	Papillomas	73
Thick lips	92	Dark skin	96
Large mouth	91	OTHER ABNORMALITIES	
Large tongue	65		
Gingival hyperplasia	69	Congenital heart defects	75

Source: Adapted from Van Eeghen et al. (45).

Table 15–2 Growth and Development in Costello Syndrome

High birth weight	Mean, 3770 g; range, 2770–4700 g
Normal birth length	Mean, 48.7 cm; range, 44–54 cm
Large birth OFC	Mean, 35.5 cm; range, 32–38.1 cm
Final height attainment	Mean, 1.38 m; range, 1.18–1.48 m
Adult OFC	Mean, 57.3 cm; range, 55.5–60 cm
IQ	Mean, 60; range, 47–85

Source: Adapted from Van Eeghen et al. (45).

a microdeletion syndrome with parental translocation could explain the occurrence of Costello syndrome in sibs. However, the possibility of genetic heterogeneity cannot be ruled out at the present time.

Hinek et al. (25) found impaired production of elastic fibers and a functional deficit of elastin-binding protein, which normally chaperones tropoelastin through secretory pathways and extracellular elastic fiber assembly. They postulated that chondroitin sulfate–dependent shedding of elastin-binding protein eliminated recycling of this tropoelastin chaperone, consequently disrupting tropoelastin secretion and extracellular elastic fiber assembly.

Tandoi et al. (42a) failed to detect functional variants in the elastin coding sequence and intron-exon boundaries, ruling out direct involvement of the gene in the pathogenesis of Costello syndrome. Perhaps the ectodermal phenotype may be caused by a later step in elastogenesis, as proposed by Hinek et al. (25).

Costello syndrome is a distinctive condition and differential diagnosis is limited. CFC syndrome shares many manifestations with Costello syndrome, but in CFC syndrome, the cranial vault is high, and other features such as bitemporal constriction, ptosis of the eyelids, and decreased or absent eyebrows should permit facial differentiation from Costello syndrome. In addition, the skin abnormalities in CFC syndrome consist of eczema, ichthyosis, and sometimes hyperkeratosis. Noonan syndrome shares some characteristics with Costello syndrome, but not a coarse facial appearance or macrocephaly (45).

MACROCEPHALY-CUTIS MARMORATA SYNDROME

The macrocephaly–cutis marmorata syndrome (OMIM 602501)[a] is characterized by macrosomia, macrocephaly, developmental delay, cutis marmorata telangiectatica congenita,[b] macular stain (nevus flammeus) of the philtrum and nose, joint laxity, hyperelastic skin, craniofacial and limb asymmetry, syndactyly of the second and third toes and/or third and fourth fingers or toes and, in some cases, postaxial polydactyly (Figs. 15–5 and 15–6). Central nervous system abnormalities besides mental deficiency include megalencephaly (hemimegalencephaly in several cases), progressive hydrocephalus that requires shunting and, in two cases, Chiari I malformation (8,21,33,44). Hypotonia is present in almost all cases and may resolve during the first

[b]The full name of the syndrome—macrocephaly-cutis marmorata telangiectatica congenita—is unwieldy and we have elected to shorten the name to "macrocephaly–cutis marmorata syndrome."

Table 15–3 Neoplasms in Costello Syndrome[a]

Neoplasm	Age	Reference
Epithelioma, neck	12 years	Martin and Jones (32)
Ganglioneuroblastoma, adrenal	17 months	Zampino et al. (46)
Schwannoma, vestibular	33 years[b]	Suri and Garrett (42)
Embryonal rhabdomyosarcoma	2 years	Kerr et al. (27)
	3 years	
Alveolar rhabdomyosarcoma	6 months	Feingold (19a)
Carcinoma, bladder	11 years	Franceschini et al. (20)
	16 years	Gripp et al. (23)

[a]In addition to the tumors listed in this table, papillomas, particularly perioral and perianal, have been recorded frequently. Other locations have included the laryngeal and facial regions, the lower eyelid, and the neck.
[b]Postmortem examination.

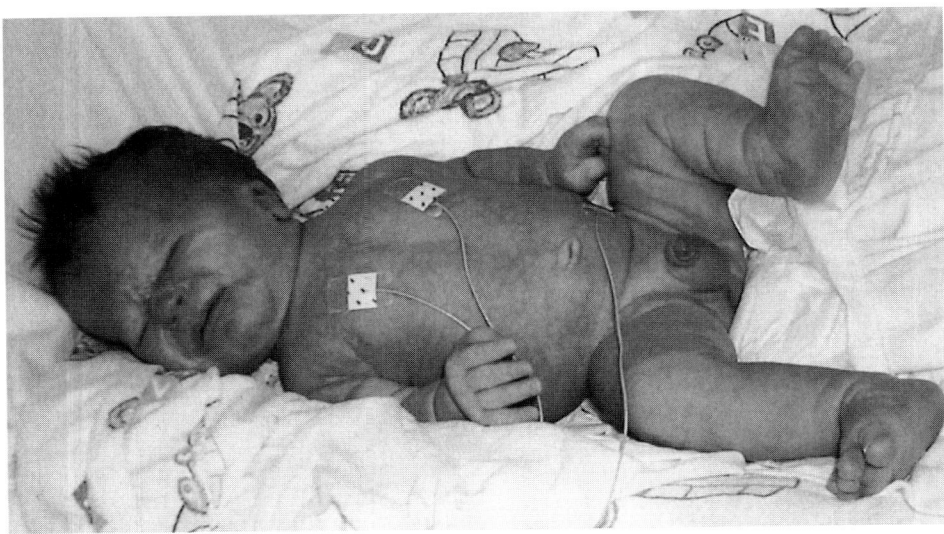

Figure 15–5 Macrocephaly–cutis marmorata syndrome. Infant with macrosomia, macrocephaly, and cutis marmorata. Patient also had neonatal hypoglycemia, polycythemia, and syndactyly of the second and third toes. Courtesy of J.M. Graham, Jr., Los Angeles, California.

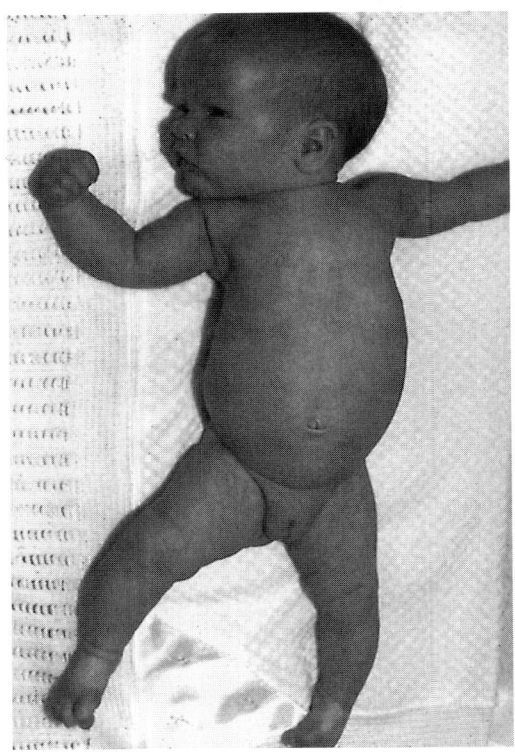

Figure 15–6 Macrocephaly–cutis marmorata syndrome. Macrocephaly and asymmetry of the limbs. Cutis marmorata was present but cannot be seen in black and white photograph.

year of life. Franceschini et al. (21) observed a case without cutis marmorata. Cherry red macules have been observed in one case (6). Moore et al. (33) noted one patient with leukemia and another with meningioma (Table 15–4). The association of arrhythmia and sudden death has been reported (45a).

The syndrome was delineated in 1996 by Toriello et al. (44) and in 1997 by Moore et al. (33) and Clayton-Smith et al. (8). Other cases have been reported since then (2,6,21,38a). Excellent reviews are those of Moore et al. (33) (13 cases), Clayton-Smith et al. (8) (9 cases), and Robertson et al. (38a) (5 cases). To date, all cases have been sporadic and expressivity has been variable. Macrosomia in otherwise normal relatives has been recorded in two families, but the significance is presently unclear (21).

Cutis marmorata telangiectatica congenita (CMTC) is nonspecific and may be found as an isolated abnormality or together with terminal transverse limb defects, aplasia cutis congenita, with double aortic arch (21), congenital glaucoma, or with various syndromes (33). Stephan et al. (41) reported the association of macrocephaly, limb asymmetry, and vascular malformations in a heterogeneous group of patients. The macrocephaly–cutis marmorata syndrome is a distinctive and easily recognizable condition (33).

Table 15–4 Features of Macrocephaly–Cutis Marmorata Syndrome

Features	Frequencies
GROWTH	
Macrocephaly	28/28
High birth weight	25/28
High birth length	8/13
NEUROLOGIC ABNORMALITIES	
Hypotonia	23/24
Developmental delay	26/26
Hydrocephalus	20/28
Chiari I malformation	2/28
VASCULAR MALFORMATIONS	
Cutis marmorata	28/28
Macular stain (nevus flammeus)	25/28
CONNECTIVE TISSUE ABNORMALITIES	
Joint laxity	23/24
Hyperelastic skin	22/24
OTHER ABNORMALITIES	
Craniofacial asymmetry	20/27
Body asymmetry	20/28
Syndactyly[a]	23/27
Postaxial polydactyly	5/28
NEOPLASIA	
Leukemia	1/28
Meningioma	1/28

[a]Second and third toes and/or third and fourth fingers or toes.

Source: Data from Moore et al. (33), Clayton-Smith et al. (8), Carcao et al. (6), and Robertson et al. (38a).

CANTÚ SYNDROME

In 1982, Cantú et al. (5) reported a distinctive syndrome in four patients: macrosomia at birth, generalized congenital hypertrichosis, coarse face, and mild osteochondrodysplasia (OMIM 239850).[a] The two sibs and two unrelated patients had cardiomegaly, narrow thorax, wide ribs, platyspondyly, hypoplastic ischium and pubic bones, small obturator foramen, coxa valga, Erlenmeyer flask–shaped long bones, and osteopenia. Two of the four patients had birthweights >4500 g.

Many cases have been reported since then (12,22,28,35,39,40), and characteristic features of 18 cases are summarized in Table 15–5. Eleven of the 18 patients were Mexican. Cantú syndrome is illustrated in Figures 15–7 to 15–9.

Initially, the two affected sibs reported by Cantú et al. (5) and a sporadic case in a consanguineous family reported by Rosser et al. (40) suggested autosomal recessive inheritance. Robertson et al. (39) performed a segregation analysis, concluding that recessive inheritance was unlikely and that autosomal dominant inheritance or a microdeletion syndrome was more likely. Lazalde et al. (28) reported an affected father and his two affected children. Male-to-male transmission was found, thus ruling out

Table 15–5 Features of Cantú Syndrome

Features	Frequencies
OVERGROWTH	
Macrosomia at birth	14/17
Macrocephaly	11/18
Congenital hypertrichosis	17/17
FACE	
Coarse appearance	18/18
Epicanthic folds	15/18
Broad nasal bridge	13/18
Small nose	6/14
Anteverted nostrils	8/14
Prominent mouth	15/17
Long philtrum	17/18
NECK, THORAX, ABDOMEN, LIMBS	
Short neck	12/18
Narrow shoulders	10/17
Narrow thorax	12/18
Umbilical hernia	4/8
Short, broad hallux	8/17
CARDIAC ABNORMALITIES	
Cardiomegaly	14/14
Congenital concentric hypertrophic cardiomyopathy	5/14
Pericardial effusion	2/14
LYMPHEDEMA	1/14
SKELETAL ABNORMALITIES	
Generalized osteopenia	8/17
Delayed bone age	5/17
Advanced bone age	1/18
Megaepiphyses	1/18
Vertical skull base, enlarged sella	11/18
Broad ribs	15/17
Vertical endplate irregularities	6/14
Platyspondyly	13/17
Ovoid vertebral bodies	5/14
Hypoplastic ischium and pubic bones	10/15
Narrow obturator foramen	11/17
Coxa valga	13/18
Metaphyseal flare with enlarged medullary canal	16/18
Transverse metaphyseal bands	7/15
Preaxial distal phalangeal hypoplasia	6/15
Broad first metatarsal	12/15

Source: Data from Cantú et al. (5), Nevin et al. (35), García-Cruz et al. (22), Rosser et al. (40), Robertson et al. (39), Concolino et al. (12), and Lazalde et al. (28).

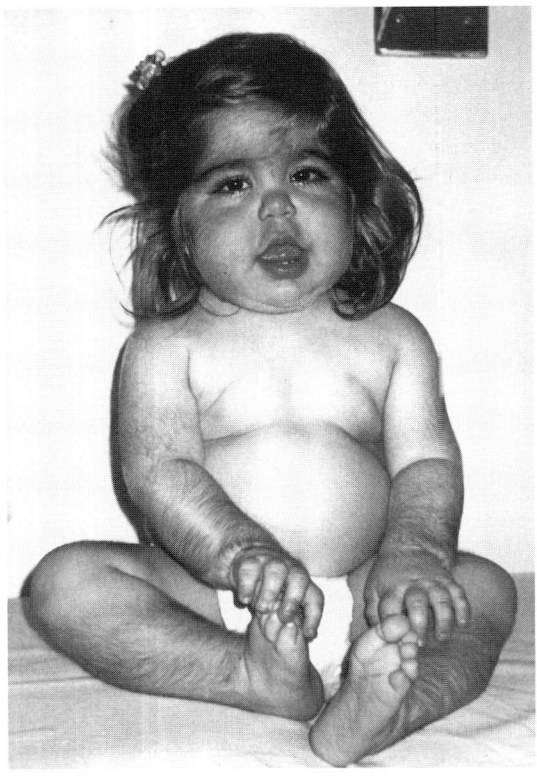

Figure 15–7 Cantú syndrome. Hypertrichosis, small nose, and flat nasal bridge. From Robertson et al. (39).

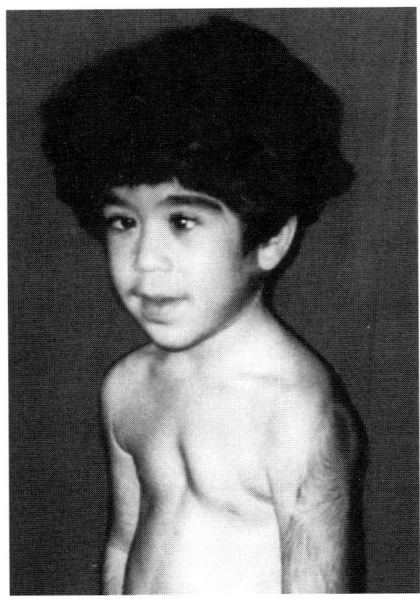

Figure 15–8 Cantú syndrome. Narrow thorax and hypertrichosis. From Concolino et al. (12).

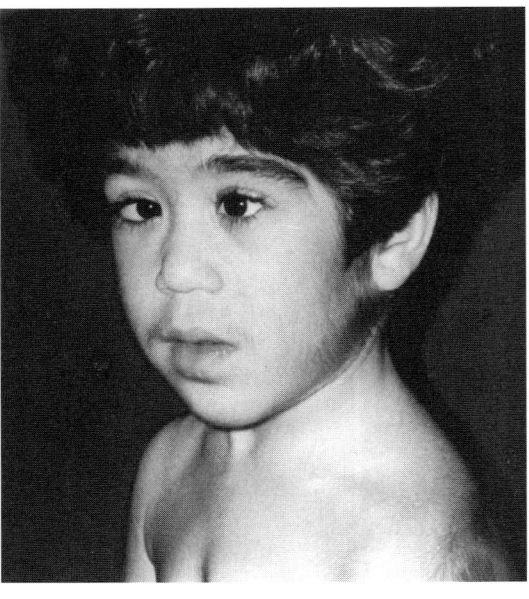

Figure 15–9 Cantú syndrome. Coarse facial appearance. From Concolino et al. (12).

X-linked inheritance. With the additional paternal age effect in sporadic cases reported by Robertson et al. (39), autosomal dominant inheritance is more firmly established. The two affected sibs noted by Cantú et al. (5) could be explained by gonadal mosaicism, although etiologic heterogeneity is possible.

Mild mental deficiency has been described in 11 patients ($n = 16$) (39). Cardiomegaly is found in virtually every case. Cardiomyopathy has been reported in five patients ($n = 14$) and may appear as a complication after puberty (22). Pericardial effusion has been noted twice ($n = 14$). One patient had cardiac problems with a PDA that required surgery in the neonatal period; symptomatic pulmonary hypertension presented in late infancy (39). Hypertrichosis is present at birth and the hair continues to grow, covering the entire body and sparing only the palms, soles, and mucosal surfaces (22).

The skeletal manifestations are variable (Table 15–5). García-Cruz et al. (22) noted that some features, such as irregularities of the articular surfaces of the vertebral bodies, became more pronounced after puberty. The patient reported by Robertson et al. (39) did not have arrested metaphyseal growth nor terminal phalangeal hypoplasia. Concolino et al. (12) re-

OTHER SYNDROMES

ported two unusual findings: advanced bone age and mega-epiphyses of long bones. Lazalde et al. (28) found thickening of the calvaria in two affected individuals in the same family.

Although macrosomia, macrocephaly, and hirsutism may occur as isolated findings or in combination with other abnormalities, all three in the same patient suggest a diagnosis of Cantú syndrome. With later developing coarse face and cardiomegaly, the diagnosis is on firm footing. The combination of hypertrichosis, coarse face, cardiac involvement, and skeletal abnormalities suggests that Cantú syndrome may be a storage disease.

NEVO SYNDROME

The syndrome was observed by Nevo et al. (36) in 1974 in three sibs among a large inbred family from Israel. Whereas Nevo and co-workers (36) described their patients as having cerebral

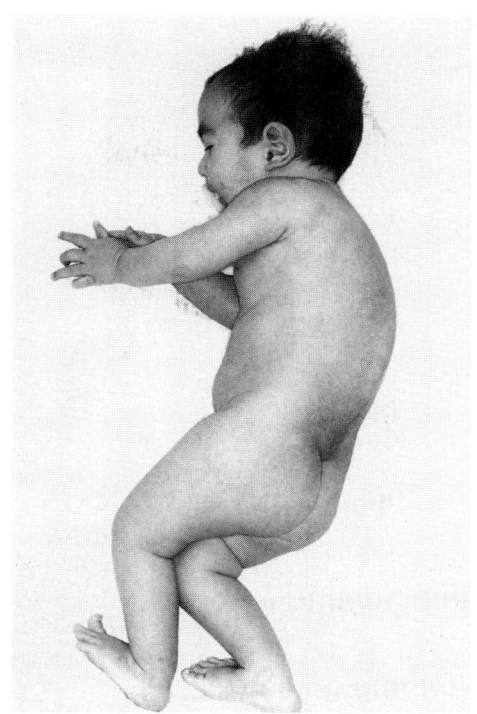

Figure 15–11 Nevo syndrome. Large, low-set ears, kyphosis, and hirsutism of lower back. From Nevo et al. (36).

gigantism, Cohen (9) pointed out that the condition was clearly at variance with cerebral gigantism and named the condition Nevo syndrome (10) (OMIM 601451).[a]

Al-Gazali et al. (1) reported two further children from two unrelated families. Hilderink and Brunner (24) observed a patient from a consanguineous Dutch family. Another patient was noted by Dumić et al. (18). To date, seven children have been reported from five families; three of these families are Arab. Autosomal recessive inheritance is clearly established.

Features of Nevo syndrome similar to those found in Sotos syndrome include intrauterine overgrowth, accelerated osseous maturation, dolichocephaly, large extremities, clumsiness, and retarded motor and speech development. Nevo syndrome has, in addition, generalized edema at birth, severe muscular hypotonia, contractures of the feet, wrist drop, and clinodactyly (Figs. 15–10 to 15–13). Large, low-set ears have been observed in most patients and cryptorchidism has been found in all males (1) (Table 15–6).

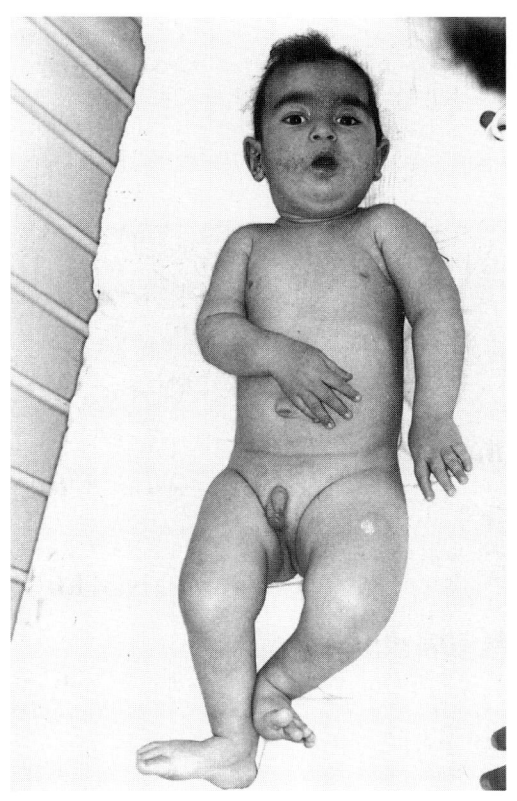

Figure 15–10 Nevo syndrome. Macrosomia, large hands and feet. From Nevo et al. (36).

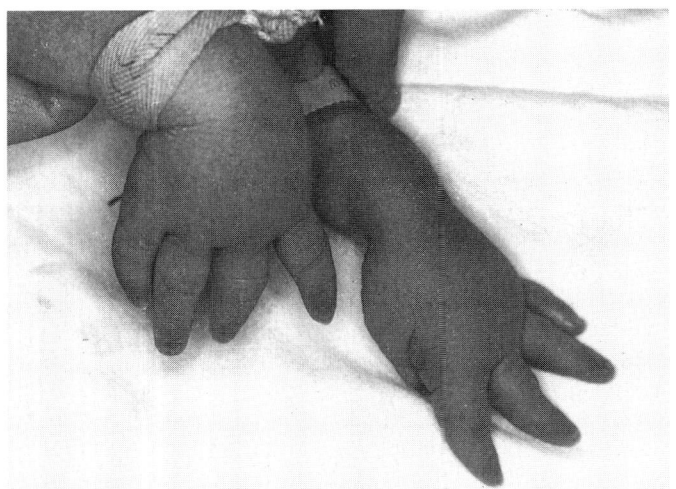

Figure 15–12 Nevo syndrome. Severe edema of hands, spindle-shaped fingers, and wrist-drop. From Nevo et al. (36).

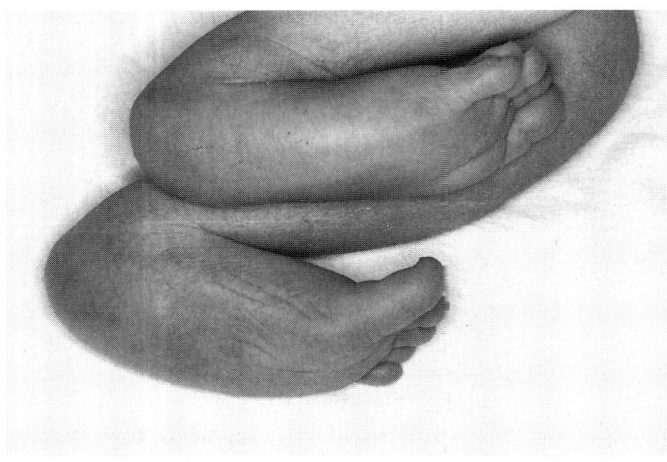

Figure 15–13 Nevo syndrome. Edema and dorsiflexion contractures of feet. From Nevo et al. (36).

Table 15–6 Findings in Nevo Syndrome

Findings	No. Affected	Findings	No. Affected
GENERAL FEATURES		**HANDS AND FEET**	
Sex	6 M:1 F	Edema	6/7
Consanguinity	6/7	Spindle-shaped fingers	6/7
Population	5 Arab; 1 Dutch; 1 Croatian	Wrist drop	7/7
Mean birth weight	3380 g (range: 2950–4150 g) (n = 6)	**SKELETAL SYSTEM**	
Mean birth length	57 cm (range: 53–62 cm) (n = 4)	Advanced bone age	5/6
		Osteoporosis	4/7
		Kyphosis	6/7
CENTRAL NERVOUS SYSTEM		**OTHER ABNORMALITIES**	
Hypotonia	7/7	Cryptorchidism	6/6 M
Developmental delay	4/7		
CRANIOFACIAL ANOMALIES			
Prominent forehead	6/7		
Large, low-set ears	6/7		
Highly arched palate	6/7		

Source: Table based on data from Nevo et al. (36), Hildeink and Brunner (24), Al-Gazali et al. (1), and Dumić et al. (18).

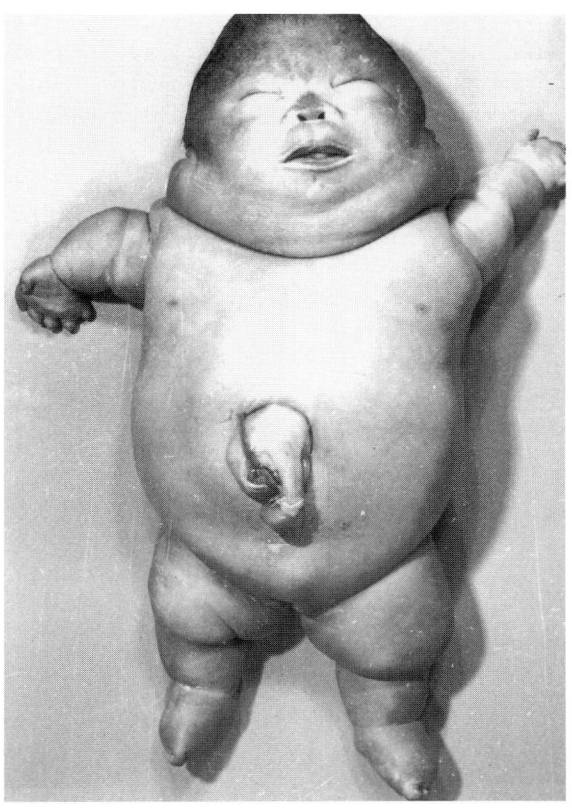

Figure 15–14 Elejalde syndrome. Fetus of 34 weeks delivered by Cesarean section weighing 4300 g. Note short limbs; acrocephalic skull; facial anomalies; excess subcutaneous tissue of neck, trunk, and limbs; and small omphalocele. From Elejalde et al. (19).

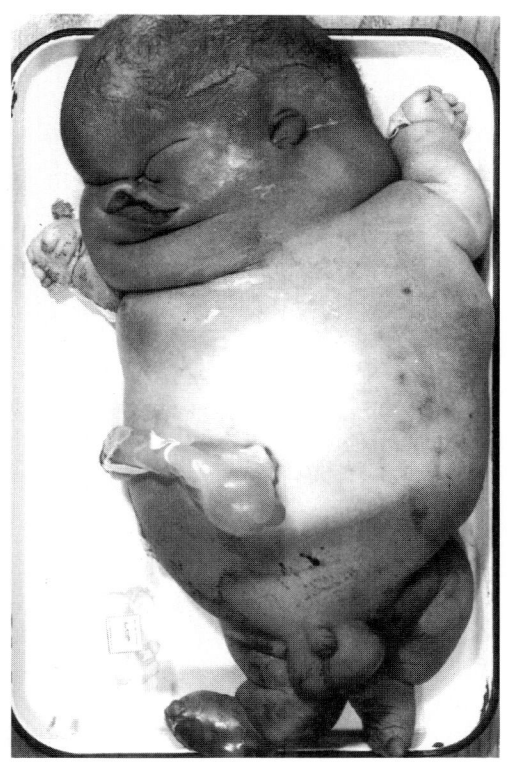

Figure 15–15 Elejalde syndrome. Second stillborn fetus weighing 7500 g. Swollen, globular body with virtual absence of the neck; short limbs; and swollen, distorted face. From Elejalde et al. (19).

ELEJALDE SYNDROME

In 1977, Elejalde and co-workers (19) described a spectacular overgrowth syndrome (**OMIM 200995**)[a] (Figs. 15–14 and 15–15).

The name Elejalde syndrome was coined by Cohen (8a) in 1986 and has been used by other authors (7,34,43). It should not be confused with neuroectodermal melanolysosomal disease, also called Elejalde syndrome (25a).

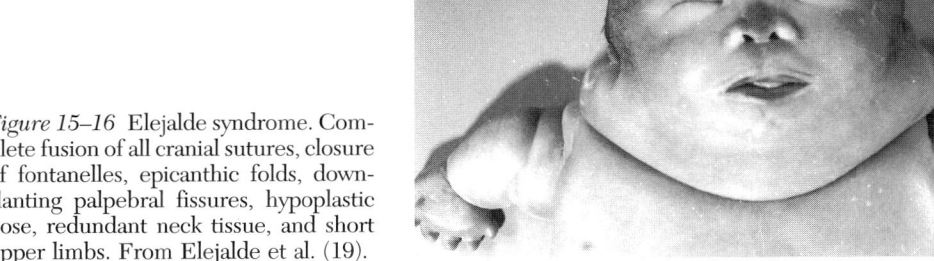

Figure 15–16 Elejalde syndrome. Complete fusion of all cranial sutures, closure of fontanelles, epicanthic folds, downslanting palpebral fissures, hypoplastic nose, redundant neck tissue, and short upper limbs. From Elejalde et al. (19).

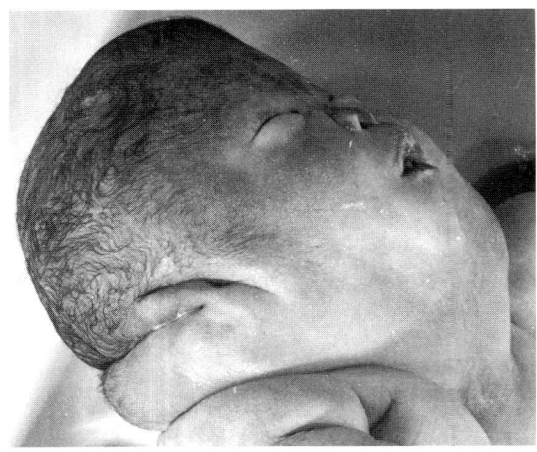

Figure 15–17 Elejalde syndrome. Craniosynostosis, rudimentary auricles, and redundant neck tissue. From Elejalde et al. (19).

Birthweights in two patients were 7,500 and 4,300 g. Features included a swollen globular body, omphalocele, short limbs, redundant neck skin, craniosynostosis, hypoplastic nose, and rudimentary auricles (Figs. 15–14 to 15–17). Three affected individuals in two sibships were recorded for which consanguinity was established. Thus, the Elejalde syndrome has autosomal recessive inheritance. Cell kinetic studies showed that fibroblasts from patients with Elejalde syndrome completed the cell cycle in 63% of the normal cell cycle time (see Fig. 1–1).

Since Elejalde's original cases were described, four other instances have been reported (7,31, 34,43). Characteristic features of the syndrome in six cases are summarized in Table 15–7.

Table 15–7 Findings in Elejalde Syndrome

Findings	No Affected
GENERAL FEATURES	
Increased birth weight	6/6
Swollen globular body	6/6
Thick skin	3/3
Excessive connective tissue	5/5
CRANIOFACIAL ANOMALIES	
Craniosynostosis	4/5
Downslanting palpebral fissures	3/3
Hypertelorism, epicanthic folds	3/3
Dysplastic ears	5/5
Hypoplastic nose	5/5
Short neck, skin folds	6/6
THORAX	
Hypoplastic lungs	4/4
ABDOMEN	
Omphalocele	4/6
Hepatomegaly	4/4
Splenic abnormality	5/6
GENITOURINARY	
Nephromegaly with cystic changes	5/6
LIMBS	
Micromelia	4/4
Polydactyly	4/6

Source: From Cohen and MacLean (11).

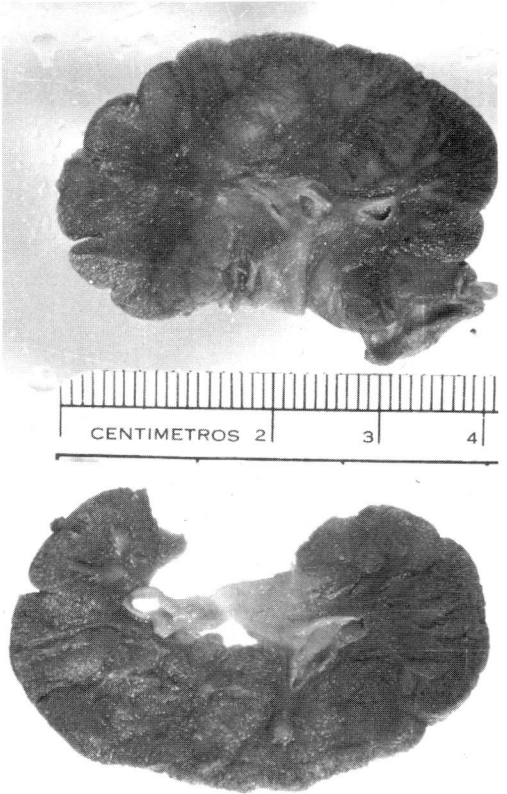

Figure 15–18 Elejalde syndrome. Enlarged kidneys with thick, fibrous capsule, lack of clearcut differentiation between cortex and medulla, and multiple cysts. From Elejalde et al. (19).

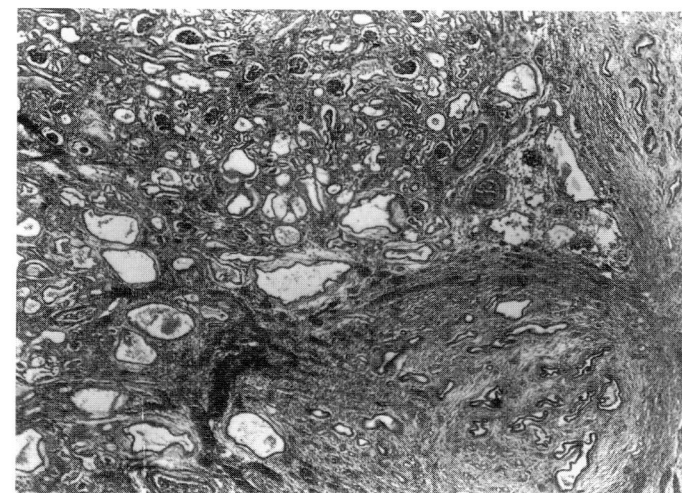

Figure 15–19 Elejalde syndrome. Histologic section of kidney showing paucity of glomeruli, multicystic dysplasia, and marked proliferation of connective tissue. From Elejalde et al. (19).

Autopsy findings (Figs. 15–18 to 15–21) showed enlarged kidneys with a thick fibrous capsule, lack of clearcut differentiation between the cortex and the medulla, and multiple cysts. Excessive connective tissue was found throughout the body, except for the central nervous system. It was most prominent subcutaneously in the media of blood vessels, in the walls of the viscera, and interstitially in organs such as the pancreas and kidneys. Perivascular proliferation

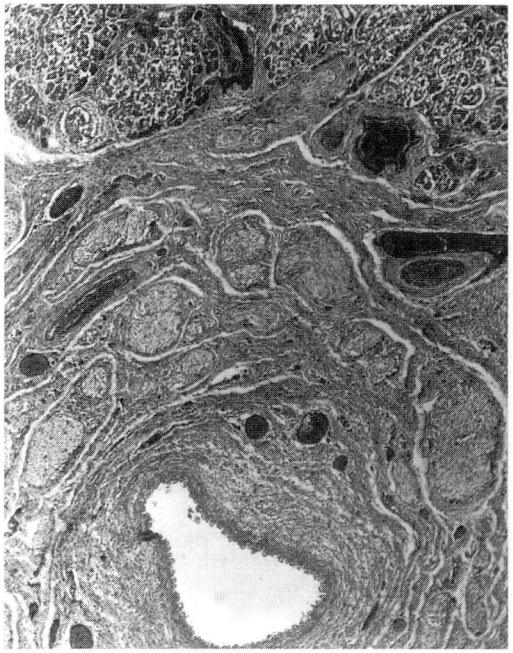

Figure 15–20 Elejalde syndrome. Histologic section of pancreas showing striking proliferation of connective tissue and nerve fibers around arteries. From Elejalde et al. (19).

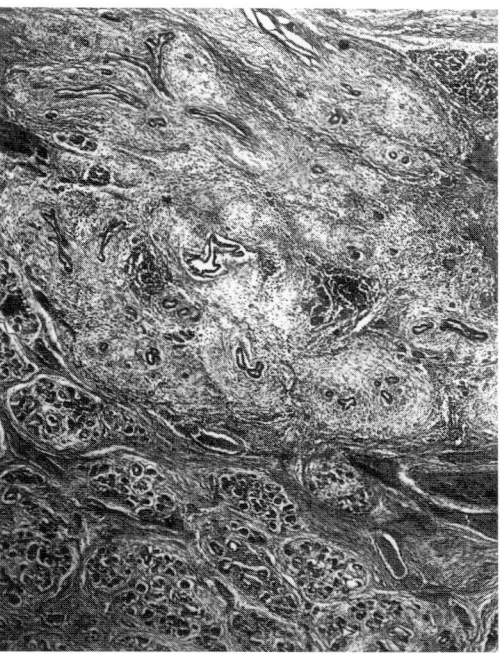

Figure 15–21 Elejalde syndrome. Histologic section of pancreas showing marked connective tissue proliferation within acini. Note dilatation of pancreatic ducts. From Elejalde et al. (19).

of nerve fibers was found in many viscera, particularly the spleen, thymus, colon, heart, and adrenal glands (19).

REFERENCES

1. Al-Gazali LI, Bakalinova D, Varady E, Scorer J, Nork M: Further delineation of Nevo syndrome. J Med Genet 34:366–370, 1997.
2. Baralle D, Firth H: A case of the new overgrowth syndrome—macrocephaly with cutis marmorata, haemangioma and syndactyly. Clin Dysmorphol 9:209–211, 2000.
3. Berberich MS, Carey JC, Hall BH: Resolution of the perinatal and infantile failure to thrive in a new autosomal recessive syndrome with the phenotype of a storage disorder and furrowing of palmar creases. Proc Greenwood Genet Ctr 10:78, 1991.
4. Borochowitz Z, Pavone L, Mazor G, Rizzo R, Dar H: New multiple congenital abnormalities: Mental retardation syndrome (MCA/MR) with facio-cutaneous-skeletal involvement. Am J Med Genet 43:678–685, 1992.
5. Cantú JM, García-Cruz D, Sánchez-Corone J, Hernandez A, Nazará Z: A distinct osteochondrodysplasia with hypertrichosis—individualization of a probable autosomal recessive entity. Hum Genet 60:36–41, 1982.
6. Carcao M, Blaser SI, Grant RM, Weksberg R, Siegel-Bartelt J: Brief clinical report. MRI findings in macrocephaly–cutis marmorata telangiectatica congenita. Am J Med Genet 76:165–167, 1998.
7. Chitty L, Keen C, Hall C: Elejalde syndrome. A detailed description of the radiological, histological and dysmorphic features. 6th Manchester Birth Defects Conference, Manchester, UK, November 1–4, 1994.
8. Clayton-Smith J, Kerr B, Brunner H, Tranebjaerg L, Magee A, Hennekam RCM, Mueller RF, Brueton L, Super M, Steen-Johnsen J, Donnai D: Macrocephaly with cutis marmorata, haemangioma and syndactyly—a distinctive overgrowth syndrome. Clin Dysmorphol 6:291–302, 1997.
8a. Cohen MM Jr: Craniosynostosis: Diagnosis, Evaluation, and Management. First edition, Raven Press, New York, 1986.
9. Cohen MM Jr: Diagnostic problems in cerebral gigantism. J Med Genet 13:80, 1976.
10. Cohen MM Jr: Overgrowth syndromes. In: *Associated Congenital Malformations*. M El-Shafie and CH Klippel eds. Williams & Wilkins, Baltimore, pp 71–104, 1981.
11. Cohen MM Jr, MacLean RE: *Craniosynostosis: Diagnosis, Evaluation, and Management*, 2nd ed. Oxford University Press, New York, 2000.
12. Concolino D, Formicola S, Camera G, Strisciuglio P: Congenital hypertrichosis, cardiomegaly, and osteochondrodysplasia (Cantú syndrome): A new case with unusual radiological findings. Am J Med Genet 92:191–194, 2000.
13. Costello JM: A new syndrome. N Z Med J 74:397, 1971.
14. Costello JM: A new syndrome: Mental subnormality and nasal papillomata. Aust Pediatr J 13:114–118, 1977.
15. Costello JM: Costello syndrome: Update on the original cases and commentary. Am J Med Genet 62:199–201, 1996.
16. Czeizel AE, Tímàr L: Hungarian case with Costello syndrome and translocation t(1;22). Am J Med Genet 57:501–503, 1995.
17. Der Kaloustian VM, Moroz B, McIntosh N, Watters AK, Blaichman S: Costello syndrome. Am J Med Genet 41:69–73, 1991.
18. Dumić M, Vukelić D, Plavsić V, Cviko A, Sokolić L, Filipović-Grčić B: Nevo syndrome. Am J Med Genet 76:67–70, 1998.
19. Elejalde BR, Giraldo C, Jimenez R, Gilbert EF: Acrocephalopolydactylous dysplasia. Birth Defects 13(3B):53–67, 1977.
19a. Feingold M: Costello syndrome and rhabdomyosarcoma. J Med Genet 36:582–583, 1999.
20. Franceschini P, Licata D, Di Cara G, Guala A, Bianchi M, Ingrosso G, Franceschini D: Bladder carcinoma in Costello syndrome: Report on a patient born to consanguineous parents and review. Am J Med Genet 86:174–179, 1999.
21. Franceschini P, Licata D, Di Cara G, Guala A, Franceschini D, Genitori L: Macrocephaly–cutis marmorata telangiectatica congenita without cutis marmorata? Am J Med Genet 90:265–269, 2000.
22. García-Cruz D, Sánchez-Corona J, Nazará Z, García-Cruz MO, Figuera LE, Castañeda V, Cantú JM: Congenital hypertrichosis, osteochondrodysplasia, and cardiomegaly: Further delineation of a new genetic syndrome. Am J Med Genet 69:138–151, 1997.
23. Gripp KW, Scott CI Jr, Nicholson L, Figueroa TE: Letter to the editor: Second case of bladder carcinoma in a patient with Costello syndrome. Am J Med Genet 90:256–259, 2000.
24. Hilderink BGM, Brunner HG: Nevo syndrome. Clin Dysmorphol 4:319–323, 1995.
25. Hinek A, Smith AC, Cutiongco EM, Callahan JW, Gripp KW, Weksberg R: Decreased elastin deposition and high proliferation of fibroblasts from Costello syndrome are related to functional deficiency in the 67-kD elastin-binding protein. Am J Hum Genet 66:859–872, 2000.
25a. Ivanovich J, Mallory S, Storer T, Ciske D, Hing A: Brief clinical report: 12-year-old male with Elejalde syndrome (neuroectodermal melanolysosomal disease). Am J Med Genet 98:313–316, 2001.
26. Johnson JP, Golabi M, Norton ME, Rosenblatt

RM, Feldman GM, Yang SP, Hall BD, Fries MH, Carey JC: Costello syndrome: Phenotype, natural history, differential diagnosis, and possible cause. J Pediatr 53:441–448.

27. Kerr B, Eden OB, Dandamudi R, Shannon N, Quarrell O, Emmerson A, Ladusans E, Gerrard M, Donnai D: Costello syndrome: Two cases with embryonal rhabdomyosarcoma. J Med Genet 35:1036–1039, 1998.

28. Lazalde B, Sánchez-Urbina R, Nuño-Arana I, Bitar WE, de la Ramírez-Duenas M: Autosomal dominant inheritance in Cantú syndrome (congenital hypertrichosis, osteochondrodysplasia, and cardiomegaly). Am J Med Genet 94:421–427, 2000.

28a. Legault L, Gagnon C, Lapointe N: Growth hormone deficiency in Costello syndrome: A possible explanation for the short stature. J Pediatr 138:151–152, 2000.

29. Lin A: Personal communication, 2001.

30. Lurie IW: Genetics of the Costello syndrome. Am J Med Genet 52:358–359, 1994.

31. Lurie IW, Lazjuk GI, Korotkova IA, Cherstvoy ED: The cerebrorenodigital syndrome: A new community. Clin Genet 39:104–113, 1991.

32. Martin RA, Jones KL: Delineation of Costello syndrome. Am J Med Genet 41:346–349, 1991.

33. Moore CA, Toriello HV, Abuelo DN, Bull MJ, Curry CJR, Hall BD, Higgins JV, Stevens CA, Twersky S, Weksberg R, Dobyns WB: Macrocephaly–cutis marmorata telangiectatica congenita: A distinct disorder with developmental delay and connective tissue abnormalities. Am J Med Genet 70:67–73, 1997.

34. Nevin NC, Herron B, Armstrong MJ: An 18 week fetus with Elejalde syndrome (acrocephalopolydactylous dysplasia). Clin Dysmorphol 3:180–184, 1994.

35. Nevin NC, Mulholland HC, Thomas PS: Congenital hypertrichosis, cardiomegaly and mild chondrodysplasia. Am J Med Genet 66:33–38, 1996.

36. Nevo S, Zelter M, Benderly A, Levy J: Evidence for autosomal recessive inheritance in cerebral gigantism. J Med Genet 11:158–165, 1974.

36a. Okamoto N, Chiyo H, Imai K, Otani K, Futagi Y: A Japanese patient with Costello syndrome. Hum Genet 93:605–606, 1994.

37. Philip N, Sigaudy S: Costello syndrome. J Med Genet 35:238–240, 1998.

38. Proud VK, Davis B, Rutledge SL, Gupyta B, Bence L, Schoyer L: Clinical phenotype and natural history of connective tissue problems in 16 individuals with Costello syndrome evaluated at the 1st International Costello Syndrome Conference, April 1999. Twenty-first David W. Smith Workshop on Malformations and Morphogenesis, La Jolla, California, August 2–5, 2000.

38a. Robertson SP, Gattas M, Rogers M, Adès LC: Macrocephaly–cutis marmorata telangiectatica: Report of five patients and a review of the literature. Clin Dysmorphol 9:1–9, 2000.

39. Robertson SP, Kirk E, Bernier F, Brereton J, Turner A, Bankier A: Congenital hypertrichosis, osteochondrodysplasia, and cardiomegaly: Cantú syndrome. Am J Med Genet 85:395–402, 1999.

40. Rosser EM, Kääriäinen H, Hurst JA, Baraitser M, Hall CM, Clayton P, Leonard JV: Three patients with the osteochondrodysplasia and hypertrichosis syndrome: Cantú syndrome. Clin Dysmorphol 7:79–85, 1998.

41. Stephan MJ, Hall BD, Smith DW, Cohen MM Jr: Macrocephaly in association with unusual cutaneous angiomatosis. J Pediatr 87:353–359, 1975.

42. Suri M, Garrett C: Costello syndrome with acoustic neuroma and cataract. Is the Costello locus linked to neurofibromatosis type 2 on 22q? Clin Dysmorphol 7:149–151, 1998.

42a. Tandoi C, Botta A, Fini G, Sangiuolo F, Novelli G, Ricci R, Zampino G, Anichini C, Dallapiccola B: Exclusion of the elastin gene in the pathogenesis of Costello syndrome. Am J Med Genet 98:286–287, 2001.

43. Thornton CM, Stewart F: Brief clinical report. Elejalde syndrome: A case report. Am J Med Genet 69:406–408, 1997.

44. Toriello H, Moore C, Dobyns W: Macrocephaly–cutis marmorata telangiectatica congenita: Description of twelve patients with this previously undescribed multiple congenital anomaly syndrome. Eur J Hum Genet 4 (Suppl 1):2, 1996.

45. Van Eeghen AM, van Gelderen I, Hennekam RCM: Costello syndrome: Report and review. Am J Med Genet 82:187–193, 1999.

45a. Yano S, Watanabe Y: Association of arrhythmia and sudden death in macrocephaly–cutis marmorata telangiectatica congenita syndrome. Am J Med Genet 102:149–152, 2001.

46. Zampino F, Mastroiacovo P, Ricci R, Zollino M, Segni G, Martini-Neri ME, Neri G: Costello syndrome: Further clinical delineation, natural history, and nosology. Am J Med Genet 47:176–183, 1993.

16

Maternal and Endocrine Effects

This chapter focuses on three maternal and endocrine effects: (a) infants of diabetic mothers; (b) persistent hyperinsulinemic hypoglycemia of infancy; and (c) infants of psoriatic mothers.

INFANTS OF DIABETIC MOTHERS

Diabetic Macrosomia

The pathogenesis of diabetic macrosomia is based on the chain of events that follows maternal hyperglycemia. The resultant fetal pancreatic hyperfunction leads to macrosomia since insulin is growth promoting. Although insulin is strongly lipotropic and some authorities (15) have claimed that diabetic macrosomia is based primarily on excessive adipose tissue, nonadipose body constituents are increased in macrosomic infants of diabetic mothers (36). Such infants have an increased number of cell nuclei in various organs, which suggests that increased protein synthesis is most likely attributable to anabolic effects of insulin other than lipogenesis (8).

Experiments with rhesus monkeys resulting in macrosomia include the administration of streptozotocin to pregnant females to produce maternal glucose intolerance (7) and direct administration of insulin to fetuses to produce hyperinsulinism (58). Both types of experiments result in macrosomia with selective organomegaly similar to that found in infants of diabetic mothers. For example, the liver, spleen, and heart show marked effects, whereas the brain and kidneys are unaffected by insulin. Morphometric and chemical analysis of the liver show fat, protein, and DNA concentrations similar to those of controls. Thus, the effect of insulin is to produce hyperplasia (without hypertrophy) of hepatocytes (52).

The frequency of macrosomic infants born to diabetic mothers varies from 7% to 19%, depending on the particular study and on the birthweight above which macrosomia is arbitrarily defined. Horger et al. (20) found that the mean birthweight of infants born to diabetic mothers is 500 g heavier than the birthweight of infants born to nondiabetic mothers. Of 352 infants of diabetic mothers in the Cleveland study (15), 85% had birthweights above the norm for gestational age. The likelihood of finding maternal diabetes mellitus increases with the degree of fetal macrosomia (20). Certainly, gestational diabetics are apt to have macrosomic infants (46,57). Long-term follow-up study indicates that a significant proportion of these mothers go on to develop symptomatic diabetes mellitus.

The size of infants born to a diabetic mother may vary with each pregnancy. Such differences are probably related to the balance between fetal pancreatic hyperfunction, on the one hand, and vascular insufficiency with placental dysfunction on the other. Hyperinsulinism tends to result in macrosomia (Fig. 16–1), while vascular insufficiency with placental dysfunction (White's class D or F diabetes) tends to result in microsomia. Adolescent obesity is more likely to occur in macrosomic infants of diabetic mothers than in macrosomic infants of normal mothers

MATERNAL AND ENDOCRINE EFFECTS

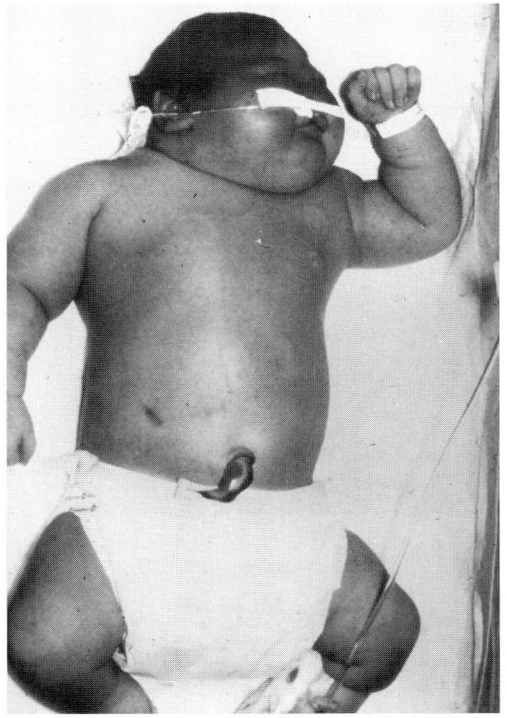

Figure 16–1 Macrosomia, holoprosencephaly, and facial dysmorphism in an infant of a diabetic mother. Courtesy of B.D. Hall, Lexington, Kentucky.

(65), which suggests that macrosomia in infants of diabetic mothers may be a predisposing factor for later obesity (8).

Congenital Anomalies

Many investigators have indicated that congenital malformations occur with increased frequency in the offspring of diabetic mothers. Methodological problems have been particularly well reviewed by Neave (37) and include inadequate sample size, improper control groups, variation in operating definitions of malformation, observer bias, and retrospective rather than prospective design.

Although a great many different anomalies have been reported in the offspring of diabetic mothers, some have been singled out as occurring with specifically higher frequency (Table 16–1), and some of these are illustrated in Figures 16–1 to 16–3. Five anomalies were observed by Neave (37) to occur with significantly greater frequency in offspring of diabetic mothers: microcephaly, ear anomalies, ventricular septal defect, single umbilical artery, and malformations of the ribs and/or vertebral column. In an epidemiologic analysis, Martínez-Frías (32) showed that (*a*) congenital heart defects were the most common malformations encountered, (*b*) caudal dysgenesis was the most characteristic, and (*c*) multiple anomalies occurred more frequently. Khoury et al. (25) assessed multiple congenital anomalies in infants of diabetic mothers to see if a "fetal diabetes syndrome" could be discerned. The clinical epidemiological study carried out by these investigators concluded that no specific pattern of anomalies was characteristic. Martínez-Frías (32a) found an increased risk for transposition of the great vessels and transposition of viscera. Ewart-Toland et al. (13) reported oculoauriculovertebral abnormalities in a craniofacially ascertained population. Hemifacial microsomia occurred in 67%, epibulbar dermoids in 24%, and vertebral anomalies in 24% ($n = 21$) of patients.

Table 16–1 Significant Malformation in Infants of Diabetic Mothers

CENTRAL NERVOUS SYSTEM	GASTROINTESTINAL ANOMALIES
Microcephaly	Neonatal small left colon
Anencephaly/spina bifida	Malrotation of bowel
Holoprosencephaly	Anal/rectal atresia
CRANIOFACIAL ANOMALIES	**GENITOURINARY ANOMALIES**
Ear anomalies	Renal agenesis
Cleft lip/palate	Multicystic dysplasia
	Hypospadias
CARDIOVASCULAR ANOMALIES	Cryptorchidism
Ventricular septal defect	
Transposition of the great vessels	**SKELETAL ANOMALIES**
Situs inversus	Caudal dysgenesis
Single umbilical artery	Rib and/or vertebral anomalies

Source: Adapted from Neave (37) and Cohen (8).

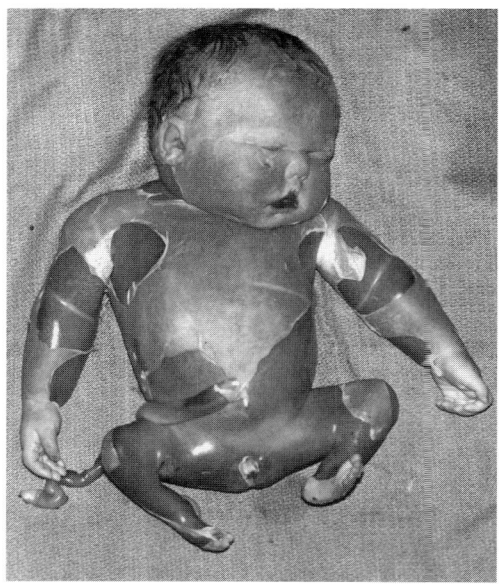

Figure 16–2 Diabetic embryopathy with caudal dysgenesis. From Cohen (8).

Neave (37) found a direct relationship between the severity of maternal diabetes and the frequency with which anomalies were observed. Because the most severe cases of diabetes are more likely to be associated with vascular insufficiency, malformations may be more common

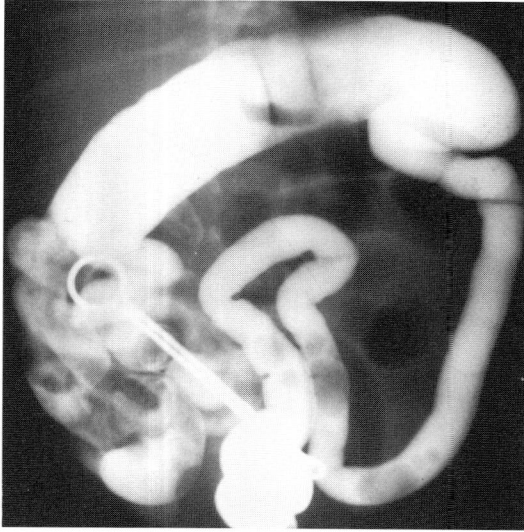

Figure 16–3 Neonatal small left colon from splenic flexure to anus. Common in both gastrointestinally symptomatic as well as asymptomatic infants of diabetic mothers. From Davis and Campbell (9).

in microsomic and normosomic infants than in macrosomic infants.

Van Allen et al. (63) indicated that with diabetic pregnancies, an increase in deformations can be expected to accompany major malformations or macrosomia.

Both macrosomia and hypoglycemia are well-recognized outcomes of gestational diabetes (46,57). The possible association of congenital anomalies with gestational diabetes had been controversial until the large, well-designed study of Martínez-Frías et al. (33). They found that gestational diabetics showed a significant risk for holoprosencephaly and anomalies of the upper and lower spine, ribs, and renal and urinary systems. Gestational diabetes is a heterogeneous disorder that includes not only gestational diabetes per se but also previously unrecognized and newly diagnosed diabetes mellitus. Thus, it is possible that the teratogenic effects encountered may be related to latent diabetes mellitus.

Teratogenicity

Many teratogenic factors have been implicated in diabetic embryopathy (Table 16–2). Pathogenesis is multifactorial and only partially understood at this writing (45,47–50). These pathogenetic factors and their modus operandi can be summarized as the result of any interference with the glycolytic pathway leading to a decreased rate of glycolysis and conversion of glucose to pyruvate (29). Pathogenetic roles are played by hyperglycemia, hypoglycemia, hypoxia, maternal vasculopathy, ketones, amino acid abnormalities, glycosylation of proteins,

Table 16–2 Teratogenic Factors in Diabetic Embryopathy

I. Carbohydrate metabolism
  a) Hyperglycemia ($\downarrow$ uptake of myoinositol)
    $\uparrow$ Sorbitol ($\downarrow$ arachidonic acid)
    $\uparrow$ Nonenzymatic glycosylation of proteins ($\downarrow$ uptake of vitamin C)
    $\uparrow$ Radical O_2 species ($\downarrow$ prostaglandins)
    $\uparrow$ Collagen ($\downarrow$ catalase)
  b) Hypoglycemia ($\downarrow$ superoxide dismutase)
II. Lipid metabolism: $\uparrow$ Ketones (hydroxybutyrate and keto-isocaproic acid)
III. Protein metabolism: $\uparrow$ Somatomedin inhibitors ($\downarrow$ insulin)
IV. Trace metals metabolism ($\downarrow$ zinc)

$\uparrow$, increased; $\downarrow$, decreased.
Source: From Kousseff (29).

hormonal imbalances, and somatomedin inhibitors (21,29,50,51).

Hyperglycemia is a major contributor to teratogenicity by several mechanisms (29): (a) decreased utilization of arachidonic acid and inhibition of the arachidonic acid cascade (17) involving deficiency of myo-inositol (3); (b) hexose monophosphate shunt activity with reduced uptake of ascorbic acid (11) and/or increased nonenzymatic glycosylation of embryonic proteins, leading to altered function (24); (c) increased production of collagen secondary to hyperglycemia metabolism of oxidative substrates with the generation of free oxygen radicals and/or decreased catalase and superoxide dismutase activity (6,12,26); and (d) abnormal levels of trace metals (17).

Monitoring Diabetic Pregnancies

Problems of pregnancy should be discussed with diabetic women before they start their families, if possible. Counseling should be given about when control is considered adequate for a pregnancy to commence. It is important to explain that insulin per se is not teratogenic. Home blood glucose monitoring and control by HbA_{1c} measurement should be carried out. Although improved first-trimester control of blood sugar is associated with a reduced frequency of anomalies (35), good control does not eliminate the possibility of malformations or macrosomia. For example, despite well-controlled diabetic pregnancies, macrosomic infants and congenital anomalies have been documented (27,47,54). Thus, an overobsessional approach to a well-controlled pregnancy should be discouraged by the physician; patients should not have to feel an overwhelming sense of guilt if these measures fail and a malformed infant is born (66).

Diabetic pregnancies and pregnancies complicated by gestational diabetes should be monitored carefully for congenital anomalies. Prenatal ultrasound examination should be directed toward detecting neural tube defects and other CNS abnormalities, cardiovascular and skeletal malformations, and renal and urinary tract defects. Fetal size should be assessed between 36–38 weeks of gestation to allow for induction of labor for the macrosomic infant before size becomes excessive and to make the obstetrician aware of the dangers that might arise during delivery. The possibility of an elective cesarean section should be considered (8).

PERSISTENT HYPERINSULINEMIC HYPOGLYCEMIA OF INFANCY

Neonatal hypoglycemia has multiple known causes (56) (Table 16–3). In normal neonates, hypoglycemia immediately after birth is associated with developmental immaturity of hepatic gluconeogenesis and ketogenesis. In addition, glycogenolysis can be compromised by peripartum stress. Thus, hypoglycemia may develop if neonatal feedings are delayed (56).

Persistent hyperinsulinemic hypoglycemia of infancy (PHHI) (OMIM 256450)[a] is a disorder of glucose metabolism in which secretion of insulin is unregulated, leading to profound hypoglycemia (2,31,41,64).[b] It occurs in about 1 per

---
[a]OMIM, On-Line Mendelian Inheritance In Man number.
[b]Persistent hyperinsulinemic hyperglycemia of infancy (PHHI) has also been called nesidioblastosis of the pancreas or familial hyperinsulinism or autosomal recessive hyperinsulinism.

Table 16–3 Causes of Neonatal Hypoglycemia

Hypoglycemia in otherwise normal infants
  Birth asphyxia
  Prematurity
  Small-for-gestational-age infants
  Large-for-gestational-age infants
  Delay in first feeding
Hyperpituitarism
Inborn errors of ketogenesis
Infants of diabetic mothers
Persistent hyperinsulinemic hypoglycemia of infancy (OMIM 256450)[a]
  High-affinity sulfonylurea receptor (SUR1) (OMIM 600509)
    Focal type
    Diffuse type
  Inwardly rectifying potassium channel subfamily J, member 11 (Kir6.2)[b] (OMIM 600937)
Autosomal dominant hyperinsulinism (OMIM 602485)
  Glucokinase (GCK) (OMIM 138079.0009)
  Glutamate dehydrogenase (GDH)[c] (OMIM 138130)
  Autosomal dominant, molecular cause unknown (OMIM 138079)

---
[a]Persistent hyperinsulinemic hypoglycemia of infancy (PHHI) is also known as nesidioblastosis of the pancreas or familial hyperinsulinism or autosomal recessive hyperinsulinism. OMIM, On-Line Mendelian Inheritance in Man number.

[b]Kir6.2 is also known as $K_{IR}6.2$ and KCNJ11.

[c]Hyperammonemia is associated with hyperinsulinism in these cases. See Yorifuji et al. (67) for an explanation of the activating mutation in GDH.

Table 16–4 Clinical Characteristics of Neonates with Focal and Diffuse Hyperinsulinism

Characteristics	Focal Hyperinsulinism ($n = 22$)	Diffuse Hyperinsulinism ($n = 30$)
M:F sex ratio	1:2	1:1.7
Birthweight >90th centile for gestational age	45%	47%
Cesarean delivery	32%	30%
Seizures	50%	53%
Loss of consciousness	23%	10%

Source: Adapted from Lonlay-Debeney et al. (31).

50,000 live births in the general population (5,55). Approximately 95% of the cases are sporadic. Some cases are autosomal recessive. In a highly consanguineous Arab population in which 51% of the births result from first cousin marriages, 1 per 2,675 newborns is affected and familial cases are common (34).

In PHHI, two histopathologic forms have been found: focal adenomatous islet cell hyperplasia and diffuse abnormalities of β-cell hyperfunction. The type and location of the pancreatic lesions can be detected by preoperative pancreatic catheterization and intraoperative histopathologic studies (31). Focal and diffuse forms of hyperinsulinism are compared in Table 16–4. Birth weights are above the 90th centile in at least 45% in both types (31) (Fig. 16–4). Partial pancreatectomy has been performed for the focal type and subtotal pancreatectomy has been attempted for the diffuse type (31 44). Infants treated for the focal type had no significant hypoglycemia, but some infants treated for the diffuse type had persistent hypoglycemia, some developed type 1 diabetes mellitus, and others developed hyperglycemia (31).

Clinical features of autosomal recessive PHHI are contrasted with those of autosomal dominant hyperinsulinism (16,31,61) in Table 16–5. Significant differences are evident in the age of onset, birthweight, and responsiveness to diet and diazoxide (61).

Malfunctioning ion channels caused by genes encoding channel proteins are termed *channelopathies*. PHHI is caused by mutations in sulfonylurea receptor (*SUR1*) (OMIM 600509), which is a member of the ATP-binding cassette superfamily. PHHI can also be caused by mutations in *Kir6.2* (OMIM 600937), which is a member of the inwardly rectifying family of potassium channels (2,26,41). These two distinct protein subunits, SUR1 and Kir6.2, map to 11p15.1 (64) and form the ATP-sensitive potas-

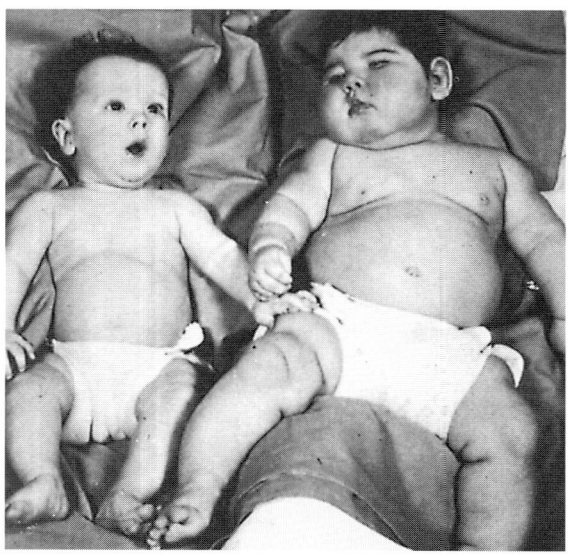

Figure 16–4 Persistent hyperinsulinemic hypoglycemia of infancy. Comparison with normal infant of same age. Courtesy of H.S. Sauls, Minneapolis, Minnesota.

Table 16–5 Clinical Features of Patients with Hyperinsulinism in Autosomal Recessive and Autosomal Dominant Types

Features	Autosomal Recessive	Autosomal Dominant
Number of cases	14	11
M:F sex ratio	1:1	1.2:1
Median age of onset	1 day	1 year
Mean birth weight	4.6 kg	3.3 kg
Responsiveness to diet and diazoxide	0%	91%

Source: Adapted from Thornton et al. (61).

sium (K_{ATP}) channels of the pancreatic β cells (10).

SUR1 is composed of two nucleotide-binding folds (NBF1 and NBF2) and two membrane-spanning domains of multiple transmembrane segments (40). A Kir channel consists of two membrane-spanning domains (M1 and M2) flanking a highly conserved pore region containing an H5 segment. The H5 and M2 segments together with the carboxy terminus hydrophilic domain are critical for potassium permeation (1).

The K_{ATP} channels are involved in glucose-mediated insulin secretion. In the fed state with high intracellular glucose, the K_{ATP} channels are inhibited, which results from a high [ATP]/[ADP] ratio that depolarizes the plasma membrane with an influx of Ca^{2+}, insulin release, and glucose uptake in the peripheral tissues. In the fasting state with low intracellular glucose, the K_{ATP} channels are open, which results from a falling [ATP]/[ADP] ratio that hyperpolarizes the plasma membrane, inhibits Ca^{2+} influx, and prevents insulin release (1,28).

Mutations in *SUR1* and *Kir6.2* alter the response of the pancreatic K_{ATP} channels to intracellular [ATP]/[ADP] levels, resulting in a constitutively depolarized state and unregulated insulin secretion. Thus, the K_{ATP} mutations account for the hyperinsulinemia and hypoglycemia found in PHHI (23,28). Over 20 *SUR1* mutations are known. They are of the missense, nonsense, deletion, insertion, and splice site types (10,38,40,59,60,64) (Table 16–6).

Table 16–6 Mutations in *SUR1*

Exon/Intron	Nucleotide Change	Codon Predicted Effect	Domain[a]
Exon 2	221G → A	Arg74Gln	Tm
Exon 3	375C → G	His125Gln	Tm
Exon 4	563A → G	Asn188Ser	Tm
Exon 6	949delC	317fs/ter	Tm
Exon 8	1216A → G	Asn406Asp	Tm
Intron 10	1630+1G → T	Aberrant splicing	Tm
Exon 12	1773C → G	Phe591Leu	Tm
Exon 13	1893delT	631fs/ter	Tm
Intron 15	2117-1G → A	Aberrant splicing	NBF1
Exon 24	2860C → T	Gln954Stop	—
Exon 28	3416C → T	Thr1139Met	Tm
Exon 29	3644G → A	Arg1215Gln	Tm
Intron 32	3992-9G → A	Aberrant splicing	NBF2
Intron 32	3992-3C → G	Aberrant splicing	NBF2
Exon 33	4058G → C	Arg1353Pro	NBF2
Exon 34	4135G → C	Gly1379Arg	NBF2
Exon 34	4144G → A	Gly1382Ser	NBF2
Exon 34	4162delTTC	Phe1388del	NBF2
Exon 34	4181G → A	Arg1394His	NBF2
Exon 35	4261C → G	Arg1421Cys	NBF2
Exon 35	4310G → A	Aberrant splicing	NBF2
Exon 37	4480C → T	Arg1494Trp	NBF2
Exon 37	4525insCGGCTT	AlaSer1509-1510ins	NBF2

Source: Data from Nestorowicz et al. (38–40), Thomas et al. (59), Dunne et al. (10), Verkarre et al. (64), and Shyng et al. (53).
[a]Tm, transmembrane domains; NBF1, nucleotide binding fold 1; NBF2, nucleotide binding fold 2.

Lonlay et al. (30) showed molecular heterogeneity in the sporadic forms of PHHI. They found loss of 11p15 alleles in the focal type but not in the diffuse type. Verkarre et al. (64) described missense mutations in the paternal allele of *SUR1* restricted to the microscopic hyperplastic lesion found in the focal type. Reduction to hemizyosity or homozygosity of the paternal defective allele and loss of the maternal allele were responsible for hyperinsulinism (64). The loss of maternal imprinted alleles at 11p15.5, including growth factors such as IGF2 and tumor suppressor genes such as *H19* and $p57^{KIP2}$, led to altered expression of these and other genes in the imprinted domain (see Chapter 2).

Mutations in the pore-forming core of Kir6.2 include a missense mutation—Leu147Pro, which disrupts the conserved α-helical second transmembrane (M2) domain, and a nonsense mutation—Tyr12Stop, which produces a truncated polypeptide that lacks the potassium pore region (39,60).

INFANTS OF PSORIATIC MOTHERS

Psoriasis is a common disorder, occurring in 2%–3% of the white population (8). Genetic factors are known to play a major role (14). Propping et al. (43) showed that infants of psoriatic mothers tend to have increased birth weights. They reported a birth weight of >4000 g in 20.4% of infants of psoriatic mothers compared to only 11.3% in a control group. Infants of psoriatic mothers averaged 3480 g and controls averaged 3340 g. Findings were independent of whether mothers developed psoriasis before or after giving birth to their children. Various factors known to influence birth weight were controlled in the study of Propping et al. (43). Specifically excluded were the height and weight of the mother, weight gain during pregnancy, mother's age, parental social class, diabetes mellitus in the mother or first-degree relatives, duration of pregnancy, sex of offspring, and mother's smoking habits during pregnancy.

Psoriasis has some metabolic similarities to diabetes mellitus and some patients have exhibited reduced glucose tolerance and hyperinsulinism following oral and intravenous glucose load (19,22), insulin resistance (4), and raised plasma growth hormone levels (42).

REFERENCES

1. Abraham MR, Jahangir A, Alekseev AE, Terzic A: Channelopathies of inwardly rectifying potassium channels. FASEB J 13:1901–1910, 1999.
2. Aguilar-Bryan L, Bryak J: ATP-sensitive potassium channels, sulfonylurea receptors, and persistent hyperinsulinemic hypoglycemia of infancy. Diabetes Rev 4:337–346, 1995.
3. Baker L, Piddington R, Goldman AS, Egler J: Diabetic embryopathy: Mechanism involves myo-inositol and arachidonic acid. Pediatr Res 20:326A, 1986.
4. Bellomo G, Fratino P, LoCurto F, Pelfini C, Vignini M, Serri F: Insulin receptors in psoriasis. In: *Psoriasis. Proceedings of the Third International Symposium.* EM Farber and AJ Cox, eds. Grune and Stratton, New York, pp. 273–274, 1982.
5. Bruining G: Recent advances in hyperinsulinism and the pathogenesis of diabetes mellitus. Curr Opin Pediatr 2:758–765, 1990.
6. Cederberg J, Eriksson UJ: Decreased catalase activity in malformation-prone embryos of diabetic rats. Teratology 56:350–357, 1997.
7. Chez, RA: Effects of maternal hyperglycemia on fetal development. Diabetics Care 3:435–436, 1980.
8. Cohen MM Jr: A comprehensive and critical assessment of overgrowth and overgrowth syndromes, in Harris H and Hirschhorn K (eds) Advances in Human Genetics. New York, Plenum Press, vol 18, Ch 4, pp 181–303; Addendum, 1989, pp 373–376.
9. Davis WS, Campbell JB: Neonatal small left colon syndrome. Am J Dis Child 129:1024–1027, 1975.
10. Dunne MJ, Kane C, Shepherd RM, Sanchez JA, James RFL, Johnson PRV, Aynsley-Green A, Lu S, Clement JP IV, Lindley KJ, Seino S, Aguilar-Bryan L: Familial persistent hyperinsulinemic hypoglycemia of infancy and mutations in the sulfonylurea receptor. N Engl J Med 336:703–706, 1997.
11. Ely JTA: Hyperglycemia and major congenital anomalies. N Engl J Med 305:833, 1981.
12. Eriksson UJ, Borg LAH: Diabetes and embryonic malformations: Role of substrate-induced free-oxygen radical production of dysmorphogenesis in cultured rat embryos. Diabetes 42:411–419, 1993.
13. Ewart-Toland A, Yankowitz J, Winder A, Imagire R, Cox VA, Aylsworth AS, Golabi M: Oculoauriculovertebral abnormalities in children of

diabetic mothers. Am J Med Genet 90:303–309, 2000.
14. Farber EM: The genetics of psoriasis. JAMA 219:1061–1064, 1972.
15. Fee SA, Weil WB Jr: Body composition of infants of diabetic mothers by direct analysis. Ann Natl Acad Sci 110:869–897, 1963.
16. Glaser B, Kesavan P, Heyman M, Davis E, Cuesta A, Buchs A, Stanley CA, Thornton PS, Permutt MA, Matschinsky FM, Herold KC: Familial hyperinsulinism caused by an activating glucokinase mutation. N Engl J Med 358:226–230, 1998.
17. Goldman AS, Baker L, Piddington R, Marx B, Herold R, Egler J: Hyperglycemia-induced teratogenesis is mediated by a functional deficiency of arachidonic acid. Proc Natl Acad Sci USA 82:8227–8231, 1985.
18. Hagay ZJ, Weiss Y, Zusman I, Peled-Kamar M, Reece EA, Erikkon UJ, Groner Y: Prevention of diabetes-associated embryopathy by overexpression of the free radical scavenger copper zinc superoxide dismutase in transgenic mouse embryos. Am J Ostet Gynecol 173:1036–1041, 1995.
19. Holtzmann H, Morsches B, Beyer J, Wenzel D, Oertel GW, Krapp R: Hyperinsulinismus und eingeschrankte Glucosetoleranz. Arch Dermatol Forsch 245:95–109, 1972.
20. Horger EO, Facog M, Miller C, Conner ED: Relation of large birthweight to maternal diabetes mellitus. Obstet Gynecol 45:150–154, 1975.
21. Horton WE Jr, Sadler TW: Effects of maternal diabetes on early embryogenesis: Alterations in morphogenesis produced by the ketone body, β-hydroxybutyrate. Diabetes 32:610–616, 1983.
22. Jucci A, Viginini M, Pelfini C, Criffo A, Fratino P: Psoriasis and insulin secretion. Arch Dermatol Res 257:239–246, 1966.
23. Kane C, Shepherd RM, Squires PE, Johnson PRV, James RFL, Milla PJ, Aynsley-Green A, Lindley KJ, Dunne MJ: Loss of functional K_{ATP} channels in pancreatic β-cells causes persistent hyperinsulinemic hypoglycemia of infancy. Nat Med 2:1344–1348, 1996.
24. Kennedy L, Baynes JW: Non-enzymatic glycosylation and the chronic complications of diabetes: An overview. Diabetologia 26:93–98, 1984.
25. Khoury MJ, Becerra JE, Cordero JF, Erickson JD: Is there a fetal diabetes syndrome? A clinical–epidemiologic assessment of patterns of birth defects associated with human teratogens. Am J Hum Genet Suppl 43:947, 1988.
26. Kitzmiller JL, Gavin LA, Gin GD, Jovanovic-Peterson L, Main EK, Zigrang WD: Preconception care of diabetes. JAMA 265:731–736, 1991.
27. Knight G, Worth RC, Ward JD: Macrosomy despite a well-controlled diabetic pregnancy. Lancet 2:1431, 1983.
28. Koster JC, Marshall BA, Ensor N, Corbett JA, Nichols CG: Targeted overactivity of β-cell K_{ATP} channels induces profound neonatal diabetes. Cell 100:645–654, 2000.
29. Kousseff BG: Gestational diabetes mellitus (Class A): A human teratogen? Am J Med Genet 83:402–408, 1999.
30. Lonlay P de, Fournet J-C, Rahier J, Gross-Morand M-S, Poggi-Travert F, Foussier V, Bonnefont J-P, Brusset M-C, Brunelle F, Robert J-J, Nihoul-Fékété C, Saudubray J-M, Junien C: Somatic deletion of the imprinted 11p15 region in sporadic persistent hyperinsulinemic hypoglycemia of infancy is specific of focal adenomatous hyperplasia and endorses partial pancreatectomy. J Clin Invest 100:802–807, 1997.
31. Lonlay-Debeney P de, Poggi-Travert F, Fournet J-C, Sempoux C, Vici CD, Brunelle F, Touati G, Rahier J, Junien C, Nihoul-Fékété C, Robert J-J, Saudubray J-M: Clinical features of 52 neonates with hyperinsulinism. N Engl J Med 340:1169–1175, 1999.
32. Martínez-Frías ML: Epidemiological analysis of outcomes of pregnancy in diabetic mothers: Identification of the most characteristic and most frequent congenital anomalies. Am J Med Genet 51:108–113, 1994.
32a. Martínez-Frías ML: Heterotaxia as an outcome of maternal diabetes: An epidemiological study. Am J Med Genet 99:142–146, 2001.
33. Martínez-Frías ML, Bermejo E, Rodríguez-Pinilla E, Prieto L, Frías JL: Epidemiological analysis of outcomes of pregnancy in gestational diabetic mothers. Am J Med Genet 78:140–145, 1998.
34. Mathew P, Young J, Abu O, Mulhern B, Hammoudi S, Hamdan J, Saadi A: Persistent neonatal hyperinsulinism. Clin Pediatr 27:148–151, 1988.
35. Miller E, Hare JW, Cloherty JP, Dunn PJ, Gleason RE, Soelder JS, Kitmiller JL: Elevated maternal hemoglobin A in early pregnancy and major congenital anomalies in infants of diabetic mothers. N Engl J Med 304:1331–1334, 1981.
36. Naeye RL: Infants of diabetic mothers: A quantitative, morphologic study. Pediatrics 35:980–988, 1965.
37. Neave C: Congenital malformation in offspring of diabetics. Perspectives Pediatr Pathol 8:213–222, 1984.
38. Nestorowiccz A, Glaser B, Wilson BA, Shyng S-L, Nichols CG, Stanley CA, Thorton PS, Permutt MA: Genetic heterogeneity in familial hyperinsulinism. Hum Mol Genet 7:1119–1128, 1998.
39. Nestorowicz A, Inagaki N, Gonoi T, Schoor K, Wilson B, Glaser B, Landau H, Stanley C, Thornton P, Seino S, Permutt M: A nonsense mutation in the inward rectifier potassium channel gene, Kir6.2 is associated with familial hyperinsulinism. Diabetes 46:1743–1748, 1997.
40. Nestorowicz A, Wilson BA, Schoor KP, Inoue H, Glaser B, Landau H, Stanley CA, Thornton

PS, Clement JP IV, Bryan J: Mutations in the sulfonylurea receptor gene are associated with familial hyperinsulinism in Ashkenazi Jews. Hum Mol Genet 5:1813–1822, 1996.
41. Permutt MA, Nestorowicz A, Glaser B: Familial hyperinsulinsim: An inherited disorder of spontaneous hypoglycemia in neonates and infants. Diabetes Rev 4:347–355, 1996.
42. Priestley GC, Gawkrodger DJ, Seth J, Going SM, Hunter JAA: Growth hormone levels in psoriasis. Arch Dermatol Res 276:147–150, 1984.
43. Propping P, Hohenschutz C, Voigtlancer V: Increased birth weight in psoriasis—another expression of a "thrifty genotype"? Hum Genet 71:92, 1985.
44. Rahier J, Sempoux C, Fournet J-C, Poggi F, Brunelle F, Nihoul-Fékété C, Saudubray J-M, Jaubert F: Partial or near-total pancreatectomy for persistent hyperinsulinaemic hypoglycaemia: The pathologist's role. Histopathology 32:15–19, 1998.
45. Reece EA, Homko CJ, Ying-King WU: Multifactorial basis of the syndrome of diabetic embryopathy. Teratology 54:171–182, 1996.
46. Sacks DA: Fetal macrosomia and gestational diabetes: What's the problem? Obstet Gynecol 81:775–781, 1993.
47. Sadler LS, Robinson LK, Msall ME: Diabetic embryopathy: Possible pathogenesis. Am J Med Genet 55:363–366, 1995.
48. Sadler TW, Denno KM, Hunter ES III: Effects of altered maternal metabolism during gastrulation and neurulation stages of embryogenesis. Maternal nutrition and pregnancy outcome. Ann NY Acad Sci 678:48–61, 1993.
49. Sadler TW, Hunter ES III, Walkan W, Horton WE Jr: Effects of maternal diabetes on embryogenesis. Am J Perinatol 5:319–326, 1988.
50. Sadler TW, Hunter ES III, Wynn RE, Phillips LS: Evidence for multifactorial origin of diabetes-induced embryopathies. Diabetes 38:70–74, 1989.
51. Schaefer UM, Songster G, Xiang A, Berkowitz K, Buchanan TA, Kjos SL: Congenital malformations in offspring of women with hyperglycemia first detected during pregnancy. Am J Obstet Gynecol 177:1165–1171, 1997.
52. Schwartz R, Susa J: Fetal macrosomia—Animal models. Diabetes Care 3:430–432, 1980.
53. Shyng SL, Ferrigui T, Shepard JB, Nestorowicz A, Glaser B, Permutt MA, Nichols CG: Functional analyses of novel mutations in the sulfonylurea receptor 1 associated with persistent hyperinsulinemic hypoglycemia of infancy. Diabetes 47:1145–1151, 1998.
54. Skyler JS, O'Sullivan MJ, Holsinger KK: The relationship between maternal hyperglycemia and macrosomia. Diabetes Care 3:433–434, 1980.
55. Stanley C: Hyperinsulinism in infants and children. Pediatr Clin North Am 44:363, 1997.
56. Stanley CA, Baker L: The causes of neonatal hypoglycemia. N Engl J Med 340:1200–1201, 1999.
57. Stephenson MJ: Screening for gestational diabetes mellitus: A critical review. J Fam Pract 37:277–283, 1993.
58. Susa JB, McCormick KL, Widness JA, Singer DB, Oh W, Adamson K, Schwartz R: Chronic hyperinsulinemia in the fetal rhesus monkey: Effects on fetal growth and composition. Diabetes 28:1058–1063, 1979.
59. Thomas PM, Cote GJ, Wohllk N, Haddad B, Mathew PM, Rabi W, Aguilar-Bryan L, Gagel RF, Bryan J: Mutations in the sulfonylurea receptor gene in familial persistent hyperinsulinemic hypoglycemia of infancy. Science 268:426–429, 1995.
60. Thomas P, Ye Y, Lightner E: Mutation of the pancreatic islet inward rectifier Kir6.2 also leads to familial persistent hyperinsulinemic hypoglycemia of infancy. Hum Mol Genet 5:1809–1812, 1996.
61. Thornton PS, Satin-Smith MS, Herold K, Glaser B, Chiu KC, Nestorowicz A, Permutt AM, Baker S, Stanley CA: Familial hyperinsulinism with apparent autosomal dominant inheritance: Clinical and genetic differences from the autosomal recessive variant. J Pediatr 132:9–14, 1998.
62. Thornton PS, Sumner AE, Ruchelli ED, Spielman RS, Baker L, Stanley CA: Familial and sporadic hyperinsulinism: Histopathologic findings and segregation analysis support a single autosomal recessive disorder. J Pediatr 199:721–724, 1991.
63. Van Allen MI, Brown ZA, Plovie B, Hanson ML, Knopp RH: Deformations in infants of diabetic and control pregnancies. Am J Med Genet 53:210–215, 1994.
64. Verkarre V, Fournet J-C, de Lonlay P, Gross-Morand M-S, Devillers M, Rahier J, Brunelle F, Robert J-J, Nihoul-Fékéte C, Saudubray J-M, Junien C: Paternal mutation of the sulfonylurea receptor (*SUR1*) gene and maternal loss of 11p15 imprinted genes lead to persistent hyperinsulinism in focal adenomatous hyperplasia. J Clin Invest 102:1286–1291, 1998.
65. Vohr BR, Lipsitt LP, Oh W: Somatic growth of children of diabetic mothers with reference to birth size. J Pediatr 97:196–199, 1980.
66. Watkins PJ: Congenital malformations and blood glucose control in diabetic pregnancy. Br Med J 284:1357–1358, 1982.
67. Yorifuji T, Muroi J, Uematsu A, Hiramatsu H, Momoi T: Hyperinsulinism-hyperammonemia syndrome caused by mutant glutamate dehydrogenase accompanied by novel enzyme kinetics. Hum Genet 104:476–479, 1999.

17

Fetal Hydrops

Most overgrowth syndromes are characterized by excessive cellular proliferation. An increase in the interstitium such as excessive fluid in fetal hydrops does not represent overgrowth per se. Nevertheless, enlargement is characteristic and the condition is well known.

Fetal hydrops results from an increase in body fluid together with a relative increase in fluid in the interstitial space (Figs. 17–1 and 17–2). When the latter is severe, free fluid may accumulate in the body cavities as well. Normal fluid distribution requires balanced osmotic and hydrostatic forces on either side of the cell membrane and an intact sodium pump. Initiating factors in hydrops include severe chronic anemia, hypoproteinemia, fetal heart failure, and obstruction of fetal circulation (3).

Fetal hydrops occurs in approximately 1 in 3000 pregnancies. About 90% of cases are of the nonimmune type and at least 80 different causes have been identified, with cardiovascular and chromosomal problems being diagnosed most frequently (2,7–10) (Table 17–1). Although some causes are responsive to in utero therapy (1), fetal hydrops mortality remains high. In particular, with cardiac anomalies, thoracic tumors, and diaphragmatic hernia, the perinatal mortality rate ranges from 80%–100% (6).

With high-resolution ultrasonography and cytogenetic techniques, it is often possible to establish a diagnosis before 20 weeks. The mean gestational age at diagnosis has fallen from 31–33 weeks during the 1970s to 24–29 weeks during the 1990s (6). Not surprisingly, a higher frequency of aneuploidy associated with fetal hydrops is diagnosed before 18 weeks than during the second half of pregnancy (5,6). In these earlier diagnosed cases, increased nuchal translu-

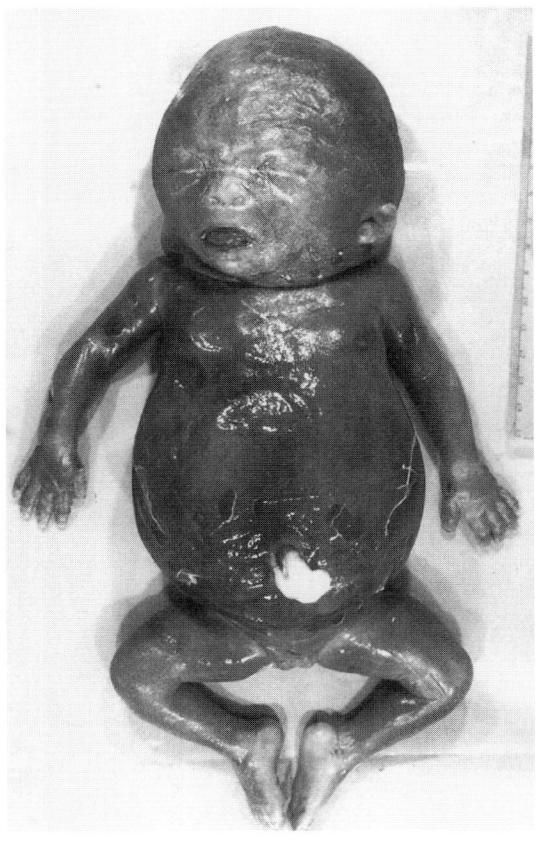

Figure 17–1 Fetal hydrops. Courtesy of M. Barr, Jr., Ann Arbor, Michigan.

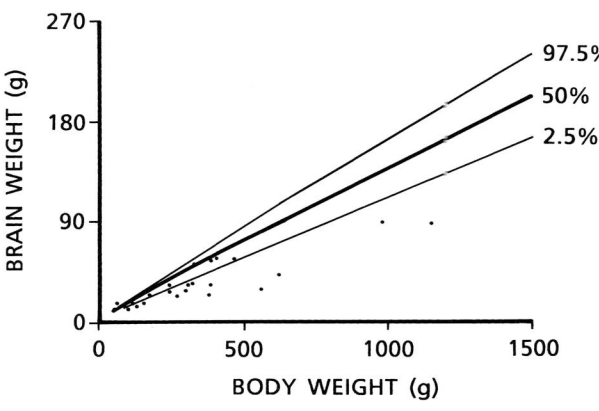

Figure 17–2 Hydrops cases caused by cervical cystic hygroma (brain weight plotted against body weight). Body weight too heavy for brain weight, i.e., 15 of 24 cases are <2.5 percentile (brain weight is too light for body weight). Courtesy of M. Barr, Jr., Ann Arbor, Michigan.

Table 17–1 Some Causes of Nonimmune Fetal Hydrops[a]

Some Causes	Some Examples
Cardiovascular	Malformations with arrhythmias
Chromosomal	Turner syndrome, trisomy 21 syndrome
Thoracic	Chondrodysplasia, cystic adenomatoid malformation, diaphragmatic hernia
Twin transfusion	Hydropic donor, hydropic recipient
Anemia	α-Thalassemia
Infection	Cytomegalovirus, parvovirus B19
Urinary tract malformation	Urethral obstruction
Genetic metabolic disorder	Lysosomal storage disorders

[a]For complete coverage, see Machin (7), Boyd and Keeling (2), Stone and Sidransky (9), and Van Maldergem et al. (10).

cency of aneuploidy associated with fetal hydrops is diagnosed before 18 weeks rather than during the second half of pregnancy. In these earlier diagnosed cases, increased nuchal translucency thickness is probably the earliest sign of fetal hydrops (6).

When fetal hydrops is recognized, amniocentesis should be considered to identify a chromosomal anomaly if present. Ultrasonography should be performed to study the rate, rhythm, and structure of the heart and to search for other structural anomalies as well. The family and obstetric history should be determined, and the mother should have an antibody screen, hemoglobin electrophoresis, and Kleihauer-Betke test for the presence of fetal blood (4).

REFERENCES

1. Ayida GA, Soothill PW, Rodeck CH: Survival in non-immune hydrops fetalis without malformation or chromosomal abnormalities after invasive treatment. Fetal Diagn Ther 10:101–105, 1995.
2. Boyd PA, Keeling JW: Fetal hydrops. J Med Genet 29:91–97, 1992.
3. Cohen MM Jr: *The Child with Multiple Birth Defects*, 2nd ed. Oxford University Press, New York, 1997.
4. Donnai D: Fetal hydrops: Mechanisms and syndromes. Proc Greenwood Genet Ctr 8:108–110, 1989.
5. Iskaros J, Jauniaux E, Rodeck C: Outcome of nonimmune hydrops fetalis diagnosed during the first half of pregnancy. Obstet Gynecol 90:321–325, 1997.
6. Jauniaux E: Diagnosis and management of early non-immune hydrops fetalis. Prenat Diagn 17: 1261–1268, 1997.
7. Machin GA: Hydrops revisited: Literature review of 1,414 cases published in the 1980s. Am J Med Genet 34:366–390, 1989.
8. Santolaya J, Alley D, Jaffe R, Warsof SL: Antenatal classifications of hydrops fetalis. Obstet Gynecol 79:256–259, 1992.
9. Stone DL, Sidransky E: Hydrops fetalis: Lysosomal storage disorders *in extremis*. In: Advances in Pediatrics, L.A. Barness, editor, Mosby, St. Louis, 1999, Vol. 46, Ch. 12, pp. 409–440.
10. Van Maldergem L, Jauniaux E, Fourneau C, Gillerot Y: Genetic causes of hydrops fetalis. Pediatrics 89:81–86, 1992.

18

Nonsyndromal Overgrowth

It is reasonably common in medical genetics, pediatric endocrinology, and child psychiatry to evaluate patients who are tall, macrocephalic, mildly retarded, and often overweight. Such patients are nonsyndromal in appearance and no specific diagnosis can be made.

NOSOLOGIC CONSIDERATIONS

Description is based on the personal observations of Neri (1,2) in about 50 patients. Features include (*a*) mild mental delay; (*b*) height or head circumference ≥75th centile; (*c*) normal chromosomes and normal *FMR1* to rule out fragile X syndrome; (*d*) exclusion of known overgrowth syndromes; and (*e*) nonspecific facial appearance (Fig. 18–1). Despite the consistency of the phenotype, nonsyndromal overgrowth is probably causally heterogeneous. Based on sporadicity, a low recurrence risk is likely, following the birth of an affected child.

PHENOTYPE

No patient has had a pattern of anomalies that suggested either a known or unknown malformation syndrome. Family histories have been noncontributory and, to date, all cases have been sporadic. Males have been affected much more commonly than females.

Birthweight is above the 75th centile in more than half the cases. Height is ≥75th centile in

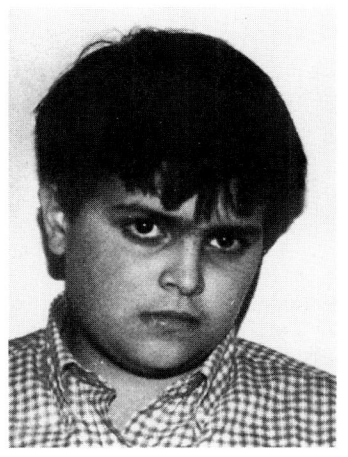 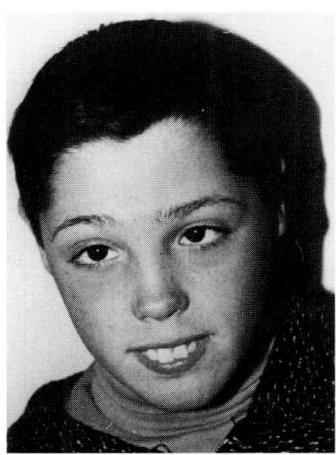 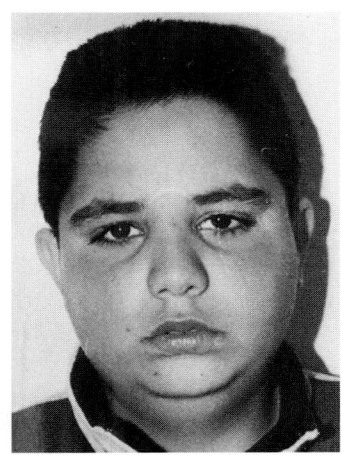

Figure 18–1 Three adolescent patients with nonsyndromal overgrowth. Note nondistinctive facial appearance.

more than half the patients, in the 75th to 97th centile in about one-third of patients, and in the 50th to 75th centile in the remaining cases. Head circumference measurements are distributed in approximately the same proportions. Bone age is advanced in nearly half the cases. Parental heights are normal and within the average range of the general population, but patient heights are greater than expected on the basis of parental heights. On the average, patients are also relatively obese.

Muscular hypotonia is found in more than 50% of patients. CT scans and MRIs of the brain are essentially normal; very mild ventriculomegaly is relatively common, but enlargement occurs in only a few instances. Several patients have been on medication for seizures. Vision and hearing are normal.

Blood levels of IGF1, IGF2, and IGFBP3[a] were assayed in some patients. IGF1 and IGFBP3 were within normal limits. IGF2 tended to exceed normal limits on the average but did not reach significance because of the small sample size.

REFERENCES

1. Neri G, Steindl K, Mazzei A, Battaglia A, Cappa M: Nonsyndromal overgrowth in males with mild psychomotor delay. Am J Med Genet 79:291–293, 1998.
2. Neri G: Personal observations, 1996–2000.

[a]IGF1 = Insulin-like growth factor 1. IGF2 = Insulin-like growth factor 2. IGFBP3 = Insulin growth factor binding protein 3.

Miscellaneous Syndromes and Conditions with Overgrowth

This chapter reviews 20 syndromes and conditions with overgrowth (Table 19–1). Many of these conditions are rare and are not likely to be of differential diagnostic concern when confronting a patient with an overgrowth syndrome. In some conditions discussed here, only a subset of patients actually exhibits overgrowth.

Several syndromes in this chapter are well delineated: Carpenter syndrome, cranioectodermal dysplasia, lipodystrophy, Marshall-Smith syndrome, and PEHO syndrome. They are included here because a subset of patients in each diagnostic category demonstrates high birth weights. In the case of Marshall-Smith syndrome, all patients show remarkably accelerated osseous maturation.

BAKKER-HENNEKAM SYNDROME

Bakker and Hennekam (2) reported two brothers with disproportionate tall stature, macrocephaly, neonatal hypotonia, developmental delay, high narrow forehead, frontal hair upsweep, ocular hypertelorism, broad short ears, and mild hypermobility of joints. During infancy and childhood, one brother's height, hand length, and foot length were above the 97th centile. The other brother's birth weight was 4650 g.

BAYOUMI SYNDROME

Bayoumi et al. (2a) reported an autosomal recessive syndrome consisting of macrocephaly, frontal bossing, hypertelorism, flat malar region, short neck, and multiple epiphyseal dysplasia. Weight and head circumference were above the 90th centile. The gene was mapped to 15q26.

CARPENTER SYNDROME

Carpenter syndrome is an autosomal recessive disorder characterized by craniosynostosis, preaxial polysyndactyly of the feet, short fingers with clinodactyly, variable soft tissue syndactyly, postaxial polydactyly in some cases, and other abnormalities such as congenital heart defects, short stature, obesity, and mental deficiency. Weight is often above average (5) and LGA infants have been noted in some instances (16).

CHORANGIOMA

Chorangioma is a vascular malformation of the placenta occurring with a frequency of about 1% of pregnancies. Small lesions are clinically silent, but large lesions carry a significant risk of perinatal morbidity and mortality. Fetal loss is primarily caused by polyhydramnios and preterm delivery. Other complications include arteriovenous shunting of fetal blood resulting in cardiomegaly, congestive heart failure, and fetal hydrops (13).

El-Haddad et al. (9) reported a male infant with fetal macrosomia who weighed 4200 g at 38 weeks of gestation and suggested that the cause could be progressive reduction in the vascularity of the placental chorangioma during fetal life, possibly by degeneration.

Table 19–1 Miscellaneous Syndromes and Conditions with Overgrowth

Bakkar-Hennekam syndrome
Bayoumi syndrome
Carpenter syndrome
Chorioangioma and fetal overgrowth
Congenital hypothyroid gigantism
Congenital muscular hypertrophy, hypertonia, and developmental retardation
Cranioectodermal dysplasia
Ectodermal overgrowth syndrome
Homfray syndrome
Lipodystrophy
Macrocephaly–autism syndrome
Macrocephaly–megalocornea syndrome
Marshall-Smith syndrome
MOMO syndrome
Ørstavik macrocephaly syndrome
PEHO syndrome
Quattrin syndrome
Richieri-Costa overgrowth syndrome
Siena-type overgrowth
Stevenson syndrome
Teebi overgrowth-microphthalmia syndrome
Transposition of the great vessels with overgrowth

CONGENITAL HYPOTHYROID GIGANTISM

Addy (1) described a single patient with congenital hypothyroidism of pituitary origin who was 57 cm long and weighed 5000 g at birth. The weight gain between the second and tenth months of life indicated considerable hyperphagia which, together with increased height, suggested abnormal hypothalamic function. Thus, in this condition, Addy postulated a defect involving both the pituitary gland and the hypothalamus.

CONGENITAL MUSCULAR HYPERTROPHY, HYPERTONIA, AND DEVELOPMENTAL RETARDATION

Cornelia de Lange (7) described three children with a distinctive condition that bears superficial resemblance to the Beckwith-Wiedemann syndrome. Findings include congenital muscular hypertrophy, hypertonia, and developmental retardation. Macroglossia and large ears were observed in two of the three patients, and overgrowth at birth was a feature in one instance. Autopsy findings in one case demonstrated polymicrogyria and a widespread porencephalic process.

CRANIOECTODERMAL DYSPLASIA

Cranioectodermal dysplasia was first described by Sensenbrenner et al. (29). The disorder was named and expanded by Leven et al. (17). Over 10 cases have been recorded and thoroughly reviewed by Cohen and MacLean (5). The syndrome consists of craniofacial, ectodermal, and skeletal abnormalities. Several children have died before 7 years of age, usually from chronic renal failure with hypertension and proteinuria resulting from tubulointerstitial nephropathy (33).

Levin et al. (17) reported five children with sagittal synostosis, dolichocephaly, sparse slow-growing hair, hypodontia and/or microdontia, narrow thorax, short limbs, and brachydactyly. Intelligence was normal. Inheritance is autosomal recessive.

Three of the five affected children had birthweights of >4000 g and one weighed >4500 g. With postnatal growth and development, weight generally varied between the third and tenth centiles, although one child was at the 50th centile. Height also varied from the third to the tenth centiles.

ECTODERMAL OVERGROWTH SYNDROME

Graham (12) observed an infant with a birthweight of 10 lb, 3 oz, macrocephaly, macroglossia, and overgrowth of skin and hair.

HOMFRAY SYNDROME

Homfray (14a) reported a newly recognized chromosomal breakage syndrome with macrocephaly, mental deficiency, dysmorphic features, and hypomelanosis of Ito. Height was at the 97th centile and bone age was advanced. Acute lymphoblastic leukemia developed at 3 years of age.

LIPODYSTROPHY

Lipodystrophy, an autosomal recessive disorder, was described independently by Berardinelli (3) and Seip (28). Features include a markedly accelerated growth rate with advanced bone age, large hands and feet, muscular hypertrophy, loss of subcutaneous fat, hyperlipemia, hepatosplenomegaly, and enlarged external genitalia. Lack of subcutaneous fat is usually evident at birth, and an occasional patient is reported with a birthweight as high as 4000 g (28).

MACROCEPHALY–AUTISM SYNDROME

Stevenson et al. (31) found macrocephaly of postnatal onset in 24% of 100 patients with autism. A family history of macrocephaly occurred in 62% of macrocephaly–autism cases. These authors also noted that patients with macrocephaly and autism tended to show lower adaptive function than autistic patients without macrocephaly. Other cases of the macrocephaly–autism syndrome have been reported by Cole and Hughes (6) and Naqvi et al. (22). Cole and Hughes (6) observed marked obesity, distinctive facial changes, and mental deficiency.

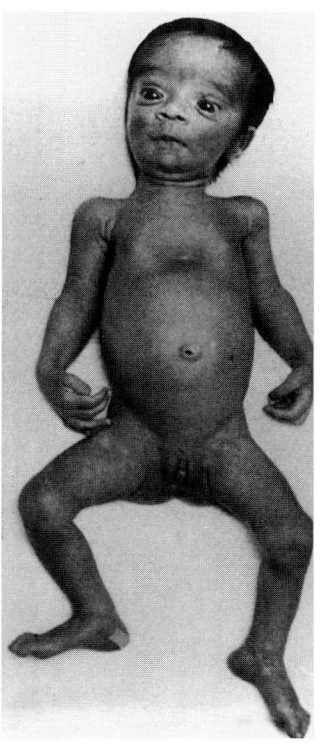

Figure 19–1 Marshall-Smith syndrome. Prominent forehead, bushy eyebrows, and bulging eyes. From Flatz and Natzschka (10).

Table 19–2 Features of the Marshall-Smith Syndrome

Finding	Frequency
GROWTH, SKELETAL	
Accelerated linear growth	2/18
Accelerated osseous maturation	18/18
Broad phalanges	17/17
Failure to thrive	11/13
PERFORMANCE	
Neurodevelopmental abnormalities	13/13
Structural brain anomalies	7/14
RESPIRATORY	
Respiratory tract abnormalities	15/18
Recurrent pneumonia	14/18
Pulmonary hypertension	4/18
Death in early infancy	10/18
CRANIOFACIAL	
Prominent forehead	15/18
Small face	12/18
Prominent eyes	17/18
Blue sclerae	11/18
Flat nasal bridge	17/18
Anteverted nares	15/16
Micrognathia	14/18
Glossoptosis	6/17
Choanal atresia/stenosis	3/17
OTHER	
Hypertrichosis	7/18
Umbilical hernia	6/18

Source: Adapted from Hoyme and Bull (15).

MACROCEPHALY–MEGALOCORNEA SYNDROME

Frydman et al. (11) observed two unrelated patients with macrocephaly, mild mental deficiency, megalocornea, large fleshy ears, and long fingers. Hypotonia, poor coordination, and swallowing difficulties were present. Birthweight was 3200 g in one patient and 4100 g in the other. Head circumference was +3.2 SD in one and +4.0 SD in the other.

Neuhauser et al. (23) reported a syndrome of megalocornea, iris hypoplasia, iridodonesis, moderate to severe mental deficiency, and EEG abnormalities. However, the patients discussed by Frydman et al. (11) appear to be distinctive.

MARSHALL-SMITH SYNDROME

Marshall et al. (19) reported a disorder characterized by accelerated osseous maturation, men-

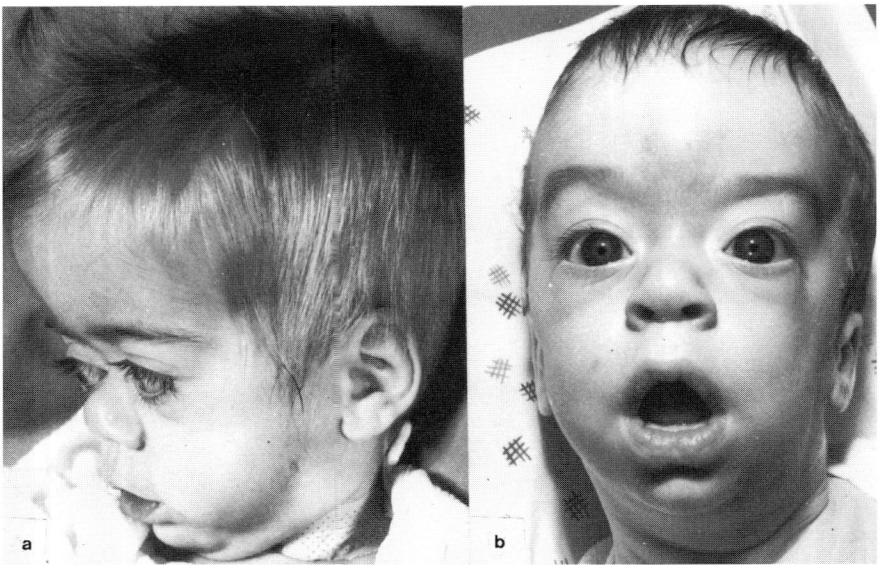

Figure 19–2 Marshall-Smith syndrome. Two patients with promient forehead, bushy eyebrows, and bulging eyes. From Marshall et al. (19).

tal deficiency, postnatal somatic retardation, characteristic facial appearance, large hands and feet, and remarkably thick proximal and middle phalanges in the hands. The syndrome has been thoroughly reviewed by Cohen (4) (Table 19–2, Figs. 19–1 to 19–4) and radiographic findings have been reviewed by Eich et al. (8).

Average birth weight is about 3300 g but weight in excess of 4500 g has been recorded (10,19). Failure to thrive, chronic respiratory distress, and an early demise have characterized many cases, but aggressive treatment may improve the prognosis (34).

Marshall-Smith syndrome is distinct from Sotos syndrome (Chapter 6) and Weaver syndrome (Chapter 7).

MOMO SYNDROME

Moretti-Ferreira et al. (21) reported two unrelated patients with *m*acrocephaly, *o*besity,

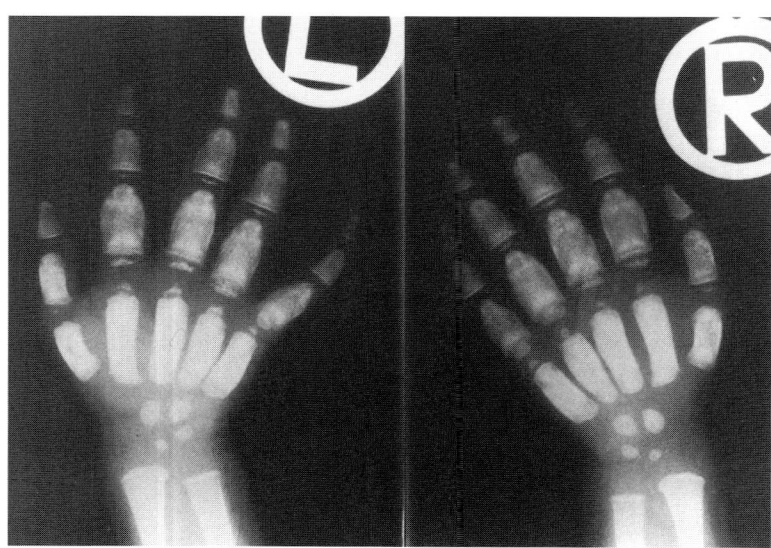

Figure 19–3 Marshall-Smith syndrome. Remarkably thick proximal and middle phalanges with great reduction in size of the terminal phalanges and distal widening of metacarpals. From Flatz and Natzschka (10).

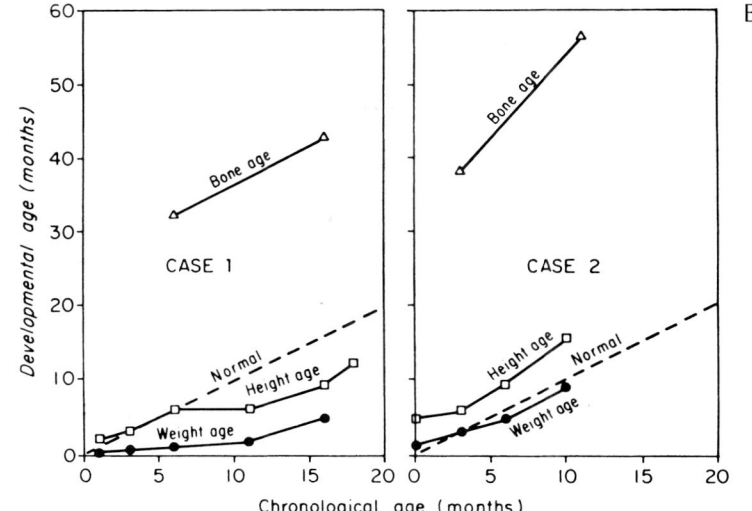

Figure 19–4 Marshall-Smith syndrome. Note remarkably advanced bone age in two patients. From Marshall et al. (19).

macrosomia, and ocular anomalies and designated the syndrome with the acronym MOMO syndrome. The height of both patients was at the 90th centile and weight and OFC were greater than the 97th centile. Other findings included mental deficiency, delayed bone age, delayed dental eruption, retinal coloboma, nystagmus, downslanting palpebral fissures, ocular hypertelorism, downturned mouth, and short neck.

ØRSTAVIK MACROCEPHALY SYNDROME

Ørstavik et al. (24) described two sisters with early postnatal macrocephaly, high broad forehead, bushy eyebrows, short philtrum, epilepsy, autistic behavior, and mental deficiency. One sister died at 5 years of age during an epileptic episode. At autopsy, brain weight was 1815 g (mean brain weight for 5 years, 1200 g).

PEHO SYNDROME

Salonen et al. (27) described a syndrome of progressive encephalopathy with edema, hypsarrhythmia, and optic atrophy and named it PEHO syndrome. Inheritance is autosomal recessive.

The mean birth weight is 3120 g ($n = 8$) and three of eight infants had birth weights between 3650 g and 4000 g (14). During infancy, height becomes −2 SD below normal and thereafter drops to −3 SD to −5 SD below normal. Head circumference drops to −2 SD below normal (27).

Infants are healthy at birth, but develop jerking of the limbs and progressive hypotonia by 2–3 weeks of age. Other findings include infantile spasms with hypsarrhythmia, arrested psychomotor development, progressive visual failure with atrophy of the optic discs, and non-pitting edema of the limbs. Facial dysmorphism consists of midface hypoplasia, epicanthic folds, protruding ear lobules, and micrognathia (27).

In autopsied cases, cerebral and cerebellar atrophy is found. Severe neuronal loss of the inner granular layer is observed in the cerebellum. Purkinje cells are reduced in number and size. The remaining cells are deformed and misaligned (14).

QUATTRIN SYNDROME

Quattrin et al. (25) described two unrelated girls who were large for gestational age—weight, length, and OFC all being greater than the 97th centile. Distinctive features consisted of macrocephaly, wide broad cheeks, ocular hypertelorism, flat nasal bridge, cardiac anomalies, vertebral defects, and initially delayed psychomotor development that improved with age.

RICHIERI-COSTA OVERGROWTH SYNDROME

Richieri-Costa et al. (26) reported a newly recognized syndrome in two sibs born to nonconsanguineous parents. Features included overgrowth in birth length but not in birth weight, mental deficiency, postnatal overgrowth craniosynostosis (in one patient), distal arthrogryposis, sacral dimple, and joint laxity.

SIENA TYPE OVERGROWTH

Mangano et al. (18) described a large family of 14 individuals who had macrosomia with or without mental deficiency but without distinctive syndromic features. The pedigree suggested autosomal dominant inheritance with phenotypic variability.

STEVENSON SYNDROME

Stevenson (30) reported two macrosomic infants with a Seckel-like facial appearance and mental deficiency. Features included delayed development, sloping forehead, prominent nasal bridge, downslanting palpebral fissures, low-set posteriorly angulated ears, extensor hand positioning, joint dislocations, thickened feet, and thickened scrotum.

TEEBI OVERGROWTH–MICROPHTHALMIA SYNDROME

Teebi et al. (32) reported an autosomal recessive syndrome in five sibs of a consanguineous mating. Findings included macrosomia, severe microphthalmia, protuberant abdomen, hepatomegaly, and respiratory infections. Three of the five sibs had cleft palate. Birth weight was 5000 g or over in two infants and over 4000 g in the other three. Death (3–180 days; mean, 67 days) occurred from massive bronchopneumonia in two infants, sudden death in two, and an overwhelming illness in one.

TRANSPOSITION OF THE GREAT VESSELS WITH OVERGROWTH

Mehrizi and Drash (20) observed that infants with complete transposition of the great vessels tended to have higher than average birth weights. Average birth weights of male and female infants with transposition were 3538 g and 3266 g, respectively, compared with 3062 g and 2835 g for a large control group. Furthermore, birth weights of infants with complete transposition of the great vessels were higher (3447 g) than the average birth weight of infants with other congenital heart defects, whether cyanotic (3157 g) or acyanotic (3162 g). None of the infants with complete transposition had signs or symptoms of heart failure and none was edematous at delivery.

The reason why infants with transposition of the great vessels are heavier than other infants is unclear. However, Mehrizi and Drash (20) noted a high frequency of diabetes mellitus in families of affected infants. Furthermore, transposition is one of the anomalies known to be associated with diabetic or prediabetic pregnancies.

REFERENCES

1. Addy DP: Congenital hypothyroid gigantism: A new diencephalic syndrome? Br Med J 2:1192–1193, 1977.
2. Bakker HD, Hennekam CM: Macrocephaly, facial abnormalities, disproportionate tall stature, and mental retardation—a sib observation. Am J Med Genet 70:312–314, 1997.
2a. Bayoumi R, Saar K, Lee Y-A, Nürnberg G, Reis A, Nur-E-Kamal M, Al-Gazali LI. Localisation of a gene for an autosomal recessive syndrome of macrocephaly, multiple epiphyseal dysplasia, and distinctive facies to chromosome 15q26. J Med Genet 38:369–373, 2001.
3. Berardinelli W: An undiagnosed endocrine—metabolic syndrome. J Clin Endocrinol 14:193–204, 1954.
4. Cohen MM Jr: A comprehensive and critical assessment of overgrowth and overgrowth syndromes. In Harris H, Hirschhorn K (eds), Advances in Human Genetics, Vol 18, New York, Plenum Press, 1989, pp 181–303, 373–375.
5. Cohen MM Jr, MacLean RE: *Craniosynostosis: Diagnosis, Evaluation, and Management*, 2nd ed. Oxford University Press, New York, 2000.
6. Cole TRP, Hughes HE: Autosomal dominant

macrocephaly: Benign familial macrocephaly or a new syndrome? Am J Med Genet 41:115–124, 1991.
7. de Lange C: Congenital hypertrophy of the muscles, extrapyramidal motor disturbance and mental deficiency. Am J Dis Child 48:243–268, 1934.
8. Eich GF, Silver MM, Weksberg R, Daneman A, Costa T: Marshall-Smith syndrome: New radiographic, clinical and pathologic observations. Radiology 181:183–188, 1991.
9. El-Haddad MA, Izquierdo L, Curet LB: Large vascular degenerating chorioangioma associated with fetal macrosomia and good fetal outcome. J SOGC 19:411–413, 1997.
10. Flatz SD, Natzschka J: Syndrom des akzelerierten Skelettreifung vom Typ Marxhall Kasuislik und Überblick. Klin Padiatr 190:592–598, 1978.
11. Frydman M, Berkenstadt M, Raas-Rothschild A, Goodman RM: Megalocornea, macrocephaly, mental and motor retardation (MMMM). Clin Genet 38:149–154, 1990.
12. Graham JM Jr: Personal communication, 1980
13. Hadi HA, Finley J, Strickland D: Placental chorioangioma: Prenatal diagnosis and clinical significance. Am J Perinatol 10:146–149, 1993.
14. Haltia M, Somer M: Infantile cerebello-optic atrophy. Neuropathology of the progressive encephalopathy syndrome with edema, hypsarrhythmia and optic atrophy (the PEHO syndrome). Acta Neuropathol 85:241–247, 1993.
14a. Homfray T. A new chromosome breakage syndrome with macrocephaly, hypomelanosis of Ito, mental retardation and dysmorphic features. 9th Manchester Birth Defects Conference, Manchester, UK, November 7–10, 2000.
15. Hoyme HE, Bull MJ: The Marshall-Smith syndrome: Natural history beyond infancy. Eighth David W. Smith Workshop on Malformations and Morphogenesis, Greenville, South Carolina, August 15–19, 1987.
16. Leonard CO: Prenatal diagnosis of the large for gestational age fetus, Ninth Annual David W. Smith Workshop on Malformations and Morphogenesis, Oakland, California, August 3–7, 1988.
17. Levin LS, Perrin JCS, Ose L, Dorst JP, Miller JD, McKusick VA: A heritable syndrome of craniosynostosis, short thin hair, dental abnormalities, and short limbs: Cranioectodermal dysplasia. J Pediatr 90:55–61, 1977.
18. Mangano L, Palmeri S, Dotti MT, Moschini F, Federico A: Macrosomia and mental retardation: Evidence of autosomal dominant inheritance in four generations. Am J Med Genet 32:67–71, 1989.
19. Marshall RE, Graham CB, Scott CR, Smith DW: Syndrome of accelerated skeletal maturation and relative failure to thrive: A newly recognized clinical growth disorder. J Pediatr 78:95–101, 1971.
20. Mehrizi A, Drash A: Birth weight of infants with cyanotic and acyanotic congenital malformations of the heart. J Pediatr 59:715–718, 1961.
21. Moretti-Ferreira D, Koiffmann CP, Listik M, Setian N, Wajntal A: Macrosomia, obesity, macrocephaly and ocular abnormalities (MOMO syndrome) in two unrelated patients: Delineation of a newly recognized overgrowth syndrome. Am J Med Genet 46:555–558, 1993.
22. Naqvi S, Cole T, Graham JM Jr: Cole-Hughes macrocephaly syndrome and associated autistic manifestations. Am J Med Genet 94:149–152, 2000.
23. Neuhauser G, Kaveggia EG, France TD, Opitz JM: Syndrome of mental retardation, seizures, hypotonic cerebal palsy and megalocorneae, recessively inherited. Z Kinderheilk 120:1–18, 1975.
24. Ørstavik KH, Strømme P, Johan Ek, Torvik A, Skjeldal OH: Macrocephaly, epilepsy, autism, dysmorphic features, and mental retardation in two sisters: A new autosomal recessive syndrome? J Med Genet 34:849–851, 1997.
25. Quattrin T, McPherson E, MacGillivray M, Afsahni E: Macrosomia, unusual facies, and early developmental delay. Dysmorphol Clin Genet 2:16–20, 1988.
26. Richieri-Costa A, Guion-Almeida ML, Cohen MM Jr: Newly recognized autosomal recessive MCA/MR/overgrowth syndrome. Am J Med Genet 47:278–280, 1993.
27. Salonen R, Somer M, Haltia M, Lorentz M, Norio R: Progressive encephalopathy with edema, hypsarrhythmia, and optic atrophy (PEHO syndrome). Clin Genet 39:287–293, 1991.
28. Seip M: Lipodystrophy and gigantism with associated endocrine manifestations. Acta Paediatr Scand 48:555–574, 1959.
29. Sensenbrenner JA, Dorgf JP, Owens RP: New syndrome of skeletal, dental, and hair anomalies. Birth Defects 11(2):372–379, 1975.
30. Stevenson RE: Large birthweight infants with Seckel facies, dislocations, and mental retardation. Birth Defects 14(6B):381–382, 1978.
31. Stevenson RE, Schroer RJ, Skinner C, Fender D, Simenson RJ: Autism and macrocephaly. Lancet 349:1744–1745, 1997.
32. Teebi AS, Al-Saleh QA, Hassoon MM, Farag TI, Al-Awadi SA: Macrosomia, microphthalmia, cleft palate and early infant death: A new autosomal recessive syndrome. Clin Genet 36:174–177, 1989.
33. Tsimaratos M, Bernard E, Sigandy S, Almahama T, Delarme A, Roquelaure B, Costet C, Antiguac C, Gubler M-C, Picon G, Philip N, Sarles J: Chronic renal failure and cranioectodermal dysplasia: A further step. Pediatr Nephrol 11:785–786, 1997.
34. Williams DK, Carlton DR, Green SH, Pearman K, Cole TRP: Marshall-Smith syndrome: The expanding phenotype. J Med Genet 34:842–845, 1997.

Index

Adenoma
  monomorphic, 79t, 91f
  papillary, 79t
Adenomatous hyperplasia, 25f
Adipose tissue, dysregulation of, 88, 90, 90f
Adrenal cortex, cytomegaly of, 23f
Adrenocortical carcinoma, 6t, 26t
AFP, 24
Allelic heterogeneity, 136
Angiomas
  cutaneous, 141
  tufted, 119, 121t
Arteriovenous malformations, 115
Astrocytoma, 5t
[ATP]/[ADP] ratio, 185
Autism. See Macrocephaly-autism syndrome

Bakker-Hennekam syndrome, 193
Bannayan-Riley-Ruvalcaba syndrome, 7, 66–67, 70f, 71f, 105t
  delineation and nomenclature, 66
  differential diagnosis, 52, 56, 71–72
  mutations, 67–69
  phenotypic features, 69–71
  PTEN mutations, 7, 68f, 69t
Bannayan-Riley-Ruvalcaba/Cowden syndrome overlap, PTEN mutations in, 69t
Bayoumi syndrome, 193
Beckwith-Wiedemann syndrome, v–vi, 4–5, 21–22f
  adenomatous hyperplasia, hilus in ovarian section, 25f
  circular indentation, posterior rim of helix, 21f
  cytomegaly of adrenal cortex, 23f
  diagnosis, differential, 26–27
  diagnostic criteria, 11, 13t
    neoplasms associated with, 6t
  diagnostic testing and recurrence risk, 18
  diaphragm, dome-shaped defect of, 19f
  earlobe groove, 20f
  and epigenetics, 12–13
  genetic and epigenetic subgroups, 14–15, 14t
  hepatoblastoma at autopsy, 5f
  historical perspective, 11
  imprinted genes implicated in, 15–17
  imprinting and, 11–12
    cancer and, 17
  incidence, 11
  kidney, 23f
  malignant/premalignant and benign tumors, 26t
  molecular genetics, 11
  natural history, 18, 19–24
    development, 19
    growth, 18–19
    neoplasia, 20, 23–24
  nephrogenic activity zones, 24f
  omphalocele and macroglossia, 12f
  pancreas, 20f
  patient evaluation
    postnatal, 24–26
    prenatal, 24
  phenotype, 11, 14–15
  renal medullary dysplasia, 24f
  Simpson-Golabi-Behmel syndrome and, 39, 43
  testis showing hyperplasia of Leydig cells, 25f
  uniparental disomy of chromosome 11p15, 21–22f
  with unknown etiologies, 17
Birthweight. See Macrosomia
Body size, increased, 5t

Café-au-lait spots, 137f, 141
  familial, 132
Calcification/calcium deposits in cerebral cortex, 117
Cantú syndrome, 171–173, 172f
  features, 171t
Capillary formation, large, 89f
Capillary malformation
  facial, 118f
  in Klippel-Trenaunay syndrome, 112–114f, 114
  in Sturge-Weber syndrome, 117, 117t, 118f, 119f

Cardiac abnormalities, 43, 172. *See also* Heart defects
Cardiovascular anomalies, 19, 62, 142–143. *See also specific topics*
Carpenter syndrome, 193
CDKN1C. *See* p57^{KIP2}
Central nervous system
    in Bannayan-Riley-Ruvalcaba syndrome, 39
    in fragile X syndrome, 155
    in neurofibromatosis, 141
    in Proteus syndrome, 97–98
    in Sotos syndrome, 53
    Weaver syndrome, 60
Cerebral cortex, calcification/calcium deposits in, 117, 120f
CFC syndrome, 169
CGG, 153, 156
Channelopathies, 184
Chorangioma, 193
Chromosomal disorders with overgrowth, 161–162, 162t, 164
Chromosome 11p15, 14, 14f, 15, 18, 19
    genes and their imprinting status on, 13f
    model for imprinted gene and imprinting center function on, 16f
    uniparental disomy, 15, 18, 21–22f
Chromosome 11p15 abnormalities, 11
Chromosome 11p15 imprinted genes, 15, 13f
Chromosome 11p15 region, 15
    model for regulation of imprinted genes in, 17
Chronic myelogenous leukemia, 141
Cognitive disability, 117
Cohen, Michael, v
Colon, small left, 182f
Connective tissue nevi. *See under* Proteus syndrome, clinical features
Conserved N-terminal region (CNTR), 143
Costello syndrome, 27, 166–168f, 169
    features, 168t
    growth and development in, 169t
    neoplasms, 169t
Cowden syndrome, 68
CpG, 135, 136
Cranioectodermal dysplasia, 194
Craniofacial features
    in Bannayan-Riley-Ruvalcaba syndrome, 70
    in Beckwith-Wiedemann syndrome, 20
    in chromosomal syndromes, 161–164
    in fragile X syndrome, 154–155, 154f
    in Marshall-Smith syndrome, 195–196, 195t
    in Perlman syndrome, 48, 48t
    in Proteus syndrome, 77t, 78t, 82f, 95, 95t, 96f, 97f, 102, 104t
    in Simpson-Golabi-Behmel, 41, 41t, 42f
    in Sotos syndrome, 54
    in Sturge-Weber syndrome, 117, 117t
    in Weaver syndrome, 60–61
Craniofacial growth, types of abnormal, 95t
Cutis marmorata telangiectatica congenita, 170
Cystadenoma, 92
    ovarian, 79t
Cystic hygroma, cervical, 190f

Cyst(s)
    inclusion, 92f
    of malformations of lung, 101f
    ovarian, 79t

del(15)(q12), 164
del(22)(q13 → qter), 164
Diabetic embryopathy, 182
    with caudal dysgenesis, 182f
    teratogenic factors in, 182t
Diabetic macrosomia, 180–181
Diabetic mothers
    congenital anomalies, 181–182
    infants of, 180–181
        macrosomia, holoprosencephaly, and facial dysmorphism, 181f
        malformation in, 181t
    teratogenicity, 182–183
Diabetic pregnancies, monitoring, 183
Diaphragm, dome-shaped defect of, 19f
Differentially methylated regions, 12
dup(4)(p16.3), 161
dup(5)(p), 161
dup(12p), 161
dup(12)(q11 → q15), 162
dup(15)(q25 → qter), 164
dup(15)(q21-qter) and dup(15)(q25-qter), 164t
Dysplasia
    See also Megaspondylodysplasia, 93f
    cranioectodermal, 194
    renal medullary, 24f

Earlobe groove, 20f
Ectodermal overgrowth syndrome, 194
Edema
    Nevo syndrome, 173
    PEHO syndrome, 197
Elejalde syndrome, 2f, 175–177f, 175–178
    findings in, 176t
"Elephant Man," 75–76, 78, 80–81
Embryopathy. *See* Diabetic embryopathy
Encephalocraniocutaneous lipomatosis (ECCL), 100–101, 105t, 132
Encephalopathy, progressive, 197
Enchondromas, 125
Enchondromatosis(es)
    classification, 127t
    Maffucci, 125, 126f, 127t, 128
    Ollier, 125, 128
Endocrine/metabolic problems, 19, 142
Epidermal nevi, 87, 88f, 97f
Epidermal nevus syndromes, 105t
Epiphyses, mottled, 63f
Ezrin, radixin, and moesin (ERM), 143

Face, 96f. *See also* Craniofacial features
Facial capillary malformation, 118f
Facial phenotype, 95, 99f
Familial lipomatosis, 105t
Fetal hydrops. *See* Hydrops, fetal
Fibroblast growth factor receptor 3 (*FGFR3*), 3–4

FMR1 gene, 152–153, 156, 157
Focal adhesion kinase (FAK), 67
Fragile X syndrome, 152
    clinical phenotype
        central nervous system and performance, 155
        connective tissue findings, 155
        craniofacial appearance, 154–155, 154f
        general features and variability, 154
        genitourinary system, 156
    diagnosis, 156
        differential, 52, 56, 156
    genetics, 152
        gene structure and protein isoforms, 152–153
        origin and effects of full mutations, 153
    guidelines for health supervision, 156–157
    macroorchidism, 155f
    prevalence, 152
    prevalence estimates, and healthy female carriers, 153t
Fungiform papillae, tongue involvement with enlarged, 35f

GEFs, Ras activation by, 135f
Gene deletions, contiguous, 136
Genes. *See also specific topics*
    modifying, 136
Genomic imprinting. *See* Imprinting
Glypicans, 38
    molecular biology, 38
GPC3 deletion mutations
    and associated clinical findings, 40t
GPC3 (glypican gene)
    molecular biology, 38–39
    mutations, 3, 39, 41
    putative role in modulating IGF2 interaction with IGF2R, 39f
GTPase activating protein (GAP), 133

H19, 15, 17
H19DMR (mouse *H19* gene), 17
Heart defects. *See also* Cardiac abnormalities
    congenital, 54, 62
Hemangiomas *vs.* vascular malformations, 5
Hemihyperplasia (hemihypertrophy), 6t, 19, 32, 34–35f, 84
    abnormalities associated with, 33t
    differential diagnosis, 104, 105
    epidemiology, 32
    etiologic considerations, 32–33
    jaws, 35f
    malignant pheochromocytoma, 36f
    nosology, 32
    pedigree in which mother has, 37f
    tongue involvement with enlarged fungiform papillae, 35f
    tumors, 33
Hemihyperplasia subsets, 4t
Hemihyperplasia/lipomatosis syndrome, 105t
Hepatoblastoma, 5f, 6t
Hepatocellular carcinoma, 6t
Heterozygosity, loss of, 135, 136

HMGIC gene, 83–84
Holoprosencephaly, 181f
Homfray syndrome, 194
Hydrops, fetal, 189–190, 189f
    caused by cervical cystic hygroma, 190f
    causes of nonimmune, 190t
Hyperglycemia, 183
Hyperinsulinism. *See also* Hypoglycemia
    in autosomal recessive and dominant types, 185t
Hyperostosis, 95, 97f
Hypoglycemia, 182
    of infancy, hyperinsulinemic, 19, 24–25, 184f
    neonatal, causes of, 183t
Hypothyroid gigantism, congenital, 194

Imprinting center and imprinted domain, 12
Insulin-like growth factor binding proteins, 83
Insulin-like growth factors, 83
    IGF2, 15, 18, 39, 39f
Intestinal type neurofibromatosis, 132

Kaposiform hemangioendothelioma, 119, 120f, 121t
    vascular lesions, 121t
Kasabach-Merritt phenomenon, 119, 121t
Kasabach-Merritt syndrome, 119
K_{ATP} channels, 185
KH domains (KH1 and KH2), 153
Kidney, 23f. *See also* Renal blastema
Klippel-Trenaunay syndrome, 84, 105, 105t, 116t
    capillary, lymphatic, and venous malformation, 112–114f
    capillary formations, 114
    diagnosis, 122
        differential, 104, 117, 122t
    etiologic considerations, 111–112, 114
    familial cases, 111–112, 114
    lateral venous anomaly, 115f
    limb enlargement, 115–116
    lymphatic malformations, 115
    lymphatic vesicles, 112f, 113f
    secondary cutaneous manifestations, 116
    varicosities, 111–112, 114–115
    vascular lesions, 121t
KvDMR1, 13, 17, 18
KvLQT1/KvLQT1-AS, 13, 16–18
Kyphosis, angular thoracic, 94f

Learning disabilities, 141
Lentigines, multiple, 132
Leptomeningeal malformation, 117
Lesions
    skin, 87
    vascular, 7f, 121t
Leukemia, 5t, 141
Lipodystrophy, 194–195
Lipomas, 88, 90, 105
    of abdomen and breast, 89f
Lipomatosis, 105, 105t
    encephalocraniocutaneous, 100–101, 105t, 132
Localized/patterned overgrowth, v
Long-chain 3-hydroxyacyl-CoA dehydrogenase deficiency (LCHAD), 70

Loss of heterozygosity (LOH), 135, 136
Lumping, problem of, 4
Lymphatic malformations, 112–114f, 115

Macrocephaly, 70, 71, 139, 166, 196
   in Bannayan-Riley-Ruvalcaba syndrome, 70–72
Macrocephaly-autism syndrome, 195
Macrocephaly-cutis marmorata syndrome, 169–170, 170f, 171t
Macrocephaly-megalocornea syndrome, 195
Macroglossia, 12f, 20
Macrosomia, 197
   diabetic, 180–181, 181f
   infant, 2–3, 19
Maffucci syndrome, 105t, 125, 126–127f
   differential diagnosis, 125, 128
   enchondromas, 125, 126f
   neoplasms, 125, 127t
   skeletal system, 125
   vascular abnormalities, 125
Malignant peripheral nerve sheath tumors (MPNSTs), 139–140
Marshall-Smith syndrome, 195–196, 195–197f, 64
   features, 195t
Megaspondylodysplasia of cervical vertebrae, 93f
Meningioma, 79t
Merrick, Joseph Carey, 75–76, 78, 80–81
Metaphyses, splayed, 63f
Moesin, 143
MOMO syndrome, 196–197
Monomorphic adenoma, 79t
Monstra per excessum, v
Mosaicism, 81, 83, 136
   clinical aspects, 100–102
   i(12p) (Pallister-Killian syndrome), 162, 162t, 163f
Mulliken classification, 5, 6t
Multiple aberration region (MAR), genes in 83–84
Muscular hypertrophy, congenital, 194
Mutations, 3–4. *See also specific topics*

Nasal bridge, bilateral hyperostoses of, 97f
Neoplasia, 4–5, 5t. *See also specific topics*
Nephroblastomatosis, 48–49
Nephrogenic activity zones, 24f
Neuroblastoma, 5t, 6t
   showing rosette formation, 63f
Neurofibromas
   isolated, 145
   multiple isolated, 145
   See also Neurofibromatosis
Neurofibromatosis, 83t, 130
   classification and types of, 130, 132–133
   diagnosis, 144–145
      differential, 145
   neurofibroma in, 80t, 130, 132–142, 137f, 140f, 144, 145
      plexiform, 136, 136t, 138f, 139, 140, 140f, 141t, 145
   NF1 gene
      molecular biology, 133–134
      mutations, 134
      pseudogenes, 135
   NF1 (type 1), 64, 75, 76, 105t, 130, 132, 134f, 137, 142f, 143f
      axillary freckling, 138f
      café-au-lait spots, 137f
      cardiovascular system, 142–143
      central nervous system, 141
      diagnosis, 144, 144t
      differential diagnosis, 145
      endocrine system, 142
      epidemiology, 133
      expressivity, 136, 136t
      eyes, 142
      features, 136t
      growth, 139
      histopathology, 140f
      Lisch nodules, 139f
      microdeletions, 135
      natural history, 137, 139
      neoplasia, 139–141
      neoplasms, 141t
      neurofibroma, 138f
      screening studies for children with proven/presumptive, 145t
      segmental *vs.* classic, 133
      skeletal system, 142
      skin, 141
      tumorigenesis, 135–136
   NF2 (type 2), 133, 143
      consensus criteria for diagnosis, 145t
      molecular biology, 143–144
      mutations, 144
      phenotype, 144
   types of, 131t, 132t
Neurofibromatosis-Noonan syndrome, 130, 132
Nevo syndrome, 52, 56, 173–174f
   findings in, 171t
Nonsyndromal overgrowth, 191f
   nosologic considerations, 191
   phenotype, 191–192
Noonan syndrome, 130, 132

Obesity, 196
Ocular anomalies, 197
OFC, 139, 197
Omphalocele, 12f
Optic atrophy, 197
Optic gliomas, symptomatic, 141
Ørstavik macrocephaly syndrome, 197
Osteosarcoma, 5t
Ovarian cysts, 92
Overgrowth, 2. *See also specific topics*
   causes, 2
   historical perspective, v, 1–2
   miscellaneous syndromes and conditions with, 194t
   mythology, 1
Overgrowth syndrome designations, 7
Overgrowth syndromes, 2. *See also specific topics*
   classification, 4, 4t
   definition, 4t

INDEX

Pallister-Killian syndrome [mosaicism, i(12p)], 162, 162t, 163f
Pancreas, 20f
Papillae, tongue involvement with enlarged fungiform, 35f
Papillary adenocarcinoma (testis), 79t
Papillary adenoma (appendix testis), 79t
Paradominant inheritance, 83
Parkes Weber syndrome, 105, 105t, 114, 116, 116t
   diagnosis, 122
      differential, 105, 122t
Parotid gland, monomorphic adenoma of, 91f
"Pederson syndrome," 103
PEHO syndrome, 197
Perlman syndrome, 26–27, 43, 47, 48f
   clinical phenotype, 47–48
   diagnosis
      differential, 49
      prenatal, 48
   etiology, 47
   features, 48t
   historical perspective, 47
   pathology, 48–49
Persistent hyperinsulinemic hypoglycemia of infancy (PHHI), 183–186
Pheochromocytoma, malignant, 36f
Phosphatase, 66, 67f
Pitt-Rogers-Danks syndrome, 161
$p57^{KIP2}$, 12, 15–18
Pregnancies
   abnormal, 3t
   Beckwith-Wiedemann syndrome and, 19
Prenatal diagnosis of large-for-gestational age fetuses, 3t
Protein tyrosine phosphatase (PTPase), 66
Proteus syndrome, 75–76, 78, 80–81
   causes of premature death, 84, 85t, 86
   clinical features, 100
      alterations in talus and navicular bones, 94f
      angular thoracic kyphosis, 94f
      central nervous system, 97–98
      chest and abdomen, 87f
      connective tissue nevi, 80t, 81f, 82f, 86–87, 86f, 87f
      connective tissue patterns, 86f, 87f, 93f
      cystadenoma of ovary, 90f
      cystic malformations of lung, 101f
      digital overgrowth, 92f
      dysregulation of adipose tissue, 88, 90, 90f
      epidermal nevi and other skin lesions, 87, 88f, 97f
      face, 96f
      facial dysmorphism, 96f
      facial phenotype, 95, 99f
      forehead with bilateral hyperostoses of nasal bridge, 97f
      hyperostosis of skull, 82f, 97f
      large capillary formation, 89f
      lipomas, 88, 89f, 90
      macrodactyly, 92f
      megaspondylodysplasia of cervical vertebrae, 93f
      mental deficiency, 95
      monomorphic adenoma of parotid gland, 91f
      ocular abnormalities, 98
      ovarian surface epithelium, inclusion cysts, and cystadenomas, 92f
      overgrowth of fingers, 93f
      papillary neoplasm, 91f
      parietal lobe, 100f
      possible findings, 76t
      pulmonary abnormalities, 99
      rectal polyposis, 101f
      renal abnormalities, 99
      skeletal abnormalities, 93, 95
      spinal cord compression, 94f
      spleen and thymus, 97
      synostosis of coronal suture, 98f
      unusual tumors, 90, 92–93
      varicose veins, 89f
      vascular malformations, 87–88
   compared with neurofibromatosis, 83t
   diagnostic criteria, 103–104, 104t
   differential diagnosis, 104–105, 105t
   etiologic considerations
      molecular speculation, 83–84
      somatic mosaicism, 81, 83
   guidelines for patient evaluation, 105t
   lumping, splitting, and, 4
   natural history, 84
   patient evaluation, guidelines for, 105–106
   phenotype, 75
   publications and the diagnosis of, 102–103
   with thrombocytopenia, splenomegaly, 100f
   uncommon and unusual findings, 77–78t
   uncommon neoplasms, 79–80t
Psoriatic mothers, infants of, 186
PTEN (gene)
   molecular biology, 66–67
   mutations, 67–69
   phosphatase and C2 domains, 67f
   regulatory network, 67f
PTEN mutations in Bannayan-Riley-Ruvalcaba syndrome and combined with Cowden syndrome, 67–69, 68f, 69t
Pulmonary embolism, 84

Quattrin syndrome, 197

Radixin, 143
Renal blastema, cytodifferentiated, 49f
Renal medullary dysplasia, 24f
Retardation, developmental, 194
Rhabdomyosarcoma, 6t
Richieri-Costa overgrowth syndrome, 198
Rosette formation, 63f

Schwannoma
   isolated, 145
   in NF2, 144
Schwannomatosis, 133, 144
Segmental neurofibromatosis, 130
Siena type overgrowth, 198

Simpson-Golabi-Behmel syndrome, 38, 41–42f, 41t
  clinical phenotype, 41, 43
  diagnosis, 43
    differential, 26, 43–44, 49, 64
  etiology, 38–39, 41
    gene mapping, 39
  historical perspective, 38
  neoplasms, 43
Skeletal findings/abnormalities, 5t, 82f, 97f
  in Cantú syndrome, 172–173
  in hemihyperplasia, 32, 33t, 35f
  in Klippel-Trenaunay syndrome, 115
  in Maffucci syndrome, 125
  in Marshall-Smith syndrome, 195–196, 195t, 196f
  in neurofibromatosis, 142
  in Proteus syndrome, 93, 95
  in Sotos syndrome, 52–53
  in Weaver syndrome, 59
Skin
  in Bannayan-Riley-Ruvalcaba syndrome, 70
  in neurofibromatosis, 141
Skin lesions, 87
Skull, hyperostosis of, 82f, 97f
Solomon syndrome. *See* Epidermal nevus syndromes
Somatic mosaicism. *See* Mosaicism
Sotos syndrome, 5, 6t, 43–44, 51, 52–55f, 54–55
  central nervous system abnormalities, 53
  clinical findings, 52t
  craniofacial features, 54
  diagnostic considerations, 52
  differential diagnosis, 56, 173
  etiologic considerations, 51
  growth and skeletal findings, 52–53
  laboratory findings, 56
  neoplasms, 55–56
  neuroimaging findings, 54t
  tumors and nontumors, 55t
Sotos syndrome cases, misdiagnosed tumors and hamartomas in, 56t
Spinal neurofibromatosis, familial, 132
Spleen, 97, 100f
Splitting, problem of, 4
Stevenson syndrome, 198
Sturge-Weber syndrome, 105, 114, 116–117, 117t, 119f
  calcification of cerebral cortex, 120f
  diagnosis, 122
    differential, 122t
  facial capillary malformation, 118f
  seizures and cognitive disability, 117
Sulfonylurea receptor (*SUR1*), 184–185
  mutations, 185t

Symmetrical lipomatosis, 105t
Syndecans, 38

Teebi overgrowth-microphthalmia syndrome, 198
Testis
  papillary adenoma/adenocarcinoma, 79t
  showing hyperplasia of Leydig cells, 25f
"Thanos syndrome," 102, 103
Thoracic kyphosis, angular, 94f
Thrombocytopenia, 100f
Thymus, 97
Tongue involvement with enlarged fungiform papillae, 35f
Transposition of the great vessels with overgrowth, 198
TSSC5/IMP1, 17
TSSC3/IPL, 16
Tufted angioma, 121t
Tumors. *See also specific topics*
  multiple, in same patient, 80t
Twins, monozygous (MZ), 17
Two-hit hypothesis, 136

Ultrasound screening, 24
Uniparental disomy (UPD), 15, 21–22f

Varicose veins, 112, 114–115
Varicosities, 111, 112, 114–115
Vascular abnormalities, 125
Vascular involvement, 5–7
Vascular lesions, 121t
  terminology, 7f, 121t
Vascular malformations, 87–88, 105, 122
  biological classification, 7t
  vascular tumors and, 119
Veins, abnormalities in, 115
Vertebrae, megaspondylodysplasia of cervical, 93f

Weaver syndrome, 43, 52, 59, 60–63f
  cardiovascular anomalies, 62
  craniofacial features, 60–61
  differential diagnosis, 62, 64
  etiologic considerations, 59
  females, 62t
  growth and skeletal findings, 59
  growth rates and parameters, 60f, 61f
  limbs, 61
  neoplasms, 61–62
  performance and central nervous system, 60
Weaver syndrome-like phenotype, 132
Wilms tumor, 5t, 6t, 33, 44, 49

Xp22, 39
Xq26, 39